Minimally Invasive Spine Surgery

Editors

ZACHARY A. SMITH
RICHARD G. FESSLER

NEUROSURGERY CLINICS OF NORTH AMERICA

www.neurosurgery.theclinics.com

Consulting Editors
RUSSELL LONSER
ISAAC YANG

April 2014 • Volume 25 • Number 2

ELSEVIER

1600 John F. Kennedy Boulevard • Suite 1800 • Philadelphia, Pennsylvania, 19103-2899

http://www.theclinics.com

NEUROSURGERY CLINICS OF NORTH AMERICA Volume 25, Number 2
April 2014 ISSN 1042-3680, ISBN-13: 978-0-323-29004-3

Editor: Jennifer Flynn-Briggs
Developmental Editor: Yonah Korngold

Neurosurgery Clinics of North America (ISSN 1042-3680) is published quarterly by Elsevier Inc., 360 Park Avenue South, New York, NY 10010-1710. Months of issue are January, April, July, and October. Business and Editorial Offices: 1600 John F. Kennedy Blvd., Suite 1800, Philadelphia, PA 19103-2899. Customer Service Office: 11830 Westline Industrial Drive, St. Louis, MO 63146. Periodicals postage paid at New York, NY, and additional mailing offices. Subscription prices are $380.00 per year (US individuals), $572.00 per year (US institutions), $415.00 per year (Canadian individuals), $711.00 per year (Canadian institutions), $525.00 per year (international individuals), $711.00 per year (international institutions), $185.00 per year (US students), and $255.00 per year (international students). International air speed delivery is included in all *Clinics* subscription prices. All prices are subject to change without notice. **POSTMASTER:** Send address changes to *Neurosurgery Clinics of North America*, Elsevier Periodicals Customer Service, 11830 Westline Industrial Drive, St. Louis, MO 63146. **Customer Service: 1-800-654-2452 (US and Canada). From outside the US and Canada, call: 1-314-453-7041. Fax: 1-314-453-5170. E-mail: JournalsCustomerService-usa@elsevier.com (for print support) and journalsonlinesupport-usa@elsevier.com (for online support).**

Reprints. For copies of 100 or more, of articles in this publication, please contact the Commercial Reprints Department, Elsevier Inc., 360 Park Avenue South, New York, NY 10010-1710. Tel. 212-633-3874; Fax: 212-633-3820; E-mail: reprints@elsevier.com.

Neurosurgery Clinics of North America is covered in *MEDLINE/PubMed (Index Medicus), EMBASE/Excerpta Medica, and Current Contents/Clinical Medicine (CC/CM).*

Printed and bound by CPI Group (UK) Ltd, Croydon, CR0 4YY

Contributors

CONSULTING EDITORS

RUSSELL LONSER, MD
Chair, Department of Neurological Surgery,
The Ohio State University, Columbus, Ohio

ISAAC YANG, MD
Assistant Professor, University of California
Los Angeles, UCLA Department of
Neurosurgery, David Geffen School of
Medicine at UCLA, UCLA Jonsson
Comprehensive Cancer Center,
Los Angeles, California

EDITORS

ZACHARY A. SMITH, MD
Assistant Professor, Department of
Neurological Surgery, Northwestern Memorial
Hospital, Feinberg School of Medicine,
Northwestern University, Chicago, Illinois

RICHARD G. FESSLER, MD, PhD
Professor, Department of Neurological
Surgery, Rush University Medical Center,
Chicago, Illinois

AUTHORS

NEEL ANAND, MD, Mch Orth
Clinical Professor of Surgery, Department of
Surgery, Director, Spine Trauma, Spine Center,
Cedars Sinai Medical Center, Los Angeles,
California

ELI M. BARON, MD
Clinical Associate Professor of Neurosurgery,
Department of Neurosurgery, Spine Center,
Cedars Sinai Medical Center, Los Angeles,
California

**BERNARD R. BENDOK, MD, MSCI, FAANS,
FACS, FAHA**
Professor of Neurological Surgery, Radiology
and Otolaryngology, Department of Neurological
Surgery; Department of Radiology; Department
of Otolaryngology, Northwestern Memorial
Hospital, Feinberg School of Medicine,
Northwestern University, Chicago, Illinois

DEAN CHOU, MD
Associate Professor, Associate Director,
Department of Neurological Surgery, UCSF
Spine Center, University of California,
San Francisco, San Francisco, California

NADER S. DAHDALEH, MD
Assistant Professor, Department of Neurological
Surgery, Feinberg School of Medicine,
Northwestern University, Chicago, Illinois

ARMEN R. DEUKMEDJIAN, MD
Chief Resident, Department of Neurosurgery &
Brain Repair, University of South Florida,
Tampa, Florida

TAREK Y. EL AHMADIEH, MD
Post Doctoral Research Fellow, Department
of Radiology, Department of Neurological
Surgery, Northwestern Memorial Hospital,
Chicago, Illinois

NAJIB E. EL TECLE, MD
Post Doctoral Research Fellow, Department of
Neurological Surgery, Northwestern Memorial
Hospital, Chicago, Illinois

RICHARD G. FESSLER, MD, PhD
Professor, Department of Neurological
Surgery, Rush University Medical Center,
Chicago, Illinois,

CARTER S. GERARD, MD
Department of Neurological Surgery, Rush
University Medical Center, Chicago, Illinois

RANDALL B. GRAHAM, MD
Resident Physician, Department of Neurological
Surgery, Feinberg School of Medicine,
Northwestern University, Chicago, Illinois

PATRICK W. HITCHON, MD
Department of Neurosurgery, Carver School of
Medicine, University of Iowa, Iowa City, Iowa

XUE YU HU, MD
Fellow, Department of Orthopaedics, Xijing
Hospital, The Fourth Military Medical
University, Shaanxi, China

SHEILA KAHWATY, PA-C
Department of Surgery, Spine Center, Cedars
Sinai Medical Center, Los Angeles, California

LARRY T. KHOO, MD
Director of Spinal Surgery, The Spine Clinic of
Los Angeles, Good Samaritan Hospital,
University of Southern California, Los Angeles,
California

CHOLL W. KIM, MD, PhD
Spine Institute of San Diego; Center for
Minimally Invasive Spine Surgery, Alvarado
Hospital and Pomerado Hospital, Palomar
Health, San Diego, California

TYLER R. KOSKI, MD
Associate Professor, Department of
Neurological Surgery, Feinberg School of
Medicine, Northwestern University, Chicago,
Illinois

ROHAN R. LALL, MD
Neurosurgery Resident, Department of
Neurological Surgery, Northwestern Memorial
Hospital, Chicago, Illinois

JI HYUN LEE, PA-C
The Spine Clinic of Los Angeles, Good
Samaritan Hospital, University of Southern
California, Los Angeles, California

XIN FENG LI, MD
Department of Orthopaedic Surgery, Renji
Hospital, Shanghai Jiaotong University School
of Medicine, Shanghai, People's Republic of
China

JOHN C. LIU, MD
Department of Neurological Surgery, Keck
School of Medicine, University of Southern
California, Los Angeles, California

PRAVEEN V. MUMMANENI, MD
Professor & Vice Chair, Co-Director,
Department of Neurological Surgery, UCSF
Spine Center, University of California, San
Francisco, San Francisco, California

JOHN E. O'TOOLE, MD
Department of Neurological Surgery, Rush
University Medical Center, Chicago, Illinois

MICHAEL S. PARK, MD
Resident Physician, Department of
Neurosurgery & Brain Repair, University of
South Florida, Tampa, Florida

BIRAJ M. PATEL, MD
Interventional Neuroradiology Fellow,
Department of Radiology, Northwestern
Memorial Hospital, Chicago, Illinois

GILAD J. REGEV, MD
Spine Surgery Unit, Departments of
Neurosurgery and Orthopaedic Surgery,
Tel Aviv Sourasky Medical Center, Tel Aviv
University, Tel Aviv, Israel

RAJIV SAIGAL, MD, PhD
Senior Resident, Department of Neurological
Surgery, University of California,
San Francisco, San Francisco, California

ZACHARY A. SMITH, MD
Assistant Professor, Department of
Neurological Surgery, Northwestern
Memorial Hospital, Feinberg School of
Medicine, Northwestern University, Chicago,
Illinois

LAURA A. SNYDER, MD
Fellow, Barrow Neurological Institute,
St. Joseph's Hospital and Medical Center,
Phoenix, Arizona; Fellow, Department of
Neurological Surgery, Rush University
Medical Center, Chicago, Illinois

JAMES A. STADLER III, MD
Resident Physician, Department of
Neurological Surgery, Feinberg School of
Medicine, Northwestern University, Chicago,
Illinois

TRENT L. TREDWAY, MD
NeoSpine, Seattle, Washington

JUAN S. URIBE, MD
Associate Professor, Director,
Department of Neurosurgery & Brain Repair,
University of South Florida, Tampa,
Florida

RISHI WADHWA, MD
Spine Fellow, Department of Neurological
Surgery, University of California,
San Francisco, San Francisco,
California

MICHAEL Y. WANG, MD, FACS
Professor, Department of Neurological
Surgery; Department of Rehabilitation
Medicine, University of Miami Miller School of
Medicine, Miami, Florida

ALBERT P. WONG, MD
Department of Neurological Surgery, Feinberg
School of Medicine, Northwestern University,
Chicago, Illinois

JIA ZHI YAN, MD
Department of Orthopaedics, Beijing Tiantan
Hospital, The Capital Medical University,
Beijing, People's Republic of China

Contents

Safe and reproducible outcomes of the lateral lumbar intervertebral fusion (LLIF) procedure rely on meticulous care and understanding of the anatomy of the lateral corridor. This review aims to describe the different important anatomic considerations when performing LLIF and offer technical notes that may help increase the safety of this procedure. The LLIF procedure is divided into 5 stages: patient positioning, abdominal wall dissection, retroperitoneal space dissection, deployment of the surgical retractors, and diskectomy. Each stage is preformed in a distinct anatomic compartment that may cause different typical complications.

The lateral transpsoas approach to the lumbar spine has become an increasingly popular method to achieve fusion. Although this approach requires less tissue dissection, a smaller incision, decreased operative time, reduced blood loss and postoperative pain, and shorter hospital stay, it carries the potential for serious neurologic and visceral complications. This article reviews these complications in detail and proposes mechanisms for their avoidance.

Posterior approaches for decompression in minimally invasive spine surgery are increasingly used for a wide range of pathology. Surgeons and patients must understand these risks in order to identify, manage, and ideally prevent complications. Technical intraoperative complications, recurrences and reoperations, infections, and medical complications associated with the surgery are considered for common posterior minimally invasive decompression procedures of the cervical and lumbar spine. Methods of possibly avoiding these complications are also discussed. This article then aggregates the relevant data to allow concise understanding of the complications associated with these procedures.

Radiation use for diagnostic and therapeutic purposes has increased in parallel with advances in minimally invasive spinal techniques and endovascular neurosurgical procedures. This change in the exposure profile of the operator and radiology personnel has raised concerns about radiation side effects and long term complications of radiation exposure. In this review, the current literature regarding risks of radiation exposure and strategies to reduce these risks are summarized. Current standards in radiation risk reduction and specific techniques that can minimize radiation exposure are also discussed.

Posterior decompressive procedures are a fundamental component of the surgical treatment of symptomatic cervical degenerative disease. Posterior approaches have the appeal of avoiding complications associated with anterior approaches such as esophageal injury, recurrent laryngeal nerve paralysis, dysphagia, and adjacent-level disease after fusion. Although open procedures are effective, the extensive subperiosteal stripping of the paraspinal musculature leads to increased blood loss, longer hospital stays, and more postoperative pain, and potentially contributes to instability. Minimally invasive access has been developed to limit approach-related morbidity. This article reviews current techniques in minimally invasive surgical management of cervical myelopathy and radiculopathy.

In the past, treatment of thoracic disc herniations has not been seen as a minimally invasive procedure. This article evaluates the progression of minimally invasive techniques for the treatment of thoracic disc herniations. Discussion of the advantages and disadvantages of the approaches is noted so that surgeons may consider them while incorporating these techniques in their practice.

Transforaminal lumbar interbody fusion (TLIF) is an important surgical option for the treatment of back pain and radiculopathy. The minimally invasive TLIF (MI-TLIF) technique is increasingly used to achieve neural element decompression, restoration of segmental alignment and lordosis, and bony fusion. This article reviews the surgical technique, outcomes, and complications in a series of 144 consecutive 1- and 2-level MI-TLIFs in comparison with an institutional control group of 54 open traditional TLIF procedures with a mean of 46 months' follow-up. The evidence base suggests that MI-TLIF can be performed safely with excellent long-term outcomes.

 Video of Mini-Open Transpedicular Corpectomy T12 Metastatic Renal Cell Cancer accompanies this article at http://www.neurosurgery.theclinics.com/

Management of spinal metastasis is a large and challenging clinical problem. For metastatic epidural spinal cord compression, a prospective, randomized, controlled trial showed the utility of circumferential surgical decompression followed by adjuvant radiotherapy. In the setting of those data, surgical techniques evolved from decompressive laminectomy only to anterior corpectomy to posterior-only transpedicular corpectomy. The transpedicular approach has recently been modernized with minimally invasive and mini-open techniques. This article presents the relevant clinical background on spinal metastasis, reviews the surgical technique for minimally invasive transpedicular corpectomy, and finally reviews relevant results in the literature.

Traditional open anterior and posterior approaches for the thoracic and thoracolumbar spine are associated with approach-related morbidity and limited surgical access to the level of abnormality. This article describes the minimally invasive anterolateral corpectomy for the treatment of spinal tumors, and reviews the current literature.

Intramedullary spinal cord tumors constitute 8% to 10% of all primary spinal cord tumors. The clinical presentation of primary spinal cord tumors is determined in part by the location of the tumor, and in nearly all clinical instances pain is the predominant presenting symptom. Motor disturbance is the next most common symptom, followed by sensory loss. Diagnosis of a primary spinal cord tumor requires a high index of suspicion based on clinical signs and symptoms, in addition to spine-directed magnetic resonance imaging.

The application of percutaneous techniques for the management of thoracolumbar fractures is gaining popularity. Short-segment or long-segment percutaneous pedicle screw fixation can be used to treat a wide variety of thoracolumbar fractures in patients who are neurologically normal. This approach provides internal fixation, allowing the fracture to heal and sparing the motion segments above and below the fracture, as the instrumentation can be removed later.

As minimally invasive surgery (MIS) has advanced to treat diverse diseases, there has been an increasing need for MIS surgery to be able to restore lumbar lordosis and treat sagittal balance abnormalities. In this article, the surgical technique and initial clinical and radiographic outcomes with a new miniopen pedicle subtraction osteotomy technique are outlined. Combining the MIS techniques of interbody fusion, percutaneous screw fixation, and facet fusion with a selective opening for the osteotomy site allows for safe and efficient deformity corrections. This technique resulted in an average increase of 29.2° of lumbar lordosis (range 17°–44°).

The lateral transpsoas approach for interbody fusion is a minimally invasive technique that has been gaining increasing popularity in the management of a variety

NEUROSURGERY CLINICS OF NORTH AMERICA

Preface

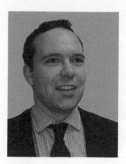
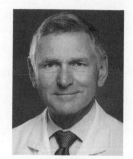

Zachary A. Smith, MD   Richard G. Fessler, MD, PhD

Editors

We are honored to edit this issue of the *Neurosurgery Clinics of North America* devoted to modern Minimally Invasive Spine Surgery. The guiding principle of these techniques is to treat effectively, and completely, a patient's pathology while minimizing injury from the surgical approach. The role minimally invasive spine surgery has grown tremendously in the last decade. While initial applications were limited to more elemental applications, such as discectomy and decompressions, modern applications have shown the tremendous range and depth of these techniques. The goal of this issue is to highlight modern minimally invasive spine surgery.

Minimally invasive spine surgery has had an extraordinary impact on patient outcomes. Patients with common degenerative pathologies, such as lumbar disk herniations or degenerative stenosis, can now be treated and discharged the same day as treatment. Furthermore, these techniques can be offered to patients with commonly accepted surgical challenges, including obesity, advanced age, and medical comorbidities. This has broadened the scope and capabilities of modern spine surgery.

Minimally invasive techniques have matured in the last decade and have been continuously refined in the hands of modern spine surgeons. With this maturation, there has been a simultaneous broadening of the scope and complexity of these techniques. Complex pathologies, such as spinal column and spine cord malignancies, spinal column trauma, and scoliosis, can now be effectively treated with minimally invasive techniques. This "second phase" of minimally invasive spine surgery has allowed us to limit approach-related morbidity in even the most complex problems encountered in spinal neurosurgery.

In this current issue, we seek to highlight the tremendous role of minimally invasive techniques in modern spine surgery. General considerations, including complication avoidance, radiation exposure, and anatomy, are considered in the initial articles. Furthermore, evidence-basis and technique are illustrated for commonly applied techniques, such as cervical foraminotomy, lumbar interbody fusion, and thoracic discectomy. Later articles are devoted to recent advances that have been applied to complex spinal pathologies. These include approaches for thoracolumbar corpectomy, intradural tumors, and complex spinal deformity.

It is our hope that this issue provides both practicing neurosurgeons and trainees an in-depth resource on this topic. We are grateful to the editors for allowing us to oversee this work, and we would like to thank the many surgeons who devoted valuable time to contribute. Last, we are indebted to our patients, who have entrusted us with their confidence.

Zachary A. Smith, MD
Department of Neurological Surgery
Northwestern University
Feinberg School of Medicine
676 N. St. Clair St., Suite 2210
Chicago, IL 60611, USA

Richard G. Fessler, MD, PhD
Department of Neurological Surgery
Rush University Medical Center
1725 W. Harrison St., Suite 855
Chicago, IL 60612, USA

E-mail addresses:
zsmithmd@gmail.com (Z.A. Smith)
rfessler@rush.edu (R.G. Fessler)

Neurosurg Clin N Am 25 (2014) xiii
http://dx.doi.org/10.1016/j.nec.2014.02.001
1042-3680/14/$ – see front matter © 2014 Published by Elsevier Inc.

Safety and the Anatomy of the Retroperitoneal Lateral Corridor with Respect to the Minimally Invasive Lateral Lumbar Intervertebral Fusion Approach

Gilad J. Regev, MD[a,b], Choll W. Kim, MD, PhD[c,d],*

KEYWORDS

- LLIF • Transpsoas approach • Retroperitoneal anatomy

KEY POINTS

- Limited visualization of the surgical field during the lateral lumbar intervertebral fusion (LLIF) procedure exposes surgeons to difficulties and dangers that do not exist when performing similar procedures in an open technique.
- Anatomic understanding of the different structures in the abdominal wall and in the retroperitoneal space and their relationship to the LLIF approach is crucial for minimizing the risk for complications.
- Conscientious evaluation of the preoperative imaging studies, proper patient position, generous use of intraoperative imaging, and a systematic approach to surgical techniques are imperative to assure safe and successful outcome.

INTRODUCTION

The lateral transpsoas approach for lumbar interbody arthrodesis is a relatively novel method for performing minimally invasive LLIFs.[1] This approach allows for a large graft to be placed at the apophyseal ring where the bone is strongest, enabling disk height restoration and deformity correction.[2–4] In addition to the advantage of avoiding manipulation of the large retroperitoneal vessels, this technique uses a small incision that avoids significant abdominal wall muscle injury.[5,6] The limited visualization of the surgical field during this procedure, however, exposes surgeons to difficulties and dangers that do not exist when doing similar procedures in an open technique. Surgeons, therefore, must rely on intraoperative fluoroscopic images and neuromonitoring guidance during certain stages of the procedure to avoid neurologic complications.[7,8]

Although LLIF gained fast and wide popularity among spine surgeons as a safe and reproducible technique for anterior spine arthrodesis, several studies challenged the safety of this procedure, reporting complication rates ranging from 6.2% to 52%.[6,9–11]

a Spine Surgery Unit, Departments of Neurosurgery and Orthopaedic Surgery, Tel Aviv Sourasky Medical Center, Tel Aviv University, Tel Aviv, Israel; b Sackler Faculty of Medicine, Tel Aviv University, Tel Aviv, Israel; c Spine Institute of San Diego, San Diego, CA, USA; d Center for Minimally Invasive Spine Surgery, Alvarado Hospital and Pomerado Hospital, Palomar Health, San Diego, CA, USA
* Corresponding author. Spine Institute of San Diego, San Diego, CA.
E-mail address: Choll@siosd.com

Neurosurg Clin N Am 25 (2014) 211–218
http://dx.doi.org/10.1016/j.nec.2013.12.001
1042-3680/14/$ – see front matter © 2014 Elsevier Inc. All rights reserved.

Anatomic understanding of the different structures in the abdominal wall and in the retroperitoneal space and their relationship to the LLIF approach is crucial for minimizing the risk for these complications. Several studies have been published in the literature regarding the morphometric measurements of these structures. Some of these studies used cadaveric specimens whereas others relied on morphometric measurements acquired by MRI studies.[12–20]

This review aims to describe the different important anatomic considerations when performing LLIF and offer technical notes that may help increase the safety of this procedure.

In order to simplify this review, the authors have divided the LLIF procedure into 5 stages; each is preformed in a distinct anatomic compartment that may cause location complications:

1. Patient positioning
2. Abdominal wall dissection
3. Retroperitoneal space dissection and anterior displacement of the peritoneum and abdominal organs
4. Transpsoas dissection and deployment of the surgical retractors
5. Diskectomy and penetration of the contralateral annulus

PATIENT POSITIONING

The importance of correct patient positioning cannot be overemphasized for the success and safety of the LLIF procedure.[12] In order to compensate for the lack of direct visualization of the operated field, the authors strongly recommend that this stage be performed by a senior surgeon or by a surgeon who is skillful and experienced in performing the procedure, because it requires multiple subtle adjustments of the surgical table under fluoroscopic guidance to achieve near-perfect anteroposterior and lateral visualization of the operated disk space and bordering vertebrae.

Among many other technical difficulties, malpositioning of patients may result in the misplacement of the surgical retractors inside the psoas muscle, which greatly increases the risk of injury to the dural sac, retroperitoneal vessels, lumbar plexus, and the psoas muscle.[12,21–26]

The retractor blades positioned inside the psoas muscle produce compression of the muscle fiber and of the adjacent nerves. This compression coupled with excessive positional stretching of the psoas and abdominal muscles can increase the intramuscular tension and may contribute to the risk of nerve injury.[27,28] Therefore, it is imperative to relax the muscle as much as possible by ensuring that the hip joint on the operated side is flexed as much as possible and that the lateral bending of the trunk is not exaggerated over what is needed to deflect the iliac wing away from the surgical corridor to the disk space.

ABDOMINAL WALL DISSECTION

The lateral abdominal wall musculature consists of 3 muscular layers: the external oblique, the internal oblique, and the transverse abdominis. Posterior to them is situated the quadratus lomborum muscle.[29,30]

Four nerves of the lumbar plexus—the subcostal, the iliohypogastric, the ilioinguinal, and the lateral femoral cutaneous nerves—travel outside the psoas in the retroperitoneum and inside the abdominal wall (**Fig. 1**). These nerves are vulnerable to injury during the early stages of the LLIF approach while accessing and dissecting the abdominal wall and retroperitoneum.[31] Injury to these nerves during laparoscopic abdominal surgery is a well-known complication that results in a full spectrum of sensory deficits (analgesia, paresthesias, and dysesthesia) at the corresponding dermatome and paresis of the abdominal wall. This may lead to an abdomen wall hernia or even a direct inguinal hernia.[32] Of the 4 nerves, the lateral femoral cutaneous nerve is the only one reported in the literature to be injured during an LLIF procedure, although nondocumented injury to the other 3 nerves have been reported by surgeons.[33]

Subcostal Nerve

The subcostal nerve originates from the T12 root and accompanies the subcostal vessels along the inferior border of the 12th rib. The nerve has a motor and a sensory component. It supplies the muscles of the anterior abdominal wall, especially the external oblique, and provides sensation to the anterior gluteal skin. If the dorsal cutaneous branch becomes injured or entrapped, this produces a posterior area of numbness with painful paresthesias, known as *nostalgia paresthetica*. When the anterior cutaneous branch is involved, this leads to an anterior area of numbness with painful paresthesias on the abdomen, known as *rectus abdominis syndrome*. Injury to the motor portion of the nerve paralyzes the muscle fibers supplied by it, thereby weakening the anterior abdominal wall.[29,34]

Iliohypogastric Nerve

The iliohypogastric nerve originates from the L1 root. It emerges from the upper lateral border of the psoas major muscle and runs obliquely

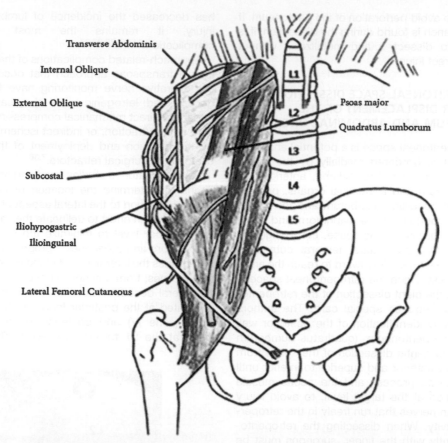

Fig. 1. Illustration demonstrating the trajectory of the 4 main nerves traveling outside the psoas muscle in the retroperitoneum along the posterior abdominal wall and within the abdominal muscles. (*From* Dakwar E, Vale FL, Uribe JS. Trajectory of the main sensory and motor branches of the lumbar plexus outside the psoas muscle related to the lateral retroperitoneal transpsoas approach. J Neurosurg Spine 2011;14:290–5; with permission.)

embedded on the retroperitoneal adipose until it reaches the anterior superior iliac spine, where it pierces the internal and external obliques. The lateral cutaneous branch of the iliohypogastric nerve provides sensation to the posterolateral gluteal skin, whereas its anterior cutaneous branch innervates the suprapubic skin.[29,35]

Ilioinguinal Nerve

Similar to the iliohypogastric nerve, the ilioinguinal nerve arises from L1 and emerges from the lateral border of the psoas major just caudal to the iliohypogastric nerve. It then passes obliquely across the quadratus lumborum and the upper part of the iliacus in the retroperitoneal space to travel within the inguinal canal, and it emerges from the superficial inguinal ring.[29,35]

Lateral Femoral Cutaneous Nerve

The lateral femoral cutaneous nerve is a purely sensory nerve. It supplies sensation to the anterolateral aspect of the thigh. The nerve originates from the L2 and L3 roots. It emerges from the lateral border of the psoas major muscle at approximately L4 and courses obliquely across the iliacus muscle toward the anterior superior iliac spine. The nerve passes through or below the inguinal ligament approximately 1 cm medial to the anterior superior iliac spine. Injury to the nerve results in a clinical presentation of impaired sensation and pain along the anterolateral aspect of the thigh, termed *meralgia paresthetica*.[29,36]

Although complications that involve the abdominal wall musculature and nerves are rare after LLIF, avoiding an extensive skin and muscle incisions (approximately 3 cm) and performing a gentle blunt dissection and spreading of the muscle fibers are keys to minimizing approach related complications during the initial stage of the procedure. The authors recommend using a surgeon's index finger and spreading with a blunt instrument (hemostat forceps or curved Mayo scissors) until the retroperitoneal space is reached. Care should be taken to avoid perforation of the peritoneum. If a nerve branch is found during the dissection, it is possible to dissect it and mobilize it without causing direct injury.

RETROPERITONEAL SPACE DISSECTION AND ANTERIOR DISPLACEMENT OF THE PERITONEUM AND ABDOMINAL ORGANS

The retroperitoneal space is a potential anatomic space that is bordered medially by the psoas muscle and the vertebral column, anteriorly by the peritoneum and abdominal organs, posteriorly by the quadratus lumborum and the iliacus muscles, superiorly by the diaphragm, and inferiorly by the pelvis. In this space, the ilioinguinal, iliohypogastric, and lateral femoral cutaneous nerves course freely downward to reach the anterior iliac crest. Once the retroperitoneal space is accessed, the blunt dissection of the retroperitoneal space requires special care. The authors suggest early identification of the posterior wall of the retroperitoneum (quadratus lumborum muscle) and gentle dissection of the space from posterior to anterior and superior to inferior until the transverse process and the psoas muscle are identified at the target level, to avoid injury to the main nerves that run freely in the retroperitoneal cavity. When dissecting the retroperitoneum bluntly with the finger, surgeons must be careful not to confuse a free running nerve in the retroperitoneal fat for an adhesion and avulse or injure it.

Patients suffering from retroperitoneal scarring and fibrosis may be at high risk for complications due to inadvertent injury to abdominal organs during the blind blunt dissection and the insertion of the expandable retractors. This condition is typical in patients with a history of diverticulitis, radiation therapy to the abdomen, or previous large abdominal/retroperitoneal surgery (nephrectomy or total colectomy). In the authors' clinical experience, an injury to the descending colon in a patient who had a history of previous urologic procedures resulted in scar formation in the retroperitoneal space. The authors, therefore, suggest considering an alternative surgical approach in these patients.

TRANSPSOAS DISSECTION AND DEPLOYMENT OF THE SURGICAL RETRACTORS

Recent studies have revealed that the most frequent complication of the lateral retroperitoneal transpsoas approach relates to injury of the lumbar plexus. Although real-time nerve monitoring has decreased the incidence of lumbar plexus injury, it remains the most common complication.[11,26–28,33,37]

Approach-related complications of the retroperitoneal transpsoas approach that occur despite intraoperative nerve monitoring have been well documented. Iatrogenic nerve injury can be secondary to direct mechanical compression, laceration, stretch/traction, or indirect ischemia caused by the insertion and deployment of the tubular dilators and surgical retractors.[7,38]

Several anatomic studies used cadaveric specimens to determine the location of the lumbar plexus in relation to the lateral aspect of the vertebral body in an effort to delineate the safe zone at each lumbar level to minimize the risk of nerve injury. Moro and colleagues[20] proposed a method that divides the lateral aspect of the vertebral body into 4 zones, from anterior to posterior. Viewed in the lateral decubitus position, the lumbar plexus is located at the posterior fourth of the vertebral body (zone IV) and posterior to the vertebral body at the L1 through L5 levels. The lumbar

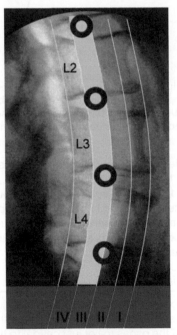

Fig. 2. Lateral radiograph of the lumbar spine demonstrating the division of the vertebral body into 4 zones (zones I–IV) from anterior to posterior. The relative safe zone (zone III) is depicted in green. The recommended safe working zones to prevent direct nerve injury have been indicated with black circles at each level. (*From* Uribe JS, Arredondo N, Dakwar E, et al. Defining the safe working zones using the minimally invasive lateral retroperitoneal transpsoas approach: an anatomic study. J Neurosurg Spine 2010;13:260–6; with permission.)

plexus nerves pass obliquely outward, behind, and through the fibers of the psoas muscle while distributing filaments to it. Progressive anterior migration of the plexus as it descends within the muscle at each disk space was noted. As a result, the L5-S1 disk space was found to be unsafe for performing LLIF as the plexus was located at zones II and III at this level. Gu and colleagues[39] studied the location of the lumbar plexus and the sympathetic trunk with reference to the superior border of the transverse process. They determined that the safe zone for making the diskectomy should be located between the plexus and the sympathetic trunk that runs along the anterior third of the vertebral bodies underneath the psoas muscle. The genitofemoral nerve, arising from the L2 and L3 nerve roots, was responsible for narrowing this safe zone at the L2-3 level. A similar observation was made by Moro and colleagues, who concluded that above the L4-5 level, the surgical safe zone narrows only at the L2-3 level by the genitofemoral nerve. Benglis and colleagues[18] also reported the progressive ventral migration of the lumbar plexus on the disk space from L1 through L5. They concluded that the risk of injury during the LLIF approach is greatest at the L4–5 level with a posteriorly positioned dilator or retractor. Uribe and colleagues[12] recommended

locating the safe zone at the midpoint of zone III at the L1 through L4 levels and between zone II and zone III at the L4-5 level (**Fig. 2**). On the contrary, Banagan and colleagues[19] identified the neural structure at risk even at zones II and III at each intervertebral level. They concluded that there is no zone of absolute safety when using the LLIF approach.

Regev and colleagues[13] determined the surgical safe zone for performing the LLIF by analyzing MRI studies from patients with normally aligned and deformed spines. They reported that lumbar scoliosis causes both the position of nerve roots and the retroperitoneal vessels to shift relative to the vertebral body. These changes are dependent on the direction of the vertebra's axial rotation.[40,41] A right scoliotic curve (counterclockwise rotation) results in a relative posterior shift of the left nerve root and anterior shift of the right vessels. A leftward rotation of the vertebra (clockwise rotation) results in a relative anterior shift of the left nerve root and posterior shift of the right vessels (**Fig. 3**).

Electrophysiologic monitoring is a necessary tool to prevent nerve injury while traversing the psoas muscle and during placement of the retractor.[7] In particular, monitoring of the psoas muscle can also yield useful information. Obtaining stimulation

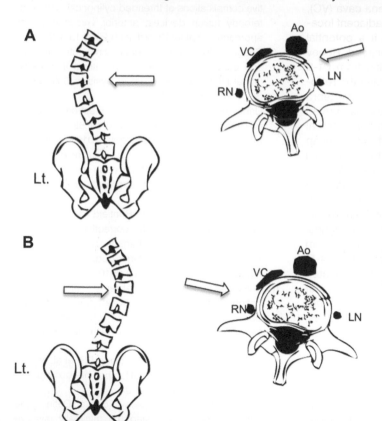

Fig. 3. (A) Dextroscoliosis with right (counterclockwise) rotation of the vertebra resulted in a relative anterior position of the right nerve root and posterior position of the left vessel and nerve root. (B) Levoscoliosis with left rotation of the vertebra (clockwise) rotation resulted in a relative anterior position of the left nerve root and a relative posterior position of the right vessel and nerve root (*arrows pointing at the concave side of the deformity*). (*From* Regev GJ, Chen L, Dhawan M, et al. Morphometric analysis of the ventral nerve roots and retroperitoneal vessels with respect to the minimally invasive lateral approach in normal and deformed spines. Spine 2009;34:1330–5.)

of muscle groups during directional electromyographic stimulation both anteriorly and posteriorly should prompt surgeons to change the dilator position to a more anterior one where only posterior stimulation provokes muscle activity. This maneuver should avoid splitting the elements of the plexus with the retractor.

DISKECTOMY AND PENETRATION OF THE CONTRALATERAL ANNULUS

Among the advantages of the LLIF approach is avoiding manipulation and retraction of the large retroperitoneal vessels, which has been related to serious vascular complication when performing the anterior lumbar interbody fusion procedure.[14,42] Although reports of vascular complication after LLIF are rare, risks of injury to the neurovascular structures that lay on the contralateral side of the disk space increase because the contralateral annulus is routinely released during the procedure by a Cobb Elevator under fluoroscopic guidance.[8] This risk is further increased in cases of degenerative scoliosis, because of the rotatory deformity of the spine that results in a relatively posterior position of the retroperitoneal vessels at the concavity of the deformity.[13]

Among the retroperitoneal vessels, it is especially important to appreciate the vena cava (VC), because its thin and friable wall and adjacent location to the right disk space make it a potential source for catastrophic bleeding if injured. Regev and colleagues[13] reported that going from L1-2 to L4-5, the degree of overlap between the retroperitoneal blood vessels and the vertebra increased progressively as the vessels moved posterior and lateral with respect to the vertebral body. As a result, the relative right side overlap of the VC increases from 10% at the L1-2 level to 22% at the L4-5. At the vertebras' left side, the relative overlap of the aorta increases from 2% at the L1-2 level to 9% at the L4-5. Hu and colleagues[16] reported on the location of the retroperitoneal vessels using Moro and colleagues' method. They found that the VC migrated from the right of zone A to the right of zone I at L4-5. In 29.2% of subjects, the VC was located completely to the right of zone I and in the rest (70.8%) was located to the right at the border between zone A and zone I. The aorta or iliac arteries, however, were found only at zone A from L1 to L5.

SUMMARY

Safe and reproducible outcomes of the LLIF procedure rely on meticulous care and understanding of the anatomy of the lateral corridor. Efficacious application of this minimally invasive technique and avoidance of potential pitfalls begins with conscientious evaluation of the preoperative imaging studies and continues in the operating room with proper patient position, generous use of intraoperative imaging, and a systematic approach to surgical techniques.

REFERENCES

1. Ozgur BM, Aryan HE, Pimenta L, et al. Extreme lateral interbody fusion (XLIF): a novel surgical technique for anterior lumbar interbody fusion. Spine J 2006;6:435–43.

2. Hollowell JP, Vollmer DG, Wilson CR, et al. Biomechanical analysis of thoracolumbar interbody constructs. How important is the endplate? Spine 1996;21:1032–6.

3. Anand N, Baron EM, Thaiyananthan G, et al. Minimally invasive multilevel percutaneous correction and fusion for adult lumbar degenerative scoliosis: a technique and feasibility study. J Spinal Disord Tech 2008;21:459–67.

4. Amin BY, Mummaneni PV, Ibrahim T, et al. Four-level minimally invasive lateral interbody fusion for treatment of degenerative scoliosis. Neurosurg Focus 2013;35. Video 10.

5. Scaduto AA, Gamradt SC, Yu WD, et al. Perioperative complications of threaded cylindrical lumbar interbody fusion devices: anterior versus posterior approach. J Spinal Disord Tech 2003;16:502–7.

6. Rodgers WB, Gerber EJ, Patterson J. Intraoperative and early postoperative complications in extreme lateral interbody fusion: an analysis of 600 cases. Spine 2011;36:26–32.

7. Uribe JS, Vale FL, Dakwar E. Electromyographic monitoring and its anatomical implications in minimally invasive spine surgery. Spine 2010;35:S368–74.

8. Regev GJ, Haloman S, Chen L, et al. Incidence and prevention of intervertebral cage overhang with minimally invasive lateral approach fusions. Spine 2010;35:1406–11.

9. Tormenti MJ, Maserati MB, Bonfield CM, et al. Complications and radiographic correction in adult scoliosis following combined transpsoas extreme lateral interbody fusion and posterior pedicle screw instrumentation. Neurosurg Focus 2010;28:E7.

10. Sofianos DA, Briseno MR, Abrams J, et al. Complications of the lateral transpsoas approach for lumbar interbody arthrodesis: a case series and literature review. Clin Orthop Relat Res 2012;470: 1621–32.

11. Pumberger M, Hughes AP, Huang RR, et al. Neurologic deficit following lateral lumbar interbody fusion. Eur Spine J 2012;21:1192–9.

12. Uribe JS, Arredondo N, Dakwar E, et al. Defining the safe working zones using the minimally invasive

lateral retroperitoneal transpsoas approach: an anatomical study. J Neurosurg Spine 2010;13: 260–6.

13. Regev GJ, Chen L, Dhawan M, et al. Morphometric analysis of the ventral nerve roots and retroperitoneal vessels with respect to the minimally invasive lateral approach in normal and deformed spines. Spine 2009;34:1330–5.

14. OuYang H, Ding Z. Research of thoracolumbar spine lateral vascular anatomy and imaging. Folia Morphol (Warsz) 2010;69:128–33.

15. Kepler CK, Bogner EA, Herzog RJ, et al. Anatomy of the psoas muscle and lumbar plexus with respect to the surgical approach for lateral transpsoas interbody fusion. Eur Spine J 2011;20:550–6.

16. Hu WK, He SS, Zhang SC, et al. An MRI study of psoas major and abdominal large vessels with respect to the X/DLIF approach. Eur Spine J 2011; 20:557–62.

17. Guerin P, Obeid I, Bourghli A, et al. The lumbosacral plexus: anatomic considerations for minimally invasive retroperitoneal transpsoas approach. Surg Radiol Anat 2012;34:151–7.

18. Benglis DM, Vanni S, Levi AD. An anatomical study of the lumbosacral plexus as related to the minimally invasive transpsoas approach to the lumbar spine. J Neurosurg Spine 2009;10:139–44.

19. Banagan K, Gelb D, Poelstra K, et al. Anatomic mapping of lumbar nerve roots during a direct lateral transpsoas approach to the spine: a cadaveric study. Spine 2011;36:E687–91.

20. Moro T, Kikuchi S, Konno S, et al. An anatomic study of the lumbar plexus with respect to retroperitoneal endoscopic surgery. Spine 2003;28:423–8 [discussion: 7–8].

21. Deukmedjian AR, Le TV, Dakwar E, et al. Movement of abdominal structures on magnetic resonance imaging during positioning changes related to lateral lumbar spine surgery: a morphometric study: clinical article. J Neurosurg Spine 2012;16: 615–23.

22. Arnold PM, Anderson KK, McGuire RA Jr. The lateral transpsoas approach to the lumbar and thoracic spine: a review. Surg Neurol Int 2012;3: S198–215.

23. Moller DJ, Slimack NP, Acosta FL Jr, et al. Minimally invasive lateral lumbar interbody fusion and transpsoas approach-related morbidity. Neurosurg Focus 2011;31:E4.

24. Santillan A, Patsalides A, Gobin YP. Endovascular embolization of iatrogenic lumbar artery pseudoaneurysm following extreme lateral interbody fusion (XLIF). Vasc Endovascular Surg 2010;44:601–3.

25. Ahmadian A, Abel N, Uribe JS. Functional recovery of severe obturator and femoral nerve injuries after lateral retroperitoneal transpsoas surgery. J Neurosurg Spine 2013;18:409–14.

26. Ahmadian A, Deukmedjian AR, Abel N, et al. Analysis of lumbar plexopathies and nerve injury after lateral retroperitoneal transpsoas approach: diagnostic standardization. J Neurosurg Spine 2013;18:289–97.

27. Houten JK, Alexandre LC, Nasser R, et al. Nerve injury during the transpsoas approach for lumbar fusion. J Neurosurg Spine 2011;15:280–4.

28. Cahill KS, Martinez JL, Wang MY, et al. Motor nerve injuries following the minimally invasive lateral transpsoas approach. J Neurosurg Spine 2012;17:227–31.

29. Dakwar E, Vale FL, Uribe JS. Trajectory of the main sensory and motor branches of the lumbar plexus outside the psoas muscle related to the lateral retroperitoneal transpsoas approach. J Neurosurg Spine 2011;14:290–5.

30. Dakwar E, Le TV, Baaj AA, et al. Abdominal wall paresis as a complication of minimally invasive lateral transpsoas interbody fusion. Neurosurg Focus 2011;31:E18.

31. Mirilas P, Skandalakis JE. Surgical anatomy of the retroperitoneal spaces, Part IV: retroperitoneal nerves. Am Surg 2010;76:253–62.

32. Korenkov M, Rixen D, Paul A, et al. Combined abdominal wall paresis and incisional hernia after laparoscopic cholecystectomy. Surg Endosc 1999; 13:268–9.

33. Knight RQ, Schwaegler P, Hanscom D, et al. Direct lateral lumbar interbody fusion for degenerative conditions: early complication profile. J Spinal Disord Tech 2009;22:34–7.

34. van der Graaf T, Verhagen PC, Kerver AL, et al. Surgical anatomy of the 10th and 11th intercostal, and subcostal nerves: prevention of damage during lumbotomy. J Urol 2011;186:579–83.

35. Klaassen Z, Marshall E, Tubbs RS, et al. Anatomy of the ilioinguinal and iliohypogastric nerves with observations of their spinal nerve contributions. Clin Anat 2011;24:454–61.

36. Murata Y, Takahashi K, Yamagata M, et al. The anatomy of the lateral femoral cutaneous nerve, with special reference to the harvesting of iliac bone graft. J Bone Joint Surg Am 2000;82:746–7.

37. Le TV, Smith DA, Greenberg MS, et al. Complications of lateral plating in the minimally invasive lateral transpsoas approach. J Neurosurg Spine 2012;16: 302–7.

38. Malham GM, Ellis NJ, Parker RM, et al. Clinical outcome and fusion rates after the first 30 extreme lateral interbody fusions. ScientificWorldJournal 2012;2012:246989.

39. Gu Y, Ebraheim NA, Xu R, et al. Anatomic considerations of the posterolateral lumbar disk region. Orthopedics 2001;24:56–8.

40. Sapkas G, Efstathiou P, Badekas AT, et al. Radiological parameters associated with the evolution of degenerative scoliosis. Bull Hosp Jt Dis 1996; 55:40–5.

41. Ploumis A, Transfeldt EE, Gilbert TJ Jr, et al. Degenerative lumbar scoliosis: radiographic correlation of lateral rotatory olisthesis with neural canal dimensions. Spine 2006;31:2353–8.

42. Guerin P, Obeid I, Gille O, et al. Safe working zones using the minimally invasive lateral retroperitoneal transpsoas approach: a morphometric study. Surg Radiol Anat 2011;33:665–71.

Minimally Invasive Lateral Transpsoas Approach to the Lumbar Spine
Pitfalls and Complication Avoidance

Randall B. Graham, MD[a],*, Albert P. Wong, MD[a],
John C. Liu, MD[b]

KEYWORDS

- Lateral transpsoas approach • Direct lateral interbody fusion • Extreme lateral interbody fusion
- Lumbar spine • Lumbosacral plexus • Surgical complications • Surgical technique

KEY POINTS

- The lateral transpsoas approach to the lumbar spine employs a true lateral position to laterally approach the midposition of the treatment disc through the psoas major muscle using fluoroscopy and tube dilators.
- The advantages to this approach include smaller incisions, less tissue dissection and blood loss, shorter operative time and hospital stay, and reduced postoperative pain.
- The main disadvantage is the fact that common fusion levels, particularly L4-5 and L5-S1, are often inaccessible.
- This approach carries a unique set of complications. The most significant of these can be divided into approach-related (eg, lumbar plexus injury, genitofemoral nerve trauma, psoas weakness, retroperitoneal hematoma, posterior abdominal wall hernias) and instrumentation-related (eg, graft subsidence, vertebral body fracture, pseudoarthrosis).

INTRODUCTION: NATURE OF THE PROBLEM

The minimally invasive lateral transpsoas approach to the lumbar spine, also known as extreme lateral interbody fusion (XLIF) or direct lateral interbody fusion (DLIF), has become an increasingly popular approach for achieving interbody fusion over the past decade.[1] This approach differs from other interbody fusion techniques in many ways. Instead of the prone or supine position, the lateral transpsoas technique employs a lateral decubitus position. The approach then utilizes a retroperitoneal dissection followed by splitting of the psoas muscle to gain access to the lateral aspect of the spine.

Reported advantages of this technique include a smaller incision and less blood loss compared with open procedures, leading to decreased operative times and shorter hospital stays as well as less postoperative pain.[2] Because the procedure utilizes a lateral (rather than anterior) retroperitoneal corridor, it also offers less risk of injury to peritoneal contents and the hypogastric sympathetic plexus when compared with more anterior minimally invasive approaches. Furthermore, the XLIF/DLIF technique has been shown to

[a] Department of Neurosurgery, Northwestern University Feinberg School of Medicine, 676 North St. Clair, #2210, Chicago, IL 60610, USA; [b] Department of Neurosurgery, Keck School of Medicine, University of Southern California, 1520 San Pablo Street, Suite 3800, Los Angeles, CA 90033, USA
* Corresponding author.
E-mail address: Randall.b.graham@gmail.com

Neurosurg Clin N Am 25 (2014) 219–231
http://dx.doi.org/10.1016/j.nec.2013.12.002
1042-3680/14/$ – see front matter © 2014 Elsevier Inc. All rights reserved.

significantly improve regional, segmental, and global coronal balance in patients with degenerative lumbar disease and has been proven to be a feasible technique for achieving fusion in adult degenerative scoliosis.[3,4] In an in vitro setting, the direct lateral approach has been proven to be biomechanically equivalent to the anterior approach.[4]

Despite these advantages, the DLIF/XLIF technique carries a unique set of complications with the potential for significant neurologic morbidity. Because the technique differs from the others, mainly in its lateral transpsoas approach to the spine, the most significant complications of the technique are approach-related.[2,5] Hardware- and instrumentation-related complications are also possible (as with any interbody fusion technique), and these will also be discussed in this article.

THERAPEUTIC OPTIONS AND SURGICAL TECHNIQUE

The lateral transpsoas procedure differs from anterior lumbar interbody fusion (ALIF), posterior lumbar interbody fusion (PLIF), and transforaminal lumbar interbody fusion (TLIF) in several important aspects (**Table 1**).[3,6–14]

While ALIF utilizes supine positioning with an anterior abdominal approach and PLIF, and TLIF uses prone positioning with posterior approaches, DLIF/XLIF is unique in that lateral decubitus positioning is used for a true lateral retroperitoneal approach to the spine. Neurologic monitoring, especially electromyography (EMG), is then employed via placement of electrodes that correspond to the L2-L5 myotomes with stimulation to confirm adequate twitch strength. This allows for accurate reproducible EMG recordings, which are mandatory throughout the DLIF/XLIF procedure, because the psoas muscle-splitting approach exposes the lumbar plexus to potential injury.[15–17]

After positioning and initiation of neurologic monitoring, a lateral radiograph is obtained to confirm a truly lateral position and to center the planned incision over the treatment level. An incision is made on the lateral aspect of the abdomen directly over the spine, and blunt dissection is used to identify a retroperitoneal corridor to the

Table 1
Comparison of surgical approaches for lumbar interbody fusion

	ALIF	PLIF	TLIF	DLIF/XLIF
Access	Open or laparoscopic	Open or minimally invasive	Open or minimally invasive	Minimally invasive
Approach	Anterior abdominal (retroperitoneal or transperitoneal)	Midline posterior incision with laminectomy/ laminotomy and nerve root retraction	Offset posterior incision with access through intervertebral foramen	Lateral retroperitoneal approach to anterior spine with specialized retractors
Advantages	• Avoids paraspinal muscle trauma • Less risk of dural tears and nerve root traction • Direct disc space visualization may allow more complete discectomy and better fusion	• Decompression allows treatment of canal pathology as well as stabilization	• Good visualization of neural elements without significant dural retraction • Provides access to posterior elements as well as disc space	• Anterior psoas dissection may reduce nerve root injury • Less blood loss and postoperative pain by avoiding paraspinal muscle trauma
Drawbacks	• Potential retraction injury to great vessels and/or peritoneal contents • Potential hypogastric plexus injury	• Significant nerve root retraction with risk of injury and dural tears • Significant paraspinal muscle dissection	• Only a partial laminectomy with less canal decompression	• Psoas dissection puts lumbar plexus at risk for injury • Decreased ability to address posterior element pathology

psoas muscle. A series of tubes and dilators are then used to direct the surgeon to the midposition of the treatment disc, taking care not to enter the peritoneal space, and the initial dilator is inserted through the psoas muscle. At this point, the fibers of the psoas muscle are separated using a system of sequential dilators, and the neural monitoring system is used to evaluate proximity to the lumbar plexus via a stimulator electrode. Stimulation typically localizes the lumbar plexus to the posterior and inferior quadrants of the dilator tubes, so the safest docking site after continued dilation to enter the disc space is a position slightly anterior to the midpoint of the disc. After the final dilator is placed, a retractor is introduced and fixed to the operating room table and then opened to reveal the disc space (**Fig. 1**).[1] Neural monitoring should then be checked again to ensure that the lumbar plexus is not being stretched across the operative field.

After the index disc has been accessed, it can be incised and removed utilizing fluoroscopy to ascertain the appropriate resection depth. After disk resection and end plate preparation, an appropriately sized interbody graft is placed. Due to the lateral approach and access, which obviates dural and nerve root retraction, DLIF/XLIF typically allows for a larger interbody implant than either PLIF or TLIF. If needed, segmental instrumentation can then be placed percutaneously from a posterior approach, which allows for an overall minimally invasive operation (**Fig. 2**).

The DLIF/XLIF approach is most commonly used for the treatment of a single disc level, although multilevel procedures are certainly feasible. The main limitation to this approach is inaccessibility of the most caudal segments. The presence of the sacrum and pelvis renders the L5-S1 disc space inaccessible from a lateral corridor, and the L4-5 interspace can be similarly obscured nearly half the time. Additionally, approaching a lumbarized sacrum has been described as a relative contraindication to this approach.[18]

CLINICAL OUTCOMES

Most DLIF/XLIF procedures are performed for degenerative conditions, including spondylolisthesis, herniated disc, degenerative disc disease, postlaminectomy kyphosis, adjacent segment disease, and degenerative scoliosis.[2] There are rare case reports of the procedure being used for treatment of spinal osteomyelitis or metastasis.[12,19]

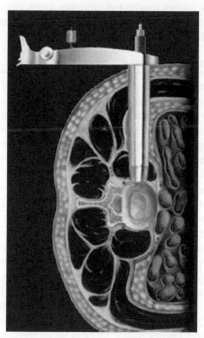

Fig. 1. Schematic of the lateral, retroperitoneal, transpsoas approach to the lumbar spine using sequential dilation and a self-retaining psoas muscle retractor. (*From* Ozgur BM, et al. Extreme Lateral Interbody Fusion (XLIF): a novel surgical technique for anterior lumbar interbody fusion. Spine J 2006;6(4):439; with permission.)

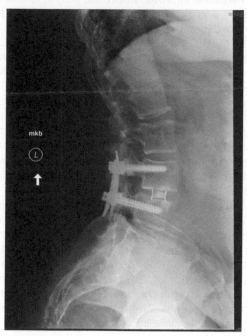

Fig. 2. Postoperative lateral radiograph demonstrating the relatively anterior placement of an interbody graft using the lateral transpsoas approach with percutaneously placed posterior segmental instrumentation at L4-5.

Several large series detailing the outcomes and complications of this approach have been published recently, the majority of these being retrospective reviews involving procedures performed at 1 to 2 levels with supplemental posterior element fixation.[9–12,14,20,21] Rodgers and colleagues[6] assessed both patient outcomes and fusion rates in 66 patients after surgery. In 1-year follow-up, 96.6% of levels were judged as fused on computed tomography (CT) scan, and nearly 90% of patients responded as "satisfied or very satisfied" on a written survey. Ozgur and colleagues[15] reported a 91% fusion rate and a favorable change in Oswestry Disability Index (ODI) in 75% of patients at 2 years after undergoing XLIF.

There have also been multiple retrospective analyses of postoperative radiographic outcomes, including both local segmental parameters and global sagittal and coronal balance. Through restoration of disc height via placement of a large interbody graft, it has been proposed that DLIF/XLIF can expand the intervertebral foramen and thus indirectly decompress the nerve roots. Olveira and colleagues[20] analyzed such indirect decompression in 15 patients undergoing XLIF for degenerative disc disease and stenosis. Using plain radiographs and magnetic resonance imaging (MRI), the authors demonstrated substantial dimensional improvement in disc height, foraminal height, and foraminal area, thus implying adequate neural decompression.

In recent years, the indications for XLIF/DLIF have expanded to include treatment of degenerative spinal deformity, which tends to involve several levels of correction and fixation. In 2008, Anand and colleagues[4] demonstrated the feasibility of XLIF for this indication in 12 patients with a mean of 3.64 corrected segments achieving an average of 13° of correction per patient. Their 2-year outcomes demonstrated a 100% fusion rate with maintenance of immediate postoperative correction.[22]

Karikari and colleagues[19] analyzed both radiographic and clinical outcomes in 22 patients treated with lateral interbody fusion for a variety of conditions (including degenerative scoliosis, tumors, thoracic disc herniations, and vertebral osteomyelitis). In those treated for degenerative scoliosis, the mean coronal Cobb angle went from 22° preoperatively to 14° postoperatively, and a substantial clinical benefit was observed in 95.5% of patients.

In a similar fashion, Dakwar and colleagues[23] reported 25 patients who underwent XLIF for thoracolumbar degenerative deformity. Although they found no significant correction in sagittal balance at 11-month follow-up, clinical outcomes were acceptable, and there were minimal long-term complications. Wang and colleagues[13] published a similar series in which a mean sagittal correction of 20° was obtained, and a fusion rate of over 97% was achieved at 2-year follow-up.

Acosta and colleagues[3] performed a thorough radiographic analysis of the changes in coronal and sagittal plane alignment following XLIF for degenerative scoliosis and noted favorable results for correction of both parameters. It was concluded that at 2-year follow-up, the direct lateral transpsoas approach (when combined with posterior segmental fixation) resulted in significant improvement in segmental, regional, and global coronal plane alignment. Although there were no statistically significant changes in global sagittal alignment or lumbar lordosis, there was a significant improvement in ODI at 2-year follow-up.[3]

COMPLICATIONS AND CONCERNS

The DLIF/XLIF technique carries a unique set of complications due to the lateral transpsoas approach utilized to access the spine. These approach-related complications include neurologic morbidity from damage to the nearby lumbar plexus, psoas weakness, and retroperitoneal complications such as hematomas and surgical hernias (**Table 2**).

Approach-Related Complications

The incidence of approach-related complications reported in the literature seems to vary significantly. The largest series of XLIF procedures was reported by Rodgers and colleagues,[12] with 600 patients and an exceedingly low (1%) approach-related complication rate and a nearly equally low (6.2%) overall complication rate. They additionally found that there was no significant difference in complication rate with obese patients.[11] Such low incidence of approach-related morbidity in these large series seems to differ widely from that reported in other smaller series published around the same time (see **Table 2**). This is likely because of differences among authors with regards to methods of reporting and tracking these complications. By far the most common reported complications to the XLIF/DLIF technique are ipsilateral anterior thigh pain and psoas major muscle weakness, both of which are likely related to splitting the psoas muscle fibers upon approaching the spine and/or minor trauma to the lumbar plexus. Anand and colleagues[22] reported these symptoms in nearly 75% of patients, while Cummock and colleagues[24] (when specifically analyzing postoperative thigh symptoms) found them in nearly two-thirds of patients. Other authors have broken down postoperative thigh/psoas symptoms into specific components (pain vs weakness vs numbness) and reported them as separate incidences. Moller and colleagues[25] reported a 36% rate of immediate postoperative psoas weakness, with 25% and 23% incidences of anterior thigh numbness and pain, respectively.

Of note, most patients who suffer from psoas and thigh-related approach complications seem to have resolution of these symptoms in long-term follow-up. Moller and colleagues[25] noted 84%, 69%, and 75% complete resolution of psoas weakness, anterior thigh numbness, and pain, respectively, at 6-month follow-up. Pumberger and colleagues[26] tracked the course of these complications at 6-week, 12-week, 6-month, and 12-month intervals and found that the incidence of anterior thigh pain, anterior thigh numbness, and psoas flexion weakness tended to diminish in a nearly linear fashion over time (see **Table 2**).

Despite reporting such a low incidence of approach-related complications in their 2 large series, Rodgers and colleagues[12] noted that, in fact, thigh pain and psoas weakness were both "nearly universal" and "always transient" in their patient population and were therefore not directly reported as approach-related complications. This likely explains the significant discrepancy of reported approach-related morbidity between their 2 large series and those of other authors.

Although less common, DLIF/XLIF also carries the risk of more permanent neurologic sequelae from its unique lateral approach (see **Table 2**). These complications are more likely caused by more severe or direct injury to the lumbar plexus, which lies underneath the psoas muscle and is at risk for traumatic injury from the surgical approach.

In a series of 58 patients treated with XLIF for degenerative conditions, Knight and colleagues[16] reported 2 patients who suffered from ipsilateral L4 distribution motor deficits that persisted 1 year postoperatively. Other studies analyzing DLIF/XLIF for degenerative conditions reported neurologic approach-related sequelae that were transient.

When utilized for degenerative scoliosis, however, the incidence of longer-lasting postoperative lumbar radiculopathy or plexopathy seems to be higher. Out of a series of 23 patients treated for adult spinal deformities, Wang and Mummaneni[13] reported a single patient who required a long-term assistive ambulatory device due to postoperative numbness, pain, and dysesthesias ipsilateral to the approach side. Tormenti and colleagues[27] reported 5 out of a series of 8 patients treated using DLIF/XLIF for adult degenerative scoliosis who had persistent sensory radiculopathy and a single patient with persistent motor radiculopathy.

Isaacs and colleagues[9] studied this particular patient population further with a prospective non-randomized analysis of 107 patients undergoing DLIF/XLIF for symptomatic adult thoracolumbar scoliosis. Similar to other studies, they found that isolated proximal hip weakness was the most common complication and was transient 86% of the time. Seven out of the 107 patients, however, suffered from severe and protracted hip weakness that persisted 6 months postoperatively.

Because the DLIF/XLIF approach involves establishing a dissection plane through the retroperitoneal space, there can be considerable manipulation of the abdominal wall and adjacent thoracoabdominal structures. Damage to these structures is thus a source of postoperative approach-related morbidity. Review of the literature reveals that these types of complications are rare, but potentially serious in that they are likely to require additional intervention (see **Table 2**).

Inadequate closure or subsequent reopening of deeper fascial layers can result in surgical hernias. This is certainly applicable in the retroperitoneal space, where visceral contents can herniate posteriorly and laterally through muscular defects. In each of their 2 large retrospective series, Rodgers and colleagues[11,12] reported single patients who had postoperative incisional hernias requiring surgical repair. In a smaller series of 30 patients, Caputo and colleagues[37] reported a similar complication in a single patient.

The dissection through the lateral abdominal wall can also damage abdominal motor nerves, leading to abdominal wall paresis and an abnormal bulging appearance.[28,35] Dakwar and colleagues first reported this complication in a retrospective review of 568 patients and found a 1.8% incidence. Similarly, Cahill and colleagues reported this finding in 5 out of 118 (4.2%) patients.

Manipulation and placement of retractors in the retroperitoneal corridor can also cause damage and hemorrhage to retroperitoneal structures. Splitting of the psoas muscle fibers can lead to a psoas hematoma, which appears to be the most common of this type of complication (see **Table 2**).[20,33] None of these isolated psoas hematomas required intervention; however, Sharma and colleagues[30] reported 1 patient out of their series of 43 who developed a retroperitoneal hemorrhage that required immediate embolization.

Although relatively remote from the DLIF/XLIF access corridor, retroperitoneal and peritoneal visceral structures are also at risk. Anand and

Table 2
Approach-related complications of DLIF/XLIF

Study	n	DLIF/XLIF Approach Complications	Rate
Anand et al,[4] 2008	12	3 thigh dysesthesias (resolved in 6 wk) 1 transient quadriceps weakness (resolved in 6 wk)	4/12 (25%)
Knight et al,[16] 2009	58	2 ipsilateral L4 nerve root injuries 6 irritation of femoral cutaneous nerve resulting in meralgia paresthetica 1 significant psoas muscle spasm extending hospital stay	9/58 (15.5%)
Anand et al,[22] 2010	28	17 thigh dysesthesias (resolved in 6 wk) Several patients with transient hip flexor weakness and pain 2 quadriceps palsies with weakness of vastus medialis (complete recovery) 1 intraoperative retrocapsular renal hematomas	20/28 (71%)
Tormenti et al,[27] 2010	8	6 sensory radiculopathies 2 motor radiculopathies 2 pleural effusions necessitating chest tube placement 1 bowel perforation	6/8 (75%)
Dakwar et al,[23] 2010	25	3 transient ipsilateral anterior thigh numbness	3/25 (12%)
Wang et al,[13] 2010	23	7 ipsilateral, pain, weakness, and dysesthesias 1 pneumothorax (requiring chest tube)	8/23 (35%)
Oliveira et al,[20] 2010	21	3 psoas weaknesses 1 psoas hematoma	4/21 (19%)
Rodgers et al,[12] 2011	600	1 incisional hernia 1 subcutaneous hematoma 3 quadriceps weaknesses 1 anterior tibialis weakness	6/600 (1%)
Rodgers et al,[11] 2010	432	4 nerve injury 1 incisional hernia	5/432 (1%)
Youssef et al,[14] 2010	84	1 ipsilateral psoas weakness and numbness	1/84 (1%)
Isaacs et al,[9] 2010	107	1 pleural effusion 1 kidney laceration 7 motor deficits 2 pleural cavity violations requiring chest tube 1 sensory deficit	12/107 (11%)
Dakwar et al,[28] 2011	568	10 abdominal paresis	10/568 (1.8%)
Moller et al,[25] 2011	53	19 subjective hip flexor weaknesses 13 new thigh/groin numbness ipsilateral to approach 12 new thigh/groin pain ipsilateral to approach	25% 23% 23%
Cummock et al,[24] 2011	59	37 thigh numbness 14 hip flexor weaknesses 4 knee extension weaknesses	37/59 (63%)
Tohmeh et al,[17] 2011	102	28 hip flexor weaknesses 18 upper medial thigh numbness 1 quadriceps weakness 1 dorsiflexion weakness	27.5% 17.6%
Pimenta et al,[29] 2011	36	5 psoas weaknesses 3 anterior thigh numbness 1 weakness of ipsilateral leg	13.8% 8.3% 2.8%

(continued on next page)

Table 2
(continued)

Study	n	DLIF/XLIF Approach Complications	Rate
Sharma et al,[30] 2011	43	15 anterior thigh pains 11 hip flexor weaknesses 4 quadriceps weaknesses 1 retroperitoneal hemorrhage	34.8% 25.6% 9.3% 2.3%
Kepler et al,[31] 2011	13	3 transient hip flexion weaknesses 1 hypoesthesia in anterior thigh	4/13 (31%)
Papanastassiou et al,[32] 2011	14	2 injuries to contralateral psoas and neural elements	2/14 (14%)
Berjano et al,[33] 2012	97	4 transient L4 distribution weaknesses 3 transient L4 distribution numbness 9 transient thigh symptoms 1 psoas hematoma	17/97 (18%)

Pumberger et al,[26] 2012	235	Sensory deficits anterior groin/thigh
		   6 wk: 70
		   12 wk: 32
		   6 mo: 14
		   12 mo: 4
		Pain anterior groin/thigh
		   6 wk: 101
		   12 wk: 39
		   6 mo: 9
		   12 mo: 2
		Psoas mechanical flexion deficits
		   6 wk: 32
		   12 wk: 9
		   6 mo: 7
		   12 mo: 4
		Lumbar plexus-related motor deficits
		   6 wk: 12
		   12 wk: 12
		   6 mo: 7
		   12 mo: 7
			
			28.7%
			13.1%
			5.7%
			1.6%
			
			41%
			16%
			3.7%
			0.8%
			
			13.1%
			3.7%
			2.9%
			1.6%
			
			4.9%
			4.9%
			2.9%
			2.9%

Sofianos et al,[5] 2012	45	10 iliopsoas weaknesses 8 anterior thigh numbness 3 quadriceps weaknesses 3 radiculopathies 1 foot drop	18/45 (40%)
Le et al,[34] 2013	71	14 transient ipsilateral thigh numbness 2 ipsilateral iliopsoas weaknesses 2 paresthesias/radiculopathy	14/71 (19.7%)
Cahill et al,[35] 2012	118	2 femoral nerve injury 5 abdominal flank bulges (injury to abdominal wall motor innervations)	1.7% 4.2%
Malham et al,[36] 2012	30	5 ipsilateral leg dysesthesias 1 ipsilateral leg motor deficit 1 bowel injury	7/30 (23%)

colleagues reported a single patient with a postoperative retrocapsular renal hematoma that tamponaded on its own. Peritoneal violation with subsequent bowel perforation is a potentially devastating complication from this approach, which has been reported twice in the literature. In their series of 8 patients undergoing multilevel lateral transpsoas approach surgery for interbody fusion for degenerative scoliosis, Tormenti and colleagues[27] reported a single patient in whom a cecal perforation occurred during the approach, requiring emergent exploratory laparotomy with bowel resection. Similarly, Malham and colleagues[36] described a patient who developed severe abdominal pain on postoperative day 3 and was found to have intraperitoneal free air; emergent laparotomy revealed injury to the descending colon adjacent to the L4-5 level. When the approach is utilized at higher levels, pleural violation and injury is possible, leading to pleural effusion or pneumothorax. This complication has been reported in multiple series of patients receiving DLIF/XLIF for treatment of thoracolumbar conditions.[9,13,27] All of these patients required temporary thoracostomy tubes.

Hardware-Related Complications

The DLIF/XLIF technique also carries the risk of fusion and hardware-related complications and failure (Table 3). The most common of such hardware-related complications appear to be interbody graft subsidence (with or without adjacent vertebral body fracture). A few of these subsidences were observed with serial radiographs with eventual fusion; however, most of them required eventual intervention. In general, minor incidentally discovered subsidences without corresponding endplate or vertebral body fracture were observed.[16,23,36] In many instances, however, subsidence presented with progressive pain and/or radiculopathy and required further intervention.

In their large series of 600 XLIF patients, Rodgers and colleagues[12] described 3 patients with postoperative graft subsidence (one with an adjacent vertebral body fracture, one with a fracture of the graft itself, and a third caused by pedicle screw violation of the endplate); all three of these patients required eventual reoperation. However, the nature of their revision surgery was not mentioned.

It is possible that graft subsidence causing symptoms represents persistent instability and/or motion at that segment. In a series of 21 patients, Olveira and colleagues[20] reported 2 patients with early postoperative graft subsidences that were discovered when the patients reported persistent pain and no improvement following standalone XLIF. Both of these patients received subsequent placement of posterior segmental instrumentation with pedicle screws across the subsidence level, resulting in eventual fusion and symptom relief in both cases. This may imply that persistent motion between the 2 vertebrae resulted in slippage of the graft and clinically manifested with recurrent symptoms that were resolved with posterior fixation. Further radiographic and biomechanical studies are needed to confirm this.

In 2 separate studies of DLIF/XLIF, Karikari and colleagues[19] reported 4 out of 66 patients and 1 out of 22 patients with cage subsidence and associated vertebral body fractures.[38] All but one of these patients required reoperation. Two of these patients presented with compression deformity in the segment rostral to the construct and received vertebroplasty or kyphoplasty augmentation at that level (Fig. 3). Another 2 presents presented with persistent movement at the treated level with cage subsidence into an adjacent vertebral body, and these were treated with pedicle screw augmentation. The authors noted that subsidence with fracture seemed to occur in patients older than 70 years (incidence of 16.7%), and it is possible that bone mineral density may play a role in the development of these complications.

As with any spinal fusion procedure, there is a risk of nonunion and pseudoarthrosis. Although reported fusion rates from DLIF/XLIF have been high as 91% to 96%,[6,15] there are rare reports of pseudoarthrosis following DLIF/XLIF in the literature. Wang and colleagues[13] described a patient with postinfectious kyphosis corrected with multilevel XLIF and posterior instrumentation who was found to have asymptomatic screw lengthening and pseudoarthrosis that was managed conservatively. Sharma and colleagues[30] reported 2 patients with pseudoarthrosis; one with a single level nonunion that required revision, and another with 4 levels of nonunion that were treated with bracing.

Adjacent segment disease and persistent stenosis are also mentioned in various series. These complications are rare, but significant in that they are likely to require reoperation.[19,20,38] Additional reports of screw pullout, intraoperative pedicle fractures, and remote vertebral fractures are mentioned in Table 3.

Prevention of Approach-Related Complications

As described previously, transient psoas weakness and anterior thigh pain are frequent complications, but are not a source of major long-term morbidity from the lateral transpsoas approach. Lasting deficits from more severe neural injury, however, are potentially devastating, and several studies have aimed to define safe working corridors to prevent such injuries.

Several cadaver studies have sought to define the anatomy of the lumbar plexus and propose safe areas for dilator placement at each level. From these studies, it has been found that the lumbosacral plexus lies within the fibers of the psoas muscle between the junction of the transverse process and the vertebral body, exiting along the medial edge of the psoas muscle.[8] The plexus is most dorsally positioned at the posterior

Table 3
Hardware-related complications of DLIF/XLIF

Study	n	DLIF/XLIF Hardware Complications	Rate
Knight et al,[16] 2009	58	1 acute graft subsidence	1/58 (1.7%)
Anand et al,[22] 2010	28	1 screw prominence 1 asymptomatic proximal screw fracture	2/28 (7.1%)
Dakwar et al,[23] 2010	25	1 graft subsidence 1 posterior instrumentation failure	2/25 (8%)
Wang et al,[13] 2010	23	1 pseudoarthrosis 1 screw pullout	2/23 (8.7%)
Oliveira et al,[20] 2010	21	1 graft subsidence 1 heterotopic bone formation 1 persistent stenosis	3/21 (14.3%)
Rodgers et al,[12] 2011	600	1 endplate fracture 1 vertebral body fracture with graft subsidence 1 osteophyte fracture 2 adjacent-level vertebral compression fractures 1 iatrogenic herniated disc 1 graft subsidence with graft fracture 1 screw fracture through endplate with graft subsidence	8/600 (1.3%)
Rodgers et al,[11] 2010	432	3 vertebral body fractures 3 posterior hardware failures	6/432 (1.4%)
Youssef et al,[14] 2010	84	1 nondisplaced bilateral pedicle fracture 1 mild endplate fracture 1 vertebral body fracture 1 graft subsidence 2 adjacent segment diseases	6/84 (7.1%)
Karikari et al,[38] 2011	66	4 graft subsidences 1 intraoperative pedicle fracture 1 remote compression fracture 1 adjacent segment disease	5/66 (7.6%)
Karikari et al,[19] 2011	22	1 graft subsidence 1 adjacent segment disease	2/22 (9.1%)
Sharma et al,[30] 2011	43 (87 levels)	18 intraoperative endplate fractures 5 pseudoarthrosis/nonunions 2 vertebral body fractures 1 malpositioned cage	26/87 (29.9%)
Kepler et al,[31] 2011	13	2 nondisplaced vertebral fractures through screw tracts	2/13 (15.4%)
Berjano et al,[33] 2012	97	2 graft subsidences	2/97 (2.1%)
Le et al,[34] 2013	71	3 dislodged lateral plates 3 vertebral body fractures	6/71 (8.5%)
Caputo et al,[37] 2012	30	1 pedicle fracture 1 symptomatic pseudoarthrosis	2/30 (6.7%)
Malham et al,[36] 2012	30	4 graft subsidences 2 reoperations (microforaminotomy, pedicle screw fixation) 1 graft breakage	7/30 (23.3%)

endplate of L1-2, and there is a trend of progressive ventral migration of the plexus at L2-3, L3-4, and L4-5.[8] When the locations of these nerves are measured relative to the center of the disc space from a lateral position (effectively simulating the position of the dilators during a lateral transpsoas approach), the intrapsoas nerves are shown to be a relatively safe distance from the center of

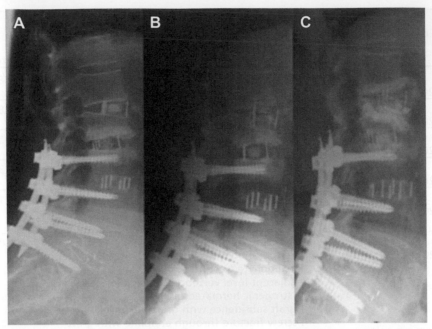

Fig. 3. Plain lateral standing lumbar radiograph of a patient with L1-2 graft subsidence and L2 compression fracture. (*A*) Immediate postoperative standing lumbar radiograph demonstrating interbody graft from XLIF at L1-2 as well as L2-3 and L3-4 and prior L3-S1 fusion. (*B*) 3-month interval radiograph demonstrating subsidence of the L1-2 cage and a compression fracture at L2. (*C*) 4-month radiograph demonstrating postvertebroplasty changes and fusion mass at L1 and L2. (*From* Karikari IO, Grossi PM, Nimjee SM, et al. Minimally invasive lumbar interbody fusion in patients older than 70 years of age: analysis of peri- and postoperative complications. Neurosurgery 2011;68(4):901; with permission.)

the disc.[39] More detailed dissection has revealed that theoretically safe corridors should avoid both the lumbar plexus and the genitofemoral nerve (**Figs. 4** and **5**), and the position of these corridors depends on the level of the approach. For higher levels (L1-2, L2-3, and L3-4), this is the mid-posterior quarter of the vertebral body, and for L4-5, the safe docking zone should be at the midpoint of the vertebral body.[40]

Electrophysiologic technology has also been developed to help avoid these complications. Real-time directionally stimulated discrete threshold electromyography (EMG) was developed in the last decade to aid in intraoperative identification of psoas nerves. This tool has allowed surgeons to determine the proximity and avoid these nerves during the approach.[41] Intraoperative monitoring studies have confirmed

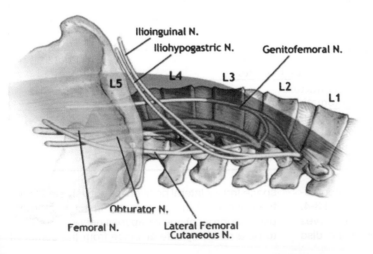

Fig. 4. Schematic of the lumbar spine, psoas muscle, and lumbar plexus from the lateral view. (*From* Uribe JS, Vale FL, Dakwar E. Electromyographic monitoring and its anatomic implications in minimally invasive spine surgery. Spine (Phila Pa 1976) 2010;35(Suppl 26):S372; with permission.)

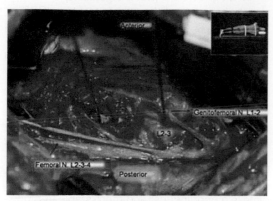

Fig. 5. Cadaveric specimen in the lateral decubitus position demonstrating markers placed relative to the genitofemoral nerve and the femoral nerve. (*From* Uribe JS, et al. Defining the safe working zones using the minimally invasive lateral retroperitoneal transpsoas approach: an anatomic study. J Neurosurg Spine 2010;13(2):263; with permission.)

previous cadaveric studies by demonstrating that most intrapsoas nerves are identified at the posterior margin of the DLIF/XLIF dilators.[17] Before the advent of this technology, postoperative neurologic sequelae from this approach were as high as 30% (with long term deficits in 10% of patients).[42] More recent series would suggest that the use of intraoperative EMG may be associated with a decreased incidence of postoperative lumbar plexopathy (see **Table 2**); however, no direct comparative studies exist. Despite this, many recent authors recommend the use of intraoperative EMG.[1,13,15–17,23]

Although the use of intraoperative EMG may be associated with reduced risk of lumbar plexus injury, this technology does not always accurately show the site of the nerves, because nerve location can be variable, thus reinforcing the need for real-time information regarding their proximity to the approach corridor.[17] Direct stimulation and visualization, as well as careful placement of this working portal, are key to avoiding nerve injury and safe performance of the lateral transpsoas approach. Additionally, the risk of stretch to the lumbar plexus can theoretically be minimized by opening the retractor blades only as much as minimally needed. This risk can also be theoretically minimized by limiting the time taken to perform the discectomy and interbody placement. By shortening the docking time, the surgeon can minimize the amount of stretch and plexus effect.

Although plexus injuries garner significant attention as approach-related complications of lateral access, visceral and vascular structures also deserve significant attention. During the initial docking, there is potential for injury to the bowel. For this reason, the trajectory and position of initial docking are critical, because even a blunt dilator can catch and damage visceral structures. Some surgeons utilize a shallow docking technique, in which the dilator is held in a position just superficial to the psoas muscle.[43] This decreases the risk of vascular and visceral injury, and the surgeon can work from the depths of this corridor, through the psoas muscle, and into the disk space. Furthermore, this suprapsoas technique can potentially aid in direct visualization of the lumbosacral plexus, thereby minimizing the postoperative neurologic morbidity discussed earlier.[43]

Although rarely described, it should be noted that anatomic injury can occur on the side contralateral to the approach. For instance, if the surgeon works with even a small degree of angulation across the disc space, the tips of the instruments can pass significantly more ventrally or dorsally than expected. Additionally, aggressive use of Cobb dilators to dissect across the contralateral ligament can lead to potential injury to the contralateral plexus or even contralateral vascular structures.[32] Careful, judicious use of these instruments is critical when dissecting across the disc space. Additionally, the surgeon should make note of the location of nearby great vessels on preoperative films.

Prevention of Hardware-Related Complications

The most frequent and morbid hardware-related complication is subsidence of the interbody graft (**Table 3**). From review of the most recent literature, symptomatic graft subsidence seems to occur when there is instability and excess movement at the treated level in the setting of standalone DLIF/XLIF.[20,38] In these cases, patients have required separate operations for posterior segmental fixation. Whether up-front construct augmentation with pedicle screws would decrease the risk of subsidence in these cases is subject for further debate and analysis.

Graft subsidence can also occur in the setting of vertebral body fracture, especially in the setting of elderly patients.[38] Meticulous preoperative planning with a thorough bone density workup can therefore be performed when there is potential for such a concern, particularly when a long construct is planned.

SUMMARY

The direct lateral transpsoas approach has gained significant recent popularity and will likely become even more popular as a method for approaching the spine to achieve interbody fusion. This technique offers favorable fusion rates and long-term clinical outcomes with less invasiveness and blood loss. Despite its relative safety, however, DLIF/XLIF carries a unique set of complications, mainly from its unique lateral transpsoas approach, which places the lumbar plexus at risk of injury. Minimizing these complications will require an even more thorough understanding of intrapsoas nerve anatomy and physiology, further development of intraoperative monitoring technology, appropriate patient selection, and appropriate preoperative planning.

REFERENCES

1. Ozgur BM, Aryan HE, Pimenta L, et al. Extreme lateral interbody fusion (XLIF): a novel surgical technique for anterior lumbar interbody fusion. Spine J 2006;6(4):435–43.
2. Arnold PM, Anderson KK, McGuire RA Jr. The lateral transpsoas approach to the lumbar and thoracic spine: a review. Surg Neurol Int 2012;3(Suppl 3):S198–215.
3. Acosta FL, Liu J, Slimack N, et al. Changes in coronal and sagittal plane alignment following minimally invasive direct lateral interbody fusion for the treatment of degenerative lumbar disease in adults: a radiographic study. J Neurosurg Spine 2011;15(1):92–6.
4. Anand N, Baron EM, Thaiyananthan G, et al. Minimally invasive multilevel percutaneous correction and fusion for adult lumbar degenerative scoliosis: a technique and feasibility study. J Spinal Disord Tech 2008;21(7):459–67.
5. Sofianos DA, Briseno MR, Abrams J, et al. Complications of the lateral transpsoas approach for lumbar interbody arthrodesis: a case series and literature review. Clin Orthop Relat Res 2012;470(6):1621–32.
6. Rodgers WB, Gerber EJ, Patterson JR. Fusion after minimally disruptive anterior lumbar interbody fusion: analysis of extreme lateral interbody fusion by computed tomography. The International Journal of Spine Surgery 2010;4(2):63–6.
7. Banagan K, Gelb D, Poelstra K, et al. Anatomic mapping of lumbar nerve roots during a direct lateral transpsoas approach to the spine: a cadaveric study. Spine (Phila Pa 1976) 2011;36(11):E687–91.
8. Benglis DM, Vanni S, Levi AD. An anatomical study of the lumbosacral plexus as related to the minimally invasive transpsoas approach to the lumbar spine. J Neurosurg Spine 2009;10(2):139–44.
9. Isaacs RF, Hyde J, Goodrich JA, et al. A prospective, nonrandomized, multicenter evaluation of extreme lateral interbody fusion for the treatment of adult degenerative scoliosis: perioperative outcomes and complications. Spine (Phila Pa 1976) 2010;35(Suppl 26):S322–30.
10. Ghahreman A, Ferch RD, Rao PJ, et al. Minimal access versus open posterior lumbar interbody fusion in the treatment of spondylolisthesis. Neurosurgery 2010;66(2):296–304 [discussion: 304].
11. Rodgers WB, Cox CS, Gerber EJ. Early complications of extreme lateral interbody fusion in the obese. J Spinal Disord Tech 2010;23(6):393–7.
12. Rodgers WB, Gerber EJ, Patterson J. Intraoperative and early postoperative complications in extreme lateral interbody fusion: an analysis of 600 cases. Spine (Phila Pa 1976) 2011;36(1):26–32.
13. Wang MY, Mummaneni PV. Minimally invasive surgery for thoracolumbar spinal deformity: initial clinical experience with clinical and radiographic outcomes. Neurosurg Focus 2010;28(3):E9.
14. Youssef JA, McAfee PC, Patty CA, et al. Minimally invasive surgery: lateral approach interbody fusion: results and review. Spine (Phila Pa 1976) 2010;35(Suppl 26):S302–11.
15. Ozgur BM, Agarwal V, Nail E, et al. Two-year clinical and radiographic success of minimally invasive lateral transpsoas approach for the treatment of degenerative lumbar conditions. SAS Journal 2010;4(2):41–6.
16. Knight RQ, Schwaegler P, Hanscom D, et al. Direct lateral lumbar interbody fusion for degenerative conditions: early complication profile. J Spinal Disord Tech 2009;22(1):34–7.
17. Tohmeh AG, Rodgers WB, Peterson MD. Dynamically evoked, discrete-threshold electromyography in the extreme lateral interbody fusion approach. J Neurosurg Spine 2011;14(1):31–7.
18. Smith WD, Youssef JA, Christian G, et al. Lumbarized sacrum as a relative contraindication for lateral transpsoas interbody fusion at L5-6. J Spinal Disord Tech 2012;25(5):285–91.
19. Karikari IO, Nimjee SM, Hardin CA, et al. Extreme lateral interbody fusion approach for isolated thoracic and thoracolumbar spine diseases: initial clinical experience and early outcomes. J Spinal Disord Tech 2011;24(6):368–75.
20. Oliveira L, Marchi L, Coutinho E, et al. A radiographic assessment of the ability of the extreme lateral interbody fusion procedure to indirectly decompress the neural elements. Spine (Phila Pa 1976) 2010;35(Suppl 26):S331–7.
21. Inamasu J, Guiot BH. Laparoscopic anterior lumbar interbody fusion: a review of outcome studies. Minim Invasive Neurosurg 2005;48(6):340–7.
22. Anand N, Rosemann R, Khalsa B, et al. Mid-term to long-term clinical and functional outcomes of minimally invasive correction and fusion for adults with scoliosis. Neurosurg Focus 2010;28(3):E6.

23. Dakwar E, Cardona RF, Smith DA, et al. Early outcomes and safety of the minimally invasive, lateral retroperitoneal transpsoas approach for adult degenerative scoliosis. Neurosurg Focus 2010;28(3):E8.

24. Cummock MD, Vanni S, Levi AD, et al. An analysis of postoperative thigh symptoms after minimally invasive transpsoas lumbar interbody fusion. J Neurosurg Spine 2011;15(1):11–8.

25. Moller DJ, Slimack NP, Acosta FL, et al. Minimally invasive lateral lumbar interbody fusion and transpsoas approach-related morbidity. Neurosurg Focus 2011;31(4):E4.

26. Pumberger M, Hughes AP, Huang RR, et al. Neurologic deficit following lateral lumbar interbody fusion. Eur Spine J 2012;21(6):1192–9.

27. Tormenti MJ, Maserati MB, Bonfield CM, et al. Complications and radiographic correction in adult scoliosis following combined transpsoas extreme lateral interbody fusion and posterior pedicle screw instrumentation. Neurosurg Focus 2010;28(3):E7.

28. Dakwar E, Le TV, Baaj AA, et al. Abdominal wall paresis as a complication of minimally invasive lateral transpsoas interbody fusion. Neurosurg Focus 2011;31(4):E18.

29. Pimenta L, Oliveira L, Schaffa T, et al. Lumbar total disc replacement from an extreme lateral approach: clinical experience with a minimum of 2 years' follow-up. J Neurosurg Spine 2011;14(1):38–45.

30. Sharma AK, Kepler CK, Girardi FP, et al. Lateral lumbar interbody fusion: clinical and radiographic outcomes at 1 year: a preliminary report. J Spinal Disord Tech 2011;24(4):242–50.

31. Kepler CK, Sharma AK, Huang RC. Lateral transpsoas interbody fusion (LTIF) with plate fixation and unilateral pedicle screws: a preliminary report. J Spinal Disord Tech 2011;24(6):363–7.

32. Papanastassiou ID, Eleraky M, Vrionis FD. Contralateral femoral nerve compression: an unrecognized complication after extreme lateral interbody fusion (XLIF). J Clin Neurosci 2011;18(1):149–51.

33. Berjano P, Balsano M, Buric J, et al. Direct lateral access lumbar and thoracolumbar fusion: preliminary results. Eur Spine J 2012;21(Suppl 1):S37–42.

34. Le TV, Burkett CJ, Deukmedjian AR, et al. Postoperative lumbar plexus injury after lumbar retroperitoneal transpsoas minimally invasive lateral interbody fusion. Spine (Phila Pa 1976) 2013;38(1):E13–20.

35. Cahill KS, Martinez JL, Wang MY, et al. Motor nerve injuries following the minimally invasive lateral transpsoas approach. J Neurosurg Spine 2012;17(3):227–31.

36. Malham GM, Ellis NJ, Parker RM, et al. Clinical outcome and fusion rates after the first 30 extreme lateral interbody fusions. ScientificWorldJournal 2012;2012:246989.

37. Caputo AM, Michael KW, Chapman TM Jr, et al. Clinical outcomes of extreme lateral interbody fusion in the treatment of adult degenerative scoliosis. ScientificWorldJournal 2012;2012:680643.

38. Karikari IO, Grossi PM, Nimjee SM, et al. Minimally invasive lumbar interbody fusion in patients older than 70 years of age: analysis of peri- and postoperative complications. Neurosurgery 2011;68(4):897–902 [discussion: 902].

39. Park DK, Lee MJ, Lin EL, et al. The relationship of intrapsoas nerves during a transpsoas approach to the lumbar spine: anatomic study. J Spinal Disord Tech 2010;23(4):223–8.

40. Uribe JS, Arredondo N, Dakwar E, et al. Defining the safe working zones using the minimally invasive lateral retroperitoneal transpsoas approach: an anatomical study. J Neurosurg Spine 2010;13(2):260–6.

41. Uribe JS, Vale FL, Dakwar E. Electromyographic monitoring and its anatomical implications in minimally invasive spine surgery. Spine (Phila Pa 1976) 2010;35(Suppl 26):S368–74.

42. Bergey DL, Villavicencio AT, Goldstein T, et al. Endoscopic lateral transpsoas approach to the lumbar spine. Spine (Phila Pa 1976) 2004;29(15):1681–8.

43. Acosta FL Jr, Drazin D, Liu JC. Supra-psoas shallow docking in lateral interbody fusion. Neurosurgery 2013;73(1 Suppl Operative):ons48–51 [discussion: ons52].

Complications Associated with Posterior Approaches in Minimally Invasive Spine Decompression

James A. Stadler III, MD[a], Albert P. Wong, MD[a],
Randall B. Graham, MD[a], John C. Liu, MD[b],*

KEYWORDS

- Minimally invasive surgery • Minimally invasive spine • Spinal decompression • Complications
- Laminectomy • Foraminotomy • Diskectomy

KEY POINTS

- Complications associated with posterior approaches for minimally invasive decompressions may be categorized as related to the intraoperative approach and decompression, need for reoperation, infections, or perioperative medical concerns.
- The incidence and nature of these complications are presented.
- Complications may be prevented with careful surgical technique.

INTRODUCTION

Minimally invasive approaches for spinal decompression are increasingly used for a wide range of degenerative pathology. These techniques have been developed to allow equivalent or improved outcomes compared with their open counterparts, with decreased iatrogenic disruption of the normal anatomy.[1] Minimally invasive spine surgeries have been associated with less morbidity and quicker return to work compared with traditional open techniques, with a similar to possibly decreased overall risk of complications.[2–7] All surgical procedures carry risk of complications, however, and the complication profile varies by procedure and approach.

Common minimally invasive posterior spine procedures include the foraminotomy, diskectomy, and laminectomy. These posterior decompressive procedures may be used in the cervical, thoracic, or lumbar spine. Cervical and thoracic approaches are used to address radiculopathy and/or myelopathy, with surgical indications and goals similar to traditional open laminectomies, diskectomies, and foraminotomies. In the lumbar spine, these same procedures are similarly used for decompression in the treatment of lumbar radiculopathy or neurogenic claudication.

Although these approaches are largely successful, it is important for surgeons and patients to understand the potential complications associated with these procedures. The learning curve for minimally invasive techniques is more significant than the open surgical correlates, and perspective on the anatomy encountered during a minimally invasive approach may be less familiar to surgeons. These factors may contribute to either intraoperative complications or to disease

Sources of Support: None.

[a] Department of Neurological Surgery, Northwestern University Feinberg School of Medicine, Chicago, IL, USA; [b] Department of Neurological Surgery, Keck School of Medicine, University of Southern California, 1200 North State Street, Suite 3300, Los Angeles, CA 90033, USA
* Corresponding author.
E-mail address: john.liu@med.usc.edu

Neurosurg Clin N Am 25 (2014) 233–245
http://dx.doi.org/10.1016/j.nec.2013.12.003

recurrence requiring reoperation. Understanding the risk of infection and medical complications associated with surgery is critical for managing patients in the postoperative period. This article presents relevant data regarding these classes of complications associated with posterior minimally invasive decompressions. A case example helps demonstrate important considerations for complication avoidance (**Figs. 1–7**).

A literature review of recent high-quality studies demonstrating complications for posterior minimally invasive spinal decompression was performed. These studies were individually reviewed for further understanding of the nature and incidence of complications. The data were further aggregated across complication classes according to spinal region (**Table 1**). Studies were included if they were designed to capture the relevant complications and sufficient data were provided to allow result aggregation. Cumulative data are shown for the cervical and lumbar regions; none of the included studies provided data regarding complications of procedures in the thoracic spine. The reported results were also compiled according to complication class (**Tables 2–5**).

INTRAOPERATIVE COMPLICATIONS

Minimally invasive approaches to spine surgery are increasingly common and surgeons are increasingly trained in these techniques. These minimally invasive approaches continue to have a steep learning curve, however, secondary to the use of long bayoneted instruments through narrow corridors, with less visualization of anatomic landmarks and the requirement for interpretation of intraoperative fluoroscopic imaging. Additionally, the surgical anatomy is encountered from a different perspective than the traditional open techniques. As a result, these procedures are associated with unique sets of intraoperative complications. Specifically, this section addresses technical complications associated with surgical approach and decompression, such as durotomy, injury to neural elements, hematoma formation, surgery performed at the incorrect level or side, and inadvertent facet fracture.

Incidence

Technical intraoperative complications have been reported in the literature as between 1.9% and 25.7%.[4,8] In a multicenter study, Matsumoto and colleagues[9] reported on a total of 5609 patients treated with a microendoscopic diskectomy or microendoscopic laminectomy/fenestration with an intraoperative complication rate of 2.2%. In another large study by Wu and colleagues,[4] an intraoperative complication rate of 1.9% was reported in 873 patients treated with a microendoscopic

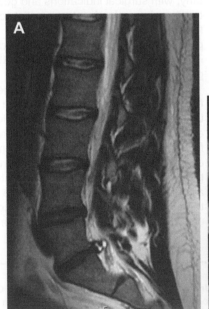
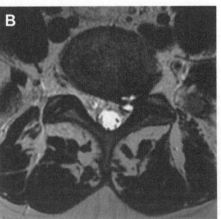

Fig. 1. Case example. The patient is a 23-year-old man presenting with signs and symptoms consistent with a left S1 radiculopathy. MRI of the lumbar spine demonstrates a left herniated disk at L5-S1, shown on (A) parasagittal and (B) axial images. After failing conservative management, he is taken for elective left L5-S1 minimally invasive microdiskectomy.

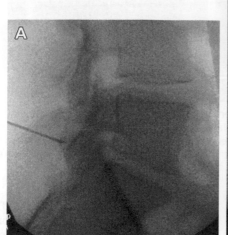
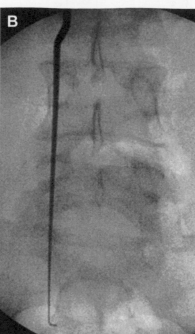

Fig. 2. Localization. (*A*) The L5-S1 interspace is appropriately identified on this localizing fluoroscopy image. The surgeon must be comfortable with fluoroscopic interpretation to ensure that the Kirschner wire, if used, is not inadvertently placed in the central canal, neural foramen, or lateral to the facet and transverse process. (*B*) Anterior-posterior fluoroscopy may help define midline prior to making incision, which is approximately 15-mm lateral from midline on the side of dominant pathology, as marked by an overlaid instrument. Careful interpretation of localizing images, with comparison to preoperative imaging and reconfirmation as needed, helps avoid operating on the incorrect side or level.

diskectomy for lumbar disk herniation. They additionally found that compared with 358 patients treated with an open procedure, the minimally invasive cohort had a shorter hospital stay, less blood loss, faster return to work, and a shorter mean operative time (see **Table 2**).

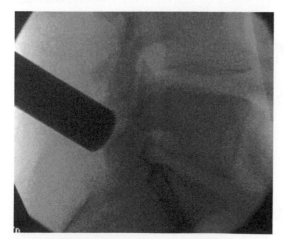

Fig. 3. Dilation. Sequential tubular dilators are placed over the appropriate disk space, and a working channel is secured.

These low rates of intraoperative morbidity in the 2 largest studies varied significantly from that reported in some of the smaller studies. Teli and colleagues[8] reported a rate of 25.7% for technical complications in a study of 70 patients. Similarly, Pao and colleagues[10] found a rate of 22.6% in 53 patients studied.

The reported complications were diverse. The most commonly reported complication was durotomy, with a rate of 2.4% (see **Table 2**). Neurologic injury was reported in 0.6% of cases and was often transient. Other complications included low rates for postoperative hematomas or seromas, inadvertent facet violation, and wrong-site surgery (see **Table 2**).

Subgroup Analysis

Within the cervical spine, minimally invasive decompressive procedures had a reported range of 2.6% to 9.8% for intraoperative complications.[11–14] Four studies, with a total of 391 patients, averaged a rate of 6.6%. Similar analysis regarding the lumbar spine yielded 23 studies with a total of 8417 patients. These studies collectively showed a complication rate of 4.4% (see **Table 1**).

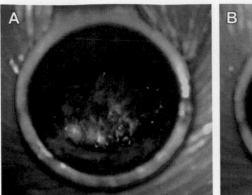
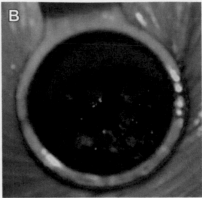

Fig. 4. Initial intraoperative approach. (*A*) After insertion of the tubular retractor and remaining soft tissue removal, the base of the spinous process and inferior laminar edge are identified. (*B*) After exposure, unilateral or bilateral decompressions may be achieved via ipsilateral laminotomy, here started with a Kerrison rongeur. Preoperative imaging may alert the surgeon to aberrant local anatomy, such as a hypertrophied facet joint, that could potentially confuse this approach.

Prevention

As with any surgical technique, use of a minimally invasive approach for posterior spinal decompression requires familiarity with the surgical anatomy and instruments. Judicious use of intraoperative fluoroscopy during the initial tubular dilation minimizes the risk of inadvertent breech of the spinal canal. Similarly, avoiding the use of Kirschner wires during localization minimizes the risk of injury to the thecal sac and underlying neurologic elements. Anatomic landmarks, often the base of the spinous process and inferior edge of the lamina, are identified to minimize disorientation and unintended removal of critical anatomy, such as the facet joint. Meticulous hemostasis, including for the dilated soft tissues on removal of the working channel, can decrease postoperative hematoma and seroma formation. Systematic and careful attention to preoperative and intraoperative imaging, with frequent confirmation of surgical anatomy during the operation, is helpful to avoid facet violation or wrong-site surgeries.

Dural tears can often be avoided with careful decompression. When able, completion of the bony drilling and decompression prior to removal of the ligamentum flavum may help avoid durotomy. A combined suction-retractor placed may facilitate diskectomy by medially displacing the traversing nerve root, and the cutting edges of Kerrison rongeurs and annulotomy knives should always be directed away from the nerve root and dura. Taking this careful approach may also help prevent injury to the underlying neural structures. This same cautious dissection should continue until the underlying pathology is removed and affected neural elements are fully decompressed.

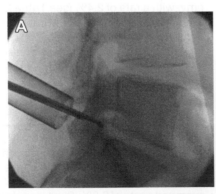
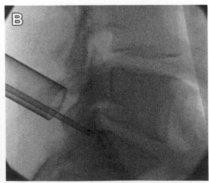

Fig. 5. Laminotomy. (*A*) The laminotomy is completed using a combination of Kerrison rongeurs and a high-speed drill. Care is taken to avoid facet joint violation, and the ligament is maintained until the bony removal is completed. (*B*) Fluoroscopic confirmation of the extent of exposure helps reassure the surgeon that access is obtained to all relevant pathology.

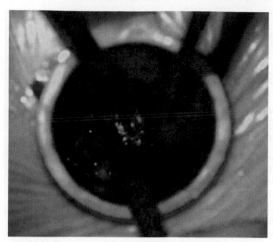

Fig. 6. Diskectomy. Disckectomy is accomplished using a combination of rongeurs and blunt instruments in standard fashion. Note the retraction of the traversing nerve root, which allows access to the disk space while protecting the nerve root and dura.

Table 1 Aggregated data regarding complications of posterior minimally invasive decompressions	
Complication	Rate
Cervical region	
Intraoperative	6.6% (26/391)
Reoperation	1.3% (5/391)
Infectious	0.5% (2/391)
Medical	0.3% (1/391)
Lumbar region	
Intraoperative	4.4% (368/8417)
Reoperation	3.5% (96/2755)
Infectious	1.4% (34/2464)
Medical	1.6% (34/2082)

When encountered, durotomies should be addressed intraoperatively to minimize risk of pseudomeningocele or cerebrospinal fluid (CSF) fistula formation. Although primary suture closure of durotomies using a knot-pushing instrument through the working channel may be accomplished, repair algorithms with blood-soaked Gelfoam, collagen matrix, fibrin glue, tight closure of the fascia, and overnight bed rest have been shown effective in preventing CSF fistulae.[15,16] Given the tamponade effect from the relatively intact paraspinal soft tissues and lack of postoperative dead space, the risk of pseudomeningocele or CSF fistula after durotomy is less significant with minimally invasive approaches than with open techniques, and CSF diversion is rarely needed for wound healing.

REOPERATION

The risk of disease recurrence or failure obtaining adequate decompression is not unique to minimally invasive procedures but is a concern for all spine surgeons. Aside from lack of improvement or even clinical worsening, patients may additionally incur the risks of reoperation. Complications in other categories significantly overlap with the need for reoperation, because events, such as CSF leaks, hematomas, or infections, may also necessitate return to the operating room.

Incidence

A total of 25 studies were identified that included reoperation statistics or were designed to capture these complications. The reported incidence of reoperation ranges from 0% to 12%.[11,13,17–22] The largest of these studies, by Wu and colleagues,[4] reported a 2.3% reoperation rate among 873 patients. In this study, 10 patients developed evidence of segmental instability and 10 other patients developed symptoms from recurrent disk herniation or regional degeneration. Another larger study by Matsumoto and colleagues[23] found a reoperation rate of 6.4% in 344 patients; the complication in all of these patients was reported as recurrent disk herniation. The rates in these larger studies compare favorably to reoperation rates reported for open surgical techniques, although direct comparison of techniques is limited.[24,25]

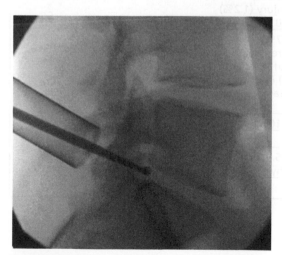

Fig. 7. Inspection. In addition to visual and tactile inspection of the nerve root, fluoroscopy may also help confirm adequate decompression prior to hemostasis, irrigation, and wound closure.

Table 2
Intraoperative complications related to approach or decompression with posterior minimally invasive decompressive surgery

Author, Year	n	Intraoperative Complications	Rate
Adamson[11] 2001[a]	100	2 Dural tears (2%) 2 Activity-related paresthesias/pain (2%) 2 Intermittent paresthesias/numbness (2%)	6/100 (6%)
Asgarzadie & Khoo,[17] 2007[b]	48	5 Dural tears (10.4%)	5/48 (10.4%)
Casal-Moro et al,[40] 2011[b]	120	5 Dural tear (3 required open surgery for sutures) (4.2%) 4 Periradicular fibrosis (3.3%) 3 Progression of diskopathy (2.5%) 3 L5 paresis (2.5%) 1 L4 paresis (0.8%) 1 Pituitary rongeur rupture (removed by open surgery) (0.8%) 1 Root puncture with microknife (0.8%) 1 Early recurrent herniation (0.8%) 1 Hernia relapse (0.8%) 1 Hernia relapse associated with periradicular fibrosis (0.8%)	21/120 (17.5%)
Castro-Menendez et al,[18] 2009[b]	50	5 Dural tears (10%) 1 Epidural hematoma causing cauda equina syndrome (2%)	6/50 (12%)
Chang et al,[41] 2009[b]	26	2 Irreparable dural tears converted to open diskectomy (7.7%) 1 Pseudomeningocele (3.8%)	3/26 (11.5%)
Garg et al,[42] 2011[b]	55	5 Dural tears (9.1%) 2 Transient S1 neuralgia (3.6%) 1 Recurrence (1.8%)	8/55 (14.5%)
Ikuta et al,[43] 2007[b]	114	12 Transient neurologic symptoms (10.5%) 6 Dural tears (5.3%) 3 Inferior facet fracture (2.6%)	21/114 (18.4%)
Jagannathan et al,[12] 2009[a]	162	9 Kyphosis (5.6%) 4 Dural tears (2.5%) 2 Nerve root injury (1.2%) 1 Hematoma (0.6%)	16/162 (9.9%)
Jhala & Mistry,[44] 2010[b]	100	7 Dural tears (7%) 5 Inadvertent removal of facet joint (5%) 4 Recurrence of herniation (3 required reoperation) (4%) 1 Nerve root damage (required conversion to open) (1%)	17/100 (17%)
Khoo & Fessler,[19] 2002[b]	25	4 Dural tears (16%)	4/25 (16%)
Lawton et al,[13] 2012[a]	38	1 CSF leak	1/38 (2.6%)
Martin-Laez et al,[20] 2012[b]	37	2 Dural tears (5.4%) 1 Radiculopathy (2.7%)	3/37 (8.1%)

(continued on next page)

Table 2
(continued)

Author, Year	n	Intraoperative Complications	Rate
Matsumoto et al,[9] 2010[b]	5609	Lumbar diskectomy (4336) 55 Dural tears (1.3%) 2 Cauda equina injury (0.05%) 4 Root injury (0.1%) 2 Hematoma (0.05%) 2 Wrong level (0.05%) 1 Wrong side (0.02%) 5 Facet fracture (0.1%) Lumbar laminectomy/fenestration (1273) 43 Dural tears (3.4%) 1 Cauda equina injury (0.08%) 4 Hematoma (0.3%) 4 Wrong level (0.3%) 2 Facet fracture (0.2%) 1 Decubitus (0.08%)	126/5609 (2.2%)
Matsumoto et al,[23] 2013[b]	344	37 Recurrent disk herniation (22 treated with revision surgery)	37/344 (10.8%)
Pao et al,[10] 2009[b]	53	5 Dural tears (9.4%) 4 Transient neuralgia (7.5%) 2 Wrong-level operations (3.8%) 1 Instability (1.9%)	12/53 (22.6%)
Perez-Cruet et al,[45] 2002[b]	150	8 Dural tears (5.3%) 1 Pseudomeningocele (0.7%)	9/150 (6%)
Podichetty et al,[46] 2006[b]	220	17 Dural tears (7.7%) 10 Hematoma or delayed wound healing (4.5%) 7 Radicular or chronic pain unchanged from preoperative level (3.2%) 1 Foot drop (0.5%)	35/220 (15.9%)
Rahman et al,[7] 2008[b]	38	2 dural tears (5.3%) 1 Synovial cyst (2.6%)	3/38 (7.9%)
Ranjan & Lath,[47] 2006[b]	107	3 Dural tears (2.8%)	3/107 (2.8%)
Righesso et al,[48] 2007[b]	21	1 Seroma (4.8%) 1 Dural tear (4.8%)	2/21 (9.5%)
Ruetten et al,[14] 2008[a]	91	3 Transient dermatome-related hypesthesia (3.3%)	3/91 (3.3%)
Shih et al,[21] 2011[b]	23	1 Dural tear (4.3%)	1/23 (4.3%)
Teli et al,[8] 2010[b]	70	8 Recurrence of herniation (11.4%) 6 Dural tears (8.6%) 2 Root injury (2.9%) 2 Worsening deficit (2.9%)	18/70 (25.7%)
Wang et al,[49] 2012[b]	151	5 Dural tears (3.3%)	5/151 (3.3%)
Wu et al,[4] 2006[b]	873	14 Dural tears (1.6%) 3 Acute hematomas of the sacrospinalis (0.3%)	17/873 (1.9%)
Xu et al,[22] 2010[b]	32	2 Dural tears (6.3%)	2/32 (6.3%)
Zhou et al,[50] 2009[b]	151	5 Recurrence of herniation (3.3%) 5 Dural tears (3.3%)	10/151 (6.6%)

[a] Denotes cervical spinal region described in studies.
[b] Denotes lumbar spinal region described in studies.

Table 3
Reoperation rates of posterior minimally invasive decompressions

Author, Year	n	Reoperation Rates and Associated Complications	Rate
Casal-Moro et al,[40] 2011[b]	120	4 Periradicular fibrosis (3.3%) 3 Progression of diskopathy (2.5%) 1 Hernia relapse (0.8%) 1 Hernia relapse associated with periradicular fibrosis (0.8%)	9/120 (7.5%)
Castro-Menendez et al,[18] 2009[b]	50	3 Clinical relapse and/or epidural fibrosis (6%) 2 Secondary lumbar instability requiring fusion (4%) 1 Epidural hematoma (2%)	6/50 (12%)
Chang et al,[41] 2009[b]	26	2 Irreparable dural tears (7.7%) 1 Reoperation for pseudomeningocele (3.8%)	3/26 (11.5%)
Garg et al,[42] 2011[b]	55	1 Recurrent disk herniation	1/55 (1.8%)
Ikuta et al,[43] 2007[b]	114	1 Cauda equina herniation (0.9%)	1/114 (0.9%)
Jagannathan et al,[12] 2009[a]	162	1 Postoperative hematoma (0.6%) 1 Deep wound infection (0.6%)	2/162 (1.2%)
Jhala & Mistry,[44] 2010[b]	100	3 Recurrent disk herniation (3%) 1 Nerve root damage (1%) 1 Débridement and interbody fusion for diskitis (1%)	5/100 (5%)
Matsumoto et al,[23] 2013[b]	344	22 Recurrent disk herniation	22/344 (6.4%)
Matsumoto et al,[9] 2010[b]	5609	Lumbar diskectomy (4336) 4 Open conversion (0.1%) Lumbar laminectomy/fenestration (1273) 2 Open conversion (0.2%)	6/5609 (0.1%)
Perez-Cruet et al,[45] 2002[b]	150	4 Recurrent disk herniation	4/150 (2.7%)
Podichetty et al,[46] 2006[b]	220	2 Facet fractures requiring later surgery (0.9%) 1 Required instrumented fusion (0.5%)	3/220 (1.4%)
Rahman et al,[7] 2008[b]	38	1 Dural tear (resulted in conversion to open)	1/38 (2.6%)
Ranjan & Lath,[47] 2006[b]	107	2 Recurrent disk herniation	2/107 (1.9%)
Righesso et al,[48] 2007[b]	21	1 Recurrent disk herniation	1/21 (4.8%)
Ruetten et al,[14] 2008[a]	91	3 Reoperations for recurrence	3/91 (3.3%)
Teli et al,[8] 2010[b]	70	8 Recurrent disk herniation	8/70 (11.4%)
Wang et al,[49] 2012[b]	151	5 Revisions (open diskectomies)	5/151 (3.3%)
Wu et al,[4] 2006[b]	873	10 Segmental instability or displacement (1.1%) 6 Recurrent herniations (0.7%) 2 Herniations at different level (0.2%) 2 Lumbar stenosis involving several segments after MED procedures (0.2%)	20/873 (2.3%)
Zhou et al,[50] 2009[b]	151	5 Revisions due to recurrence of herniation	5/151 (3.3%)

[a] Denotes cervical spinal region described in studies.
[b] Denotes lumbar spinal region described in studies.

Table 4
Infectious complications of posterior minimally invasive decompressions

Author, Year	n	Infectious Complications	Rate
Adamson[11] 2001[a]	100	1 Superficial wound infection	1/100 (1%)
Casal-Moro et al,[40] 2011[b]	120	1 Diskitis	1/120 (0.8%)
Castro-Menendez et al,[18] 2009[b]	50	2 Superficial wound infections	2/50 (4%)
Chang et al,[41] 2009[b]	26	2 Superficial wound infections	2/26 (7.7%)
Jagannathan et al,[12] 2009[a]	162	1 Deep wound infection	1/162 (0.6%)
Jhala & Mistry,[44] 2010[b]	100	4 Diskitis	4/100 (4%)
Perez-Cruet et al,[45] 2002[b]	150	1 Superficial wound infection	1/150 (0.7%)
Podichetty et al,[46] 2006[b]	220	3 Superficial wound infection (1.4%) 1 Diskitis (0.5%) 1 Epidural abscess (0.5%)	5/220 (2.3%)
Rahman et al,[7] 2008[b]	38	1 Superficial wound infection	1/38 (2.6%)
Ranjan & Lath,[47] 2006[b]	107	1 Superficial wound infection (0.8%) 1 Diskitis (0.8%)	2/107 (1.9%)
Teli et al,[8] 2010[b]	70	1 Spondylodiskitis	1/70 (1.4%)
Wang et al,[49] 2012[b]	151	3 Spinal spondylodiskitis	3/151 (2%)
Wu et al,[4] 2006[b]	873	5 Diskitis (0.6%) 4 Superficial wound infection (0.5%)	9/873 (1%)
Zhou et al,[50] 2009[b]	151	3 Vertebral/disk infection	3/151 (2%)

[a] Denotes cervical spinal region described in studies.
[b] Denotes lumbar spinal region described in studies.

The number of studies with no reported cases of reoperation tended to include a smaller population, with an average study population of 43 patients; this suggests that these studies may not have been large enough to capture a rare need for reoperation. As with all complications, reporting bias may further limit incidence estimations.

Recurrent disk herniation was the most common indication for reoperation, with a rate of 2%. Across studies, conversion to open procedures was noted in 0.4% of cases. Postoperative

Table 5
Medical complications of posterior procedures

Author, Year	n	Medical Complications	Rate
Casal-Moro et al,[40] 2011[b]	120	1 DVT	1/120 (0.8%)
Garg et al,[42] 2011[b]	55	4 Temporary urinary retention	4/55 (7.3%)
Jagannathan et al,[12] 2009[a]	162	1 MI	1/162 (0.6%)
Khoo & Fessler,[19] 2002[b]	25	5 Medical complications (unspecified)	5/25 (20%)
Podichetty et al,[46] 2006[b]	220	6 Urinary retention (2.7%) 1 Prolonged nausea (0.5%) 1 Atelectasis (0.5%) 1 MI (0.5%) 1 Pneumonia (0.5%) 1 CHF exacerbation (0.5%) 1 Pneumonia and cerebrovascular accident (0.5%)	12/220 (5.4%)
Shih et al,[21] 2011[b]	23	3 Urinary retention	3/23 (13%)
Wu et al,[4] 2006[b]	873	7 Acute urinary retention (0.8%) 2 Acute gastritis (0.2%)	9/873 (1.0%)

[a] Denotes cervical spinal region described in studies.
[b] Denotes lumbar spinal region described in studies.

instability was also found in 0.4% and often required subsequent spinal fusion. Less common indications for reoperation included fibrosis, durotomy or CSF leak, hematoma, and infection.

Subgroup Analysis

In 4 studies of cervical procedures, with a total of 391 patients, reoperation rates were reported between 0% and 3.2%; the average across these studies was 1.3%.[11–14] Within the lumbar spine, 21 studies reported an average reoperation rate of 3.5% in 2755 patients, with rates ranging from 0% to 12% (see **Table 1**).

Prevention

Although there are no perfect techniques to avoid recurrence of disk herniation, aggressive diskectomy may reduce the rate of revision diskectomies.[26] Cautioning patients to avoid excessive physiologic loads on the decompressed spinal regions in the early postoperative course may help avoid recurrent herniation. Recurrent disk herniation may be more common in patients with larger initial annular defects, so preoperative counseling of patients should be guided based on individual imaging findings and surgeon experience.[24,27]

Minimally invasive techniques inherently disrupt less surrounding tissue and, therefore, may inherently decrease postoperative fibrosis or segmental instability, but complications were noted across several studies and should be considered if patients have persistent or worsening symptoms. Careful attention to minimize ligamentous and facet disruption may further mitigate the risks of postoperative scarring and instability. Because reoperation rates are at least partially driven by associated complications, such as CSF leaks or infections, avoidance of these also helps decrease the need for further surgery.

INFECTIOUS COMPLICATIONS

Surgical site infections are a common concern for any spine surgery and seem multifactorial in etiology. Infections complicate 0.7% and 12% of all spine surgeries, although estimates of infection rates are generally limited by the retrospective nature of most studies.[28–30] Risk factors for infection are similarly difficult to quantify. Although decompressive procedures may have an infection rate of less than 1%, instrumented fusions seem to have a higher rate.[31] Patient factors, such as diabetes, obesity, smoking, malignancy, radiation exposure, and prior surgery, further influence infectious risk, although understanding of the relative contributions of these concerns is limited.[28–35]

O'Toole and colleagues[31] reported an overall infection rate of 0.22% in a retrospective study of 1338 patients after both instrumented and noninstrumented minimally invasive spine surgery. Rates of infection in minimally invasive procedures may be lower than in open surgery for several reasons: tubular retractors limit deep tissue exposure, local contamination by the surgical team and instruments are similarly limited, skin edge contact after retractor insertion is minimal, incisions are generally smaller, and postoperative dead space is decreased due to less tissue disruption.[31] Although direct comparison is lacking, the low infection rate after minimally invasive approaches seems to offer a significant advantage compared with similar open procedures.

Incidence

In this analysis, 25 studies with a total of 2855 patients were identified as including sufficiently extractable data to consider postoperative infections after posterior minimally invasive spinal decompressions. In these studies, the overall infection rate was 1.2%, with a range of 0% to 7.7%. Similar to other complications, studies that reported no infections tended to include smaller populations (see **Table 4**).

The reported infections were generally divided between diskitis/spondylodiskitis and superficial wound infections, with rates of 0.7% and 0.5% respectively. There was 1 reported epidural abscess and 1 unspecified deep infection. Collective review of the included studies did not provide adequate data to allow analysis of causative organisms or associated risk factors.

Subgroup Analysis

Within the studies of minimally invasive cervical decompressions, 2 infections were reported in 391 patients, for an average rate of 0.5% with a range of 0% to 1.0%. A slightly higher rate was found in the 21 studies focused on lumbar procedures, with 34 infections in 2464 patients yielding an average rate of 1.4%. The reported infection rate in these studies ranged from 0% to 7.7% (see **Table 4**).

Prevention

Smaller incisions and the lack of postoperative dead space help minimize the risk of infection after minimally invasive spine surgery. Although infection rates after minimally invasive surgeries for spinal decompression are low, efforts to minimize risk are appropriate. Preoperative antibiotics are routinely administered to all patients. After insertion of the tubular retractor, the skin edge and superficial soft tissues do not require further manipulation until wound closure. Meticulous attention to proper sterile technique offers significant protection against postoperative infection. Postoperatively, the wound is kept clean and dry while healing, and both patients and clinicians remain vigilant for early signs of infection to allow prompt treatment. Consultation of infectious disease specialists may be indicated for complex individual cases or system-wide concerns.

Patient factors weigh significantly on infectious risk. Patients with known comorbidities that may increase infection risk should be appropriately advised preoperatively, and elective surgery should be postponed if a patient has an active infectious concerns. Wound healing benefits from appropriate nutrition and vitamin supplementation may be particularly helpful in higher-risk populations. Postoperative glycemic control has been demonstrated to aid wound healing in multiple surgical populations and is likely appropriate for these patients as well.[28–30,32–35]

MEDICAL COMPLICATIONS

Significant medical complications fortunately are rare after minimally invasive spine surgeries. The rate of medical complications of spine surgery in general varies widely according to the patient population and extent of surgical intervention. Incidence of medical morbidity is known to increase with advanced age, complex surgical correction of spinal deformities, greater number of levels treated, preoperative medical diagnoses, and obesity.[36–38] Although minimally invasive surgeries result in decreased intraoperative blood loss and less physiologic stress than open procedures, these procedures are performed most frequently for patients with degenerative spine disease, a population with frequent medical comorbidities, such as cardiovascular disease or diabetes.[10,39] Patient death is rare, but these complications can add significant length to hospitalizations and are distressing to patients and surgeons when they occur.

Incidence

Collectively, 21 studies, including 2473 patients, were identified to include sufficient data for analysis of medical complications. Review of these studies yielded 35 medical complications, for an overall rate of 1.4% and reported rates ranging from 0% to 20%. The largest of these studies, by Wu and colleagues,[4] identified 9 complications in 873 patients, for a rate of 1.0% (see **Table 5**).

The most frequent medical complication in these studies was postoperative urinary retention.

This was noted for 20 patients, which comprised 0.8% of patients. Cardiovascular complications affected 4 patients, or 0.2%, with 3 cases of myocardial infarction (MI) and 1 congestive heart failure (CHF) exacerbation. The remaining complications were diverse and included gastritis, deep vein thrombosis, atelectasis, pneumonia, excessive nausea, and 1 stroke associated with a case of pneumonia.

Subgroup Analysis

In 4 studies of posterior minimally invasive cervical decompression, with a total of 391 patients, 1 MI was described, for an overall estimated rate of 0.3% for medical complications. Within the lumbar spine group, 17 studies showed a total of 34 medical complications in 2082 patients, for an average rate of 1.6% and a range of 0% to 20% (see **Table 1**).

Prevention

Although minimally invasive techniques tend to induce less physiologically stress than comparable open approaches, all patients should nonetheless undergo routine medical evaluation prior to elective spinal operations, with medical optimization as indicated. Patients should thoroughly understand the medical risks of general anesthesia, and care should be coordinated between the surgical, anesthesiology, and preoperative medical teams to address medical comorbidities or unique concerns for each case. Intraoperative blood loss has been consistently showed to be less in minimally invasive cohorts relative to similar open surgical groups, but operative time is frequently increased; this difference decreases with surgeon experience.

The most common medical complication after minimally invasive spine surgery, postoperative urinary retention, is multifactorial, but is likely decreased in the minimally invasive population compared with patients undergoing traditional open operations given decreased postoperative narcotic usage and the avoidance of muscle relaxants during surgery.[21] Foley catheterization can often be avoided given the short duration of many decompression procedures. Postoperatively, prompt recognition of urinary retention allows timely management, with urologic consultation, if indicated, and potential avoidance of compounding complications.

SUMMARY

Complications associated with posterior minimally invasive decompression of the spine can be categorized as intraoperative technical complications, reoperation, infections, or perioperative medical complications. A compilation of complications as reported in the literature allows better understanding of the rates and nature of these events. Aggregated analysis of these studies allows estimation, then, of these complications across a larger population. Understanding of the complications, combined with careful surgical technique, may help avoid adverse outcomes.

REFERENCES

1. Fessler RG, O'Toole JE, Eichholz KM, et al. The development of minimally invasive spine surgery. Neurosurg Clin N Am 2006;17(4):401–9.

2. Kazemi N, Crew LK, Tredway TL. The future of spine surgery: new horizons in the treatment of spinal disorders. Surg Neurol Int 2013;4(Suppl 1): S15–21.

3. Hsieh PC, Koski TR, Sciubba DM, et al. Maximizing the potential of minimally invasive spine surgery in complex spinal disorders. Neurosurg Focus 2008; 25(2):E19.

4. Wu X, Zhuang S, Mao Z, et al. Microendoscopic discectomy for lumbar disc herniation: surgical technique and outcome in 873 consecutive cases. Spine 2006;31(23):2689–94.

5. Smith ZA, Fessler RG. Paradigm changes in spine surgery: evolution of minimally invasive techniques. Nat Rev Neurol 2012;8(8):443–50.

6. German JW, Adamo MA, Hoppenot RG, et al. Perioperative results following lumbar discectomy: comparison of minimally invasive discectomy and standard microdiscectomy. Neurosurg Focus 2008;25(2):E20.

7. Rahman M, Summers LE, Richter B, et al. Comparison of techniques for decompressive lumbar laminectomy: the minimally invasive versus the "classic" open approach. Minim Invasive Neurosurg 2008;51(2):100–5.

8. Teli M, Lovi A, Brayda-Bruno M, et al. Higher risk of dural tears and recurrent herniation with lumbar micro-endoscopic discectomy. Eur Spine J 2010; 19(3):443–50.

9. Matsumoto M, Hasegawa T, Ito M, et al. Incidence of complications associated with spinal endoscopic surgery: nationwide survey in 2007 by the Committee on Spinal Endoscopic Surgical Skill Qualification of Japanese Orthopaedic Association. J Orthop Sci 2010;15(1):92–6.

10. Pao JL, Chen WC, Chen PQ. Clinical outcomes of microendoscopic decompressive laminotomy for degenerative lumbar spinal stenosis. Eur Spine J 2009;18(5):672–8.

11. Adamson TE. Microendoscopic posterior cervical laminoforaminotomy for unilateral radiculopathy: results of a new technique in 100 cases. J Neurosurg 2001;95(Suppl 1):51–7.

12. Jagannathan J, Sherman JH, Szabo T, et al. The posterior cervical foraminotomy in the treatment of cervical disc/osteophyte disease: a single-surgeon experience with a minimum of 5 years' clinical and radiographic follow-up. J Neurosurg Spine 2009;10(4):347–56.

13. Lawton CD, Smith ZA, Lam SK, et al. Clinical outcomes of microendoscopic foraminotomy and decompression in the cervical spine. World Neurosurg 2012. [Epub ahead of print].

14. Ruetten S, Komp M, Merk H, et al. Full-endoscopic cervical posterior foraminotomy for the operation of lateral disc herniations using 5.9-mm endoscopes: a prospective, randomized, controlled study. Spine 2008;33(9):940–8.

15. Chou D, Wang VY, Khan AS. Primary dural repair during minimally invasive microdiscectomy using standard operating room instruments. Neurosurgery 2009;64(5 Suppl 2):356–8 [discussion: 358–9].

16. Ruban D, O'Toole JE. Management of incidental durotomy in minimally invasive spine surgery. Neurosurg Focus 2011;31(4):E15.

17. Asgarzadie F, Khoo LT. Minimally invasive operative management for lumbar spinal stenosis: overview of early and long-term outcomes. Orthop Clin North Am 2007;38(3):387–99 [abstract vi–vii].

18. Castro-Menendez M, Bravo-Ricoy JA, Casal-Moro R, et al. Midterm outcome after microendoscopic decompressive laminotomy for lumbar spinal stenosis: 4-year prospective study. Neurosurgery 2009;65(1):100–10 [discussion: 110; quiz: A112].

19. Khoo LT, Fessler RG. Microendoscopic decompressive laminotomy for the treatment of lumbar stenosis. Neurosurgery 2002;51(Suppl 5):S146–54.

20. Martin-Laez R, Martinez-Agueros JA, Suarez-Fernandez D, et al. Complications of endoscopic microdiscectomy using the EASYGO! system: is there any difference with conventional discectomy during the learning-curve period? Acta Neurochir 2012;154(6):1023–32.

21. Shih P, Wong AP, Smith TR, et al. Complications of open compared to minimally invasive lumbar spine decompression. J Clin Neurosci 2011;18(10): 1360–4.

22. Xu BS, Tan QS, Xia Q, et al. Bilateral decompression via unilateral fenestration using mobile microendoscopic discectomy technique for lumbar spinal stenosis. Orthop Surg 2010;2(2): 106–10.

23. Matsumoto M, Watanabe K, Hosogane N, et al. Recurrence of lumbar disc herniation after microendoscopic discectomy. J Neurol Surg A Cent Eur Neurosurg 2013;74(4):222–7.

24. Lee JK, Amorosa L, Cho SK, et al. Recurrent lumbar disk herniation. J Am Acad Orthop Surg 2010;18(6):327–37.

25. Ambrossi GL, McGirt MJ, Sciubba DM, et al. Recurrent lumbar disc herniation after single-level lumbar discectomy: incidence and health care cost analysis. Neurosurgery 2009;65(3):574–8 [discussion: 578].

26. McGirt MJ, Eustacchio S, Varga P, et al. A prospective cohort study of close interval computed tomography and magnetic resonance imaging after primary lumbar discectomy: factors associated with recurrent disc herniation and disc height loss. Spine 2009;34(19):2044–51.

27. McGirt MJ, Ambrossi GL, Datoo G, et al. Recurrent disc herniation and long-term back pain after primary lumbar discectomy: review of outcomes reported for limited versus aggressive disc removal. Neurosurgery 2009;64(2):338–44 [discussion: 344–5].

28. Pull ter Gunne AF, Cohen DB. Incidence, prevalence, and analysis of risk factors for surgical site infection following adult spinal surgery. Spine 2009;34(13):1422–8.

29. Pull ter Gunne AF, Hosman AJ, Cohen DB, et al. A methodological systematic review on surgical site infections following spinal surgery: part 1: risk factors. Spine 2012;37(24):2017–33.

30. McDermott H, Bolger C, Humphreys H. Postprocedural discitis of the vertebral spine: challenges in diagnosis, treatment and prevention. J Hosp Infect 2012;82(3):152–7.

31. O'Toole JE, Eichholz KM, Fessler RG. Surgical site infection rates after minimally invasive spinal surgery. J Neurosurg Spine 2009;11(4):471–6.

32. Junker T, Mujagic E, Hoffmann H, et al. Prevention and control of surgical site infections: review of the Basel Cohort Study. Swiss Med Wkly 2012;142: w13616.

33. Schuster JM, Rechtine G, Norvell DC, et al. The influence of perioperative risk factors and therapeutic interventions on infection rates after spine surgery: a systematic review. Spine 2010; 35(Suppl 9):S125–37.

34. Silber JS, Anderson DG, Vaccaro AR, et al. Management of postprocedural discitis. Spine J 2002; 2(4):279–87.

35. van Middendorp JJ, Pull ter Gunne AF, Schuetz M, et al. A methodological systematic review on surgical site infections following spinal surgery: part 2: prophylactic treatments. Spine 2012;37(24):2034–45.

36. Proietti L, Scaramuzzo L, Schiro GR, et al. Complications in lumbar spine surgery: A retrospective analysis. Indian J Orthop 2013;47(4):340–5.

37. Zheng F, Cammisa FP Jr, Sandhu HS, et al. Factors predicting hospital stay, operative time, blood loss, and transfusion in patients undergoing revision posterior lumbar spine decompression, fusion, and segmental instrumentation. Spine 2002;27(8): 818–24.

38. Cassinelli EH, Eubanks J, Vogt M, et al. Risk factors for the development of perioperative complications in elderly patients undergoing lumbar decompression and arthrodesis for spinal stenosis: an analysis of 166 patients. Spine 2007;32(2):230–5.

39. Shamji MF, Cook C, Pietrobon R, et al. Impact of surgical approach on complications and resource utilization of cervical spine fusion: a nationwide perspective to the surgical treatment of diffuse cervical spondylosis. Spine 2009;9(1):31–8.

40. Casal-Moro R, Castro-Menendez M, Hernandez-Blanco M, et al. Long-term outcome after microendoscopic diskectomy for lumbar disk herniation: a prospective clinical study with a 5-year follow-up. Neurosurgery 2011;68(6):1568–75 [discussion: 1575].

41. Chang SS, Fu TS, Liang YC, et al. Results of microendoscopic discectomy performed in the 26 cases with a minimum 3 years follow-up. Chang Gung Med J 2009;32(1):89–97.

42. Garg B, Nagraja UB, Jayaswal A. Microendoscopic versus open discectomy for lumbar disc herniation: a prospective randomised study. J Orthop Surg 2011;19(1):30–4.

43. Ikuta K, Tono O, Tanaka T, et al. Surgical complications of microendoscopic procedures for lumbar spinal stenosis. Minim Invasive Neurosurg 2007; 50(3):145–9.

44. Jhala A, Mistry M. Endoscopic lumbar discectomy: experience of first 100 cases. Indian J Orthop 2010;44(2):184–90.

45. Perez-Cruet MJ, Foley KT, Isaacs RE, et al. Microendoscopic lumbar discectomy: technical note. Neurosurgery 2002;51(Suppl 5):S129–36.

46. Podichetty VK, Spears J, Isaacs RE, et al. Complications associated with minimally invasive decompression for lumbar spinal stenosis. J Spinal Disord Tech 2006;19(3):161–6.

47. Ranjan A, Lath R. Microendoscopic discectomy for prolapsed lumbar intervertebral disc. Neurol India 2006;54(2):190–4.

48. Righesso O, Falavigna A, Avanzi O. Comparison of open discectomy with microendoscopic discectomy in lumbar disc herniations: results of a randomized controlled trial. Neurosurgery 2007; 61(3):545–9 [discussion: 549].

49. Wang M, Zhou Y, Wang J, et al. A 10-year follow-up study on long-term clinical outcomes of lumbar microendoscopic discectomy. J Neurol Surg A Cent Eur Neurosurg 2012;73(4):195–8.

50. Zhou Y, Wang M, Wang J, et al. Clinical experience and results of lumbar microendoscopic discectomy: a study with a five-year follow-up. Orthop Surg 2009;1(3):171–5.

Minimizing Radiation Exposure in Minimally Invasive Spine Surgery
Lessons Learned from Neuroendovascular Surgery

Najib E. El Tecle, MD[a], Tarek Y. El Ahmadieh, MD[a],
Biraj M. Patel, MD[b], Rohan R. Lall, MD[a],
Bernard R. Bendok, MD, MSCI[c,d,e,*], Zachary A. Smith, MD[c]

KEYWORDS

- Radiation exposure • Radiation avoidance • As low as reasonably achievable
- Neuroendovascular surgery • Spine surgery • Minimally invasive spine surgery

KEY POINTS

- Increased radiation exposure is largely due to increased used of radiation for therapeutic and diagnostic purposes.
- Minimizing radiation exposure can be achieved by controlling radiation doses, limiting time of exposure, maintaining distance from the source, shielding, and appropriate engineering.
- Minimally invasive spinal surgery is associated with high levels of radiation exposure, which warrants abiding by radiation exposure precautions.
- Cone beam computed tomography reduces the surgeon's exposure while increasing the patient exposure.
- Neuronavigation is an increasingly popular radiation-free technique, which can be used in certain cases of minimally invasive spinal procedures.

INTRODUCTION

Radiation use for diagnostic and therapeutic purposes has significantly increased over the past several decades. Techniques that rely on radiation for image guidance such as minimally invasive spine surgery and neurointerventional surgery have resulted in less morbidity and improved outcomes for select patients, but the issue of operator and personnel exposure remains a concern.[1,2] Protective technologies and policies continue to evolve to meet the protection needs. Incorporating these policies and technologies into practice is a challenge.

In light of the available data regarding radiation exposure, national and international organizations

[a] Department of Neurological Surgery, Northwestern Memorial Hospital, 633 North St Clair, Suite 1800, Chicago, IL 60611, USA; [b] Department of Radiology, 676 N. St. Clair Street, Suite 800, Chicago, IL 60611, USA; [c] Department of Neurological Surgery, Northwestern Memorial Hospital, Feinberg School of Medicine, Northwestern University, 676 North St Clair, Suite 2210, Chicago, IL 60611, USA; [d] Department of Radiology, Northwestern Memorial Hospital, Feinberg School of Medicine, Northwestern University, 676 North St Clair, Suite 2210, Chicago, IL 60611, USA; [e] Department of Otolaryngology, Northwestern Memorial Hospital, Feinberg School of Medicine, Northwestern University, 676 North St Clair, Suite 2210, Chicago, IL 60611, USA
* Corresponding author. Department of Neurological Surgery, Feinberg School of Medicine, Northwestern University, 676 North St Clair, Suite 2210, Chicago, IL 60611.
E-mail address: bbendok@nmff.org

Neurosurg Clin N Am 25 (2014) 247–260
http://dx.doi.org/10.1016/j.nec.2013.12.004
1042-3680/14/$ – see front matter © 2014 Elsevier Inc. All rights reserved.

have recognized radiation risk from occupational exposure as a significant hazard to health care professionals. Particularly in specialties such as spine surgery and neurointerventional surgery, operators who are susceptible to increased radiation exposure consider that the large number of procedures they perform can benefit from other experiences in the operative field or the angiography suite.[3] Knowledge acquired in one field or the other can help promote radiation safety among neurosurgeons in general and make the operative setting a safer environment for the patient, the surgeon, and the operating room (OR) personnel (**Box 1**).

REGULATORY PROCESSES IN RADIATION PROTECTION

An increasing number of radiation-related procedures as well as an increasing number of involved personnel led to the institution of federal and international regulations aiming to control radiation exposure. As a result of international collaboration, the International Commission on Radiological Protection issued the As Low As Reasonably Achievable (ALARA) principle, which is a regulatory requirement aiming to minimize radiation exposure by using all reasonable methods. All operators using ionizing radiation are advised to abide by this principle.

> **Box 1**
> **Summary of general recommendations for radiation exposure reduction**
>
> Wear protective devices (lead apron, thyroid shield, leaded glasses, leaded gloves)
>
> Use the hands-off technique
>
> Keep X-ray tube under the patient table
>
> Use time-distance-shielding principle: minimize time, maximize distance, use shielding
>
> Stand by the detector opposite to the X-ray source
>
> Wear dosimeter
>
> Use fluoroscope in automatic mode
>
> Establish a radiation exposure profile of your operating room and take advantage of the room design when feasible
>
> Use shielding even when using cone beam computed tomography scan
>
> Beware of a false sense of safety while wearing protective equipment

KEY CONCEPTS IN RADIATION PHYSICS

Radiation comprises energetic particles or energy waves traveling in space. When these particles or waves have enough energy to liberate electrons from atoms or molecules, this is known as ionizing radiation. Radiation propagates in a forward linear direction in air. At the air-matter interface, physical phenomena such as absorption, reflection, refraction, and scattering may occur, possibly leading to secondary sources of radiation. Many variables can be used to quantify radiation exposure. The most common methods of measuring radiation in medicine include absorbed dose and equivalent dose, which are measured in Gray and Sievert, respectively. One Gray and 1 Sievert both correspond to the absorption of 1 J of energy per kilogram of matter. However, the Sievert is corrected to express the equivalent dose for a fixed mass of biological tissue.

BIOLOGICAL EFFECTS OF RADIATION

Ionizing radiation damages cells by incurring direct injuries to DNA molecules or by inducing free radicals, which may affect DNA as well as other cellular structures. Low-dose radiation is usually believed to cause stochastic effects such as mutations, which may result in cancer, and hereditary diseases. However, data regarding low-dose radiation exposure remain limited because most low-dose human ionizing radiation risk estimates come from studies conducted on atomic bomb survivors in Japan.

Large doses of radiation might also cause stochastic effects; however, they are more likely to induce direct necrosis or fibrotic changes. Documented radiation effects range from skin irritation to instantaneous death. Mild radiation sickness necessitates a dose that is 10 times higher than US radiation workers' annual limit.[4] Organs that are particularly sensitive to radiation include skin, the eyes, and most mucosal membranes. Acute radiation doses delivered to skin during a single procedure or closely spaced procedures may induce skin erythema at a dose of 2 Gy, permanent epilation at a dose of 7 Gy, and delayed skin necrosis at 12 Gy. Secondary ulceration may occur at 24 Gy.[5–7] Eye exposure may cause cataract if 2 Gy of radiation is received in a short period or if 4 Gy is received in less than 3 months. Cataract may occur as a delayed effect if 5.5 Gy is received in more than 3 months.[5–7]

SOURCES OF RADIATION

In its 2008 report to the United Nations General Assembly, the United Nations Scientific Committee on the Effects of Atomic Radiation classified radiation exposure into 2 major types: public exposure and occupational exposure.[8] Public exposures were divided into those resulting from natural sources such as cosmic radiation, man-made sources such as nuclear power production, historical situations, and exposure from accidents. Occupational exposures were divided into natural sources such as cosmic ray exposures of aircrew or space crew and man-made sources such as medical uses of radiation.

GENERAL RECOMMENDATIONS FOR MINIMIZING RADIATION EXPOSURE

In light of the increased use of radiation in daily medical practice, abiding by the ALARA principle has become mandatory. Observing this principle entails applying several strategies to limit radiation exposure.

Controlling Radiation Doses

Radiation dose received by a biological tissue is the major determinant of histopathologic outcomes. Therefore, controlling radiation doses is the most important step in the process of avoiding side effects. This process can be achieved via optimizing image capturing algorithms and avoiding unnecessary radiographic studies.[9] For example, new fluoroscopy algorithms are optimized to benefit from the evolution of detectors, which diminishes the amount of radiation needed without compromising the clinical sensitivity or specificity of the study.

A good planning of radiographic shots can help control doses of radiation by minimizing the number of unnecessary shots. For example, fluoroscopy technicians should make sure they have an adequate setting before taking the shot, thus minimizing the number of repeated unnecessary exposures. Ideally, only 1 shot would be taken per procedure step. In deformity cases, radiation doses can be controlled via preoperative planning, resulting in fewer radiographs taken during surgery.

Limiting Time of Exposure

Another factor that correlates with the absorbed dose is the time of exposure. Limiting exposure time depends on good operator training and also on limiting the number of shots taken during the procedure. Exposure time is particularly important in fluoroscopic procedures; certain procedures such as coiling necessitate videolike image acquisition. Operators of fluoroscopic machines, whether in the OR or in the interventional suite, should try to take the least number of views to minimize exposure.

Time of exposure can also be limited by stepping out of the room or standing behind a shield when feasible. For example, during neurointerventional surgery, an automatic drug delivery system, which can inject contrast at preset rates, allows the personnel to step out of the room while the angiogram is being performed. Although this strategy might not be a possibility when an aneurysm is being coiled, avoiding unnecessary radiation during simple angiograms might significantly limit the total exposure time.

Time of exposure can also be analyzed from the larger perspective of lifetime exposure. From this perspective, it is the role of regulatory authorities to ensure that lifetime exposure of health care professionals does not exceed maximal allowed doses.

Maintaining Distance from Source of Radiation

Energy carried by radiation per unit surface is inversely proportional to the square of the distance traveled between the source and the detector. This finding means that energy carried by radiation decreases rapidly with distance from the source. Therefore, maintaining distance from the source helps achieve better radiation protection. In addition to attenuation caused by the distance, air between the source and the operator or the patient can also provide minimal shielding, which helps decrease the energy of radiation. Consequently, maximizing the distance between the source and the operator, the patient, or the personnel, when feasible, can help reduce the amount of radiation received. Although there is no agreement on how much distance is enough, from a physics point of view, even minimal distances can significantly affect radiation exposure.

This goal can also be achieved by stepping out of the room or by stepping back from the radiation field during spine surgeries. Other minor steps that can be taken include using a Kocher to hold the Jamshidi needle as seen in **Fig. 1**.

Shielding

Shielding minimizes radiation exposure by ensuring that radiation is absorbed before it reaches sensitive biological tissue. Shielding depends both on the physical nature of the offending particle and the shield. For example, whereas for α particles keratin on top of the skin provides enough shielding, γ rays necessitate dense metallic shielding such as lead. Dense metal shields, such as lead, provide more efficient

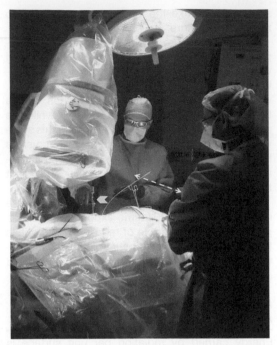

Fig. 1. The surgeon and first assistant are maintaining distance (*dashed arrow*) from the radiation source. They are wearing leaded gloves and leaded protective eyewear. Notice that the Jamshidi needle is being held by a Kocher (*small arrow*) to maintain the surgeon's hand outside the radiation field.

shielding than other types of shields, such as glass. For this purpose, leaded transparent materials have been developed and are available for use in protective eyewear and mobile shields. Shielding also depends on the shield thickness; when an energetic particle is traveling through a shield, it is more likely to be absorbed when the lead is thick enough. Shielding types and their uses are discussed later.

Collimation

Whereas shielding consists of blocking radiation before it reaches the physician, collimation consists of blocking radiation before going out of the source. Collimation can be performed when the operator does not need to visualize the whole field and has been shown to significantly decrease radiation exposure.[4,10] A recent study also showed that collimation maintains image quality.[11] Collimation is available in most modern machines and is beneficial to both the patient and the surgeon. Collimation can prove particularly beneficial in interventional neurosurgery. For example, during coiling, the surgeon can minimize radiation exposure by collimating the field to view the aneurysm and nearby vessels.

Engineering Controls

ORs as well as neurointerventional suites can be customized to minimize radiation exposure from secondary sources. From the design of facilities and equipment to the room setup, minimizing scattering as well as minimizing reflections are engineering challenges that can optimize this environment for use of radiation for medical purposes. This situation is achieved by abiding to several engineering principles: first, increasing absorbing surfaces to minimize reflections or scattering; second, making free space available to ensure the possibility of fitting mobile shields; and third, by providing roof-suspended radiation shields.

RADIATION EXPOSURE TO THE OPERATOR

There are 3 sources of radiation exposure to the operator: primary beam exposure, scattered radiation from the patient, and X-ray tube leakage.[12] The beam of radiation is most intense on the side entering the patient and significantly decreased on the image receptor side of the patient. Scattered radiation is a result of X-ray beam interactions with patient tissues. These Compton interactions are greatest near the beam entrance and lower on the exiting side of the patient, because most of the radiation is absorbed by the patient. The image receptor (image intensifier [C-arm unit] or digital image detector [neurointerventional suite]) contains lead shielding to act as a barrier for both primary and scattered radiation. Hence, it is advisable that operators work on the image receptor side whenever possible to decrease exposure. In addition, using collimators to exclude the operators' hands/fingers from the radiation beam can also reduce exposure.

Even although there is protective lead lining the X-ray tubes, radiation leakage is a known occurrence in fluoroscopy units in which radiation emanates not only in the primary beam but also in other directions. Therefore, routine maintenance is mandatory to evaluate for and minimize any tube leaks.

Operators should keep track of radiation exposure with the use of thermoluminescent dosimetry badges, typically worn at the waist level under the apron and at the thyroid level over the lead shield. The International Commission on Radiological Protection recommends that the effective dose be limited to 20 mSv/y averaged over 5 consecutive years, with no single year exceeding 50 mSv.[4]

RADIATION EXPOSURE TO THE PATIENT

X-ray tube voltage and current, automatic brightness control (ABC), collimation, beam filtration, use of pulsed fluoroscopy mode, and magnification are various parameters of the fluoroscopy unit that affect radiation dose to the patient. The voltage (kVp) and current (mA) are controlled by the ABC subsystem to produce enough radiation to produce an acceptable image at the image receptor (typically 60–120 kVp). The patient dose is directly proportional to the tube current and beam-on time. The former is out of the operator's control, for the most part. However, the total beam-on time can be controlled by the operator and should be minimized as practically possible.

Collimators allow operators to focus in on the area of interest and reduce radiation exposure to the areas that are not of clinical interest. As mentioned earlier, collimation also decreases operators' exposure to scatter radiation. The interventional units are also equipped with equalization filters, more commonly known as soft cones, which are lead-impregnated acrylic or rubber filters, which reduce patient dose.

Beam filters are thin metal (aluminum or copper) filters, which are located between the exit port and collimator. These filters reduce patient dose by absorbing low-energy X-rays that are insufficient to penetrate the patient and thus are not useful in image production.

Pulsed fluoroscopy mode, found on more recent interventional units, has decreased patient and operator radiation doses. Instead of producing X-rays continuously, the X-ray tube is pulsed on for several milliseconds and then turned off until the next frame is acquired.[12] Lowering the frame rate helps reduce radiation dose, although at the expense of temporal resolution.

Although magnification helps sort out minute details, it does so at the expense of higher patient dose. With increased magnification, the total brightness gain decreases and the resulting image is dimmer.[12] The ABC subsystem compensates for this situation by increasing the patient entrance dose. Therefore, the magnification function should be used when it is absolutely necessary.

CURRENT PRACTICES IN RADIATION PROTECTION

Various devices were developed to minimize radiation exposure and ensure a safe environment for both the operator and the patient. The armamentarium includes aprons, thyroid shields, eyewear, and protective gloves, as well as mobile shields.

Lead Aprons

Protective shielding is essential and should be mandatory when X-ray units are in function. Protective aprons typically consist of 0.5 mm of lead or lighter-weight lead equivalent material; thicknesses ranging from 0.25 to 1 mm lead equivalent are available. A 0.5-mm lead equivalent usually attenuates 90% of the radiation that strikes it. Various lead apron styles exist on the market, including a wrap-around style consisting of a skirt and vest, front coverage aprons, and aprons that wrap around the body. The advantage of the vest and kilt garment is that is allows the weight to be distributed to the hips, instead of concentrated to the upper back.[13] Lead aprons should be fitted to the individual so that there are no gaps in appropriate coverage (**Fig. 2**). Shielding material should be scanned under fluoroscopy on a yearly basis to scan for holes and reduced shielding integrity.

Evidence supporting the use of aprons while operating X-ray machines is overwhelming. However, problems with the use of lead apron have also been reported. In 1992, Moore and colleagues[14] conducted a study of 688 radiologists to assess the effect of wearing lead aprons on back pain. Fifty-two percent of radiologists using lead aprons for more than 10 hours a week suffered from back pain, compared with only 40% among those who wore their lead aprons for less than 10 hours. The results did not reach statistical significance. Other issues with the use of lead aprons include discomfort of the operator, especially in long procedures. However, other studies have documented an increase in orthopedic problems that are related to long-term use of heavy aprons.[15] Composite materials are currently used to reduce the weight of aprons; aprons made of tungsten, barium, or other material provide similar safety to that offered by lead, at less than 30% the weight.[16,17]

Thyroid Collars

Thyroid collars are recommended for operators receiving more than 4 mSv of radiation on collar radiation monitors (see **Fig. 2**B).[13] The Cardiovascular and Interventional Radiology Society of Europe and the Society of Interventional Radiology recommend that all operators wear a thyroid shield.[18] However, the National Academy of Sciences and National Research Council note that use of thyroid collars in personnel older than 40 years becomes less important, because radiation-induced thyroid cancer is reduced significantly with age.

Means other than thyroid collars exist to decrease the radiation dose received by the thyroid. For example, disposable protective patient drapes with a metallic element have been shown to decrease the operator dose substantially, with reported reductions of 12-fold to the eyes, 26-fold to the thyroid, and 29-fold to the hands.[19]

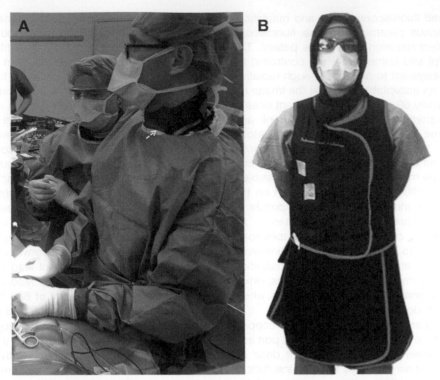

Fig. 2. (*A*) Surgeon wearing the thyroid collar. (*B*) Surgeon wearing complete radiation protection costume: lead apron, thyroid collar, and leaded eyewear.

Protective Eyewear

New data regarding radiosensitivity of the lens suggest that cataract might occur at doses lower than the previously set threshold of 150 mSv per year.[20–22] This finding emphasizes the importance of eye protection among exposed physicians. Currently, protective shielding of the eyes can be achieved through either leaded eyewear or suspended shields (**Fig. 3**A). Regular protective glasses have a 0.75 mm lead equivalent thickness, which provides an attenuation of 95% of incident X-rays.

An important factor that should be considered is eye exposure to scattered radiation from the head and from the sides. Without protective side shields, leaded glasses reduce eye exposure by a factor of 2 to 3 only.[23] It is therefore important to consider wearing a lead cap to protect from back-scattered radiation. Studies evaluating the effect of lead caps are scarce. However, in 2003, Kuon and colleagues[24] assessed the benefit of wearing a lead cap in interventional cardiology and found that caps might provide significant attenuation of radiation.

Lead Gloves

Cases of skin damage have been reported on multiple occasions in physicians who routinely place their hands into the primary beam.[13] Protective lead gloves can be useful during fluoroscopic procedures (see **Fig. 3**B). The standard heavy glove is used in routine gastrointestinal fluoroscopic examinations but may not be practical for sterile procedures in the neurointerventional suite or the OR. For that reason, lead-impregnated thin sterile gloves are available, which may be helpful during certain maneuvers. For instance, during cross-compression of the contralateral cervical carotid artery to maximize opacification of the anterior communicating artery, thin sterile lead gloves help reduce radiation exposure to the operator's hand during digital subtraction angiography. Thin lead gloves have been shown to attenuate approximately 50% of X-rays. Therefore, it is best practice to make use of thin sterile lead gloves to minimize direct exposure of the operator's hand to the primary X-ray beam, whenever possible. However, in the particular case of leaded gloves, previous studies have shown a possible increase in radiation exposure associated with a false sense of security.[25,26] Therefore, it is important to abide by the standard rules of security even when protective tools are available.

Mobile Lead Shields

Mobile lead shields should also be used for radiation protection for the operators, nurses, or

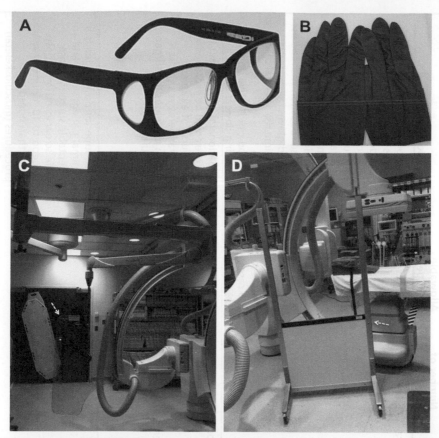

Fig. 3. Protective eyewear (*A*) with side protection are important tools to decrease eye radiation exposure. Leaded gloves (*B*) provide hands protection especially in procedures that necessitate handling of tools directly in the radiation field. Ceiling-mounted (*arrow*) (*C*) shields and mobile shields (*arrow*) (*D*) provide protection to the operating surgeon and the personnel. ([A] *Courtesy of* Universal Medical, Inc., Norwood, MA; with permission.)

anesthesiology personnel in the room (see **Fig. 3**C, D). These shields are available in various sizes and can be positioned in any part of the interventional suite or OR. Also available are table drape shields, that help reduce radiation exposure to the operator's lower extremities and further decrease scatter radiation exposure.

NUANCES IN SPINE SURGERY RADIATION EXPOSURE

Spine surgery is characterized by high radiation exposure. Fluoroscopically assisted thoracolumbar pedicle screw placement, for example, was found to expose the surgeon to significantly greater radiation levels than any other nonspinal musculoskeletal procedure that involves the use of the fluoroscope.[27] Dose rates up to 10 to 12 times greater were reported.[2] Despite general concerns regarding radiation exposure in spine surgery, it was recently shown that, in general, fluoroscopic dosage to the spine surgeon remains

lower than the annual maximum allowed limit if the surgeon abides by radiation safety rules.[28] Different aspects of radiation exposure in spinal surgery have been investigated; in particular, the type of procedure, as well as the used image acquisition modality, were evaluated in multiple prospective studies.

Minimally Invasive Spinal Surgery and Radiation Exposure

Interest in minimally invasive approaches in spine surgery has considerably increased over the past 2 decades. However, as well as increased use of radiation in minimally invasive procedures, there has been an escalating concern of increased radiation exposure to both the patient and the surgeon. Several prospective studies have attempted to quantify radiation exposure risk form minimally invasive surgeries (**Table 1**).[2,27,29–42]

Lumbar procedures were among the most investigated because of their prevalence. In

Table 1
Radiation exposure in various fluoroscopically guided spine procedures

Procedure	Author/y	Radiation Dose	Number of Assessed Cases	Number of Allowable Cases per Year	Conclusion
Vertebroplasty	Kruger & Faciszewski,[29] 2003	Whole body: 1.44 mSv/vertebra Hand: 2.04 mSv/vertebra	69 procedures	34 cases	Reduction caused by shielding ranges from 42.9% to 86.1%
	Kallmes et al,[30] 2003	Hand, syringe: 1 mSv/case Hand, injector: 0.55 mSv/case	39 procedures	500 injections (syringe)	Dose is decreased with use of injection device
	Harstall et al,[31] 2005	Thyroid: 0.052 mSv/vertebra Eye: 0.02 mSv/vertebra Hand: 0.107 mSv/vertebra	32 procedures	—	The annual risk of developing fatal cancer is very low. Lifetime morbidity is high to very high
	Synowitz & Kiwit,[32] 2006	Hand, unprotected: 1.81 mSv Hand: protected: 0.49 mSv	41 procedure	300 procedures (unprotected) >1000 procedures protected	75% dose reduction with the use of lead gloves The lifetime risk for fatal cancer is 0.04%
	Fitousi et al,[33] 2006	Eyes: 0.328 mGy/case Hand: 1.661 mGy/case	11 procedures	150 cases 229 cases	Reduction of effective dose by shielding devices by >75%
Kyphoplasty	Mroz et al,[34] 2008	Whole body: 0.248 mSv/vertebra Eye: 0.271 mSv/vertebra Hand: 1.744 mSv/vertebra	27 patients	300 cases for the hand	Occupational exposure limit to the eye could be exceeded over the course of a career
	Schils et al,[35] 2013	Left finger: 0.272 mSv (direct injection) vs 0.04 mSv (cement delivery system) Right wrist: 0.028 mSv (direct injection) vs 0.143 mSv	20 patients	O-ARM (Medtronic, Minneapolis, MN, USA) allows the surgeon to work lower than the limit of exposure	New intraoperative injection system decreases the surgeon's exposure
Pedicle screw insertion	Jones et al,[27] 2000	Eye: 0.56 µGy/image Thyroid: 0.81 µGy/image	140 patients	—	Source-superior position leads to minimal patient's dose and an acceptable surgeon's dose
	Rampersaud et al,[2] 2000	Thyroid: 0.083 mSv/min Ventral waist: 0.533 mSv/min Hand: 0.582 mSv/min	6 cadavers	—	Pedicle screw insertion exposes surgeon to 10–12 times higher doses than nonspinal procedures (musculoskeletal)
	Ul Haque et al,[36] 2006	Thyroid and eye: 0.109 mSv/case	14 procedures × 23 screws per procedure	Lifetime dose limit surpassed after <10 y of exposure	Rate of thyroid malignancies that can be related to radiation exposure is increased among orthopedic surgeons

Procedure	Study	Measurement	Sample	Maximum cases	Comments
MIS TLIF	Bindal et al,[37] 2008	Waist (protected): 0.27 mSv/case; Neck (unprotected): 0.32 mSv/case; Hand: 0.76 mSv/case	24 patients	194 cases for the torso; 166 cases for the thyroid; 664 cases for the hand	Annual occupational exposure limit could be exceeded
	Kim et al,[38] 2008	Fluoroscopy: 0.124 mSv; Navigation: undetectable	8 cadavers	—	Navigation leads to virtually no exposure to the surgeon and team
Lateral lumbar interbody fusion (LLIF)	Taher et al,[39] 2013	Chest (protected): 0.44 mRem/procedure; Thyroid: 2.19 mRem/procedure; Eye: 2.64 mRem/procedure	18 procedures	2700 procedure	More than 2700 LLIF can be performed annually with the adequate precautions
Minimally invasive microdiscectomy (MIS) vs open microdiscectomy	Mariscalco et al,[40] 2011	Whole body: 0.0021 (open) vs 0.0308 (MIS); Thyroid/eye: 0.0016 (open) vs 0.0172 (MIS); Hand: 0.0020 (open) vs 0.0445 (MIS)	10 (open) vs 10 (MIS)	1623 case (MIS); 8720 cases (MIS); 11,235 cases (MIS)	Radiation exposure is 10–20 times higher during MIS
Percutaneous endoscopic lumbar diskectomy (PELD)	Ahn et al,[41] 2013	Whole body: 0.1718 mSv/level; Thyroid: 0.0785 mSv/level; Hand: 0.7318 mSv/level	30 procedures	683 cases for hands	Use of adequate equipment is essential, because without protection 291 PELD exposes the surgeon to the maximal allowable dose
Mixed cases (O-ARM)	Nottmeier et al,[42] 2013	At OR table: 176 mRem/spin; At 3 to 4 m (10–13 ft) from gantry: 0.7–3.6 mRem/spin	25 patients/124 screws		Radiation scatter to OR personnel from O-ARM is minimal

2008, Bindal and colleagues[37] studied surgeon and patient exposure in minimally invasive transforaminal lumbar interbody fusion (TLIF). These investigators evaluated radiation exposure during 24 consecutive procedures (33 levels) performed by a single surgeon. The mean fluoroscopy time was 1.69 minutes per case, with mean exposure to hands reaching 76 mRem, mean exposure to the chest under the apron reaching 27 mRem, and mean exposure to the unprotected thyroid reaching 32 mRem. Patient exposure was noticed to vary with position and reached 59.5 mGy in the anteroposterior plane and 78.8 in the lateral plan. This study concluded that annual allowed limit could be exceeded if a large number of fluoroscopically guided procedures are performed. Kim and colleagues[38] assessed the effect of using navigation-assisted fluoroscopy on radiation exposure during TLIF. These investigators performed a combined cadaveric (18 cadavers) and human (18 patients) study comparing navigation-assisted fluoroscopy with standard intraoperative fluoroscopy. Although procedure time was similar between the 2 groups, the total fluoroscopy time was higher in the fluoroscopy group when compared with the navigation-assisted group (41.9 seconds vs 28.7 seconds, $P = .042$). Radiation exposure was undetectable in the navigation-assisted group, whereas, on average, 12.4 mRem was delivered to the surgeon during a unilateral fluoroscopy-guided, TLIF procedure. Although this study shows interesting results, assessment of postoperative outcomes in a study comparing navigation-assisted TLIF with fluoroscopy-based TLIF still needs to be performed in order to show that both procedures have similar clinical outcomes and that decreased radiation exposure does not come at the expense of procedure quality and patient outcomes.

Radiation exposure in minimally invasive surgery (MIS) for lumbar microdiskectomy (MD) was also evaluated. In 2011, Mariscalco and colleagues[40] conducted a prospective case control study, during which they compared radiation exposure in 10 minimally invasive lumbar MDs with radiation exposure in 10 open lumbar diskectomies. MIS was shown to expose the surgeon to 10-fold to 20-fold more radiation than the open lumbar MD. Yet, Mariscalco and colleagues calculated that despite this higher exposure, a surgeon can perform up to 8720 MIS safely each year.

A more recent study assessed radiation exposure during percutaneous endoscopic lumbar diskectomy (PELD).[41] Three surgeons were followed during 30 consecutive PELDs over a 3-month period. High levels of radiation were detected without shielding; a surgeon performing PELDs without protection was found to reach the maximum allowable dose in only 291 procedures per year. With protection, this number increased to 683, the number of procedures at which the surgeon exceeds the radiation exposure limit for the hands.

Taher and colleagues evaluated radiation exposure in lateral lumbar interbody fusion (LLIF). These investigators showed that lateral positioning of the patient and hands-on use of fluoroscopic imaging during LLIF may increase the surgeon's radiation exposure. Higher body mass index was also found to increase patient exposure. However, other factors such as number of fused levels and the technical difficulty of surgeries did not significantly increase the amount of radiation needed. The conclusion was that up to 2700 LLIF procedures might be performed safely per year.

Fitousi and colleagues[33] studied patient and staff dosimetry during vertebroplasty. In this study, hand exposure during a single procedure was found to reach 1.7 mGy, whereas eye exposure was found to reach 0.3 mGy. The total number of safe vertebroplasties that can be performed before reaching the yearly maximal dose threshold was estimated to be 150 cases only, which is the lowest number of procedures reported to be safe by a study. Fitousi and colleagues also evaluated the effect of mobile shielding, which was shown to decrease 75% of the effective dose received by the surgeon. Other investigators who also evaluated radiation exposure during vertebroplasty include Kurger and colleagues, Kallmes and colleagues, Harstall and colleagues, and Synowitz and colleagues.[29–32] These investigators all found a significant risk of radiation exposure and recommended appropriate protection. In particular, Harstall and colleagues found a lifetime risk of cancer of 0.04%. Kallmes and colleagues found that use of an automated injection device helps decrease radiation dose.

Similarly, Mroz and colleagues[34] assessed radiation exposure from kyphoplasty and found that exposure to the operator's hands during a single procedure might reach 1.7 mGy and radiation exposure to the eyes might reach 0.3 mGy. These investigators concluded that total exposure to the hands and eyes could easily exceed occupation exposure limit if no shielding is used.

Imaging Modality

Modifying the image acquisition process during minimally invasive spinal surgery was proposed as a possible strategy to minimize radiation expose. Among others, use of three-dimensional

(3D) image guidance and neuronavigation were promoted as possible solutions to the radiation exposure problem.

3D image guidance has been successfully used for accurate instrumentation placement in the cervical, thoracic, and lumbar spine. Cone beam computed tomography (CBCT) has been designed to provide a safer image acquisition tool for the surgeon (**Fig. 4**). However, CBCT was reported to have similar scattering to a standard 64-slice computed tomography (CT) scanner.[43] In 2 recent studies, Nottmeier and colleagues[44] evaluated surgeon exposure while performing a 3D image-guided spinal surgery. In their first study, they assessed radiation in a single surgeon after performing 25 miscellaneous spinal surgeries and concluded that no radiation exposure to the surgeon occurs in CBCT 3D imaging-guided spinal surgery when the surgeon is standing behind a lead shield at 3 m (10 feet) from the device. In their second study, Nottmeier and colleagues[42] attempted to quantify radiation exposure to medical staff by measuring radiation at 5 unshielded locations in the OR. Radiation scatter from the O-ARM was found to be minimal at a distance of 1.8 m (6 feet) from the device. A more recent cadaveric study by Tabaraee and colleagues[45] also attempted to compare radiation exposure from the use of O-ARM with the use of C-ARM (Phillips, Eindhoven, The Netherlands). This study involved 4 surgeons, who placed 80 pedicle screws using the O-ARM and 80 pedicle screws using the C-ARM. Breach rate, setup time, average total time, and radiation exposure were evaluated. This study as well as other reported studies found that O-ARM and C-ARM had similar breach rates and average total surgery time.[46] However, the setup time was longer for the O-ARM group (529 seconds vs 297 seconds), whereas radiation exposure in the O-ARM group was significantly

lower (undetected) for the surgeon and significantly higher for the cadaver. Other teams also reported similar results, Abdullah and colleagues[47] conducted a prospective clinical study of 10 patients and found that radiation exposure to the surgical team during routine use of O-ARM is minimal; the number of necessary procedures to reach occupational exposure limits was calculated to be 1,130,071. Although CBCT significantly decreases exposure to the surgeon and the OR staff, an analysis of patient radiation exposure form the O-ARM using phantom models and ion chambers showed a significant increase in patient exposure. During 1 spin of the O-ARM, the patient is exposed to radiation equal to 47% to 83% of the exposure sustained from a regular 64-slice CT scan.[43] Furthermore, this exposure also depends on the used imaging mode (eg, using the standard 3D mode rather than the high-definition 3D mode helps reduce radiation by up to 40%).[42] Other studies also reported increased patient radiation exposure from O-ARM use.[45]

Neuronavigation was also described as a potential tool that can be used to minimize radiation exposure to both the patient and the surgeon. Neuronavigation has potentially zero or minimal radiation exposure.[38] A recent review of neuronavigation in minimally invasive spine surgery found 52 PubMed listed articles describing diverse tools and innovative techniques that can be used in spinal surgeries.[48] However, neuronavigation still has several limitations: a major drawback, for example, is the error resulting from positioning difference between the time of imaging and during the surgery. Particularly the distortion of the interspinous regions can be augmented in situations such as deformity or posttraumatic spinal instability. Despite current limitations of neuronavigation, refinements in image-guidance technologies might progressively allow for better outcomes

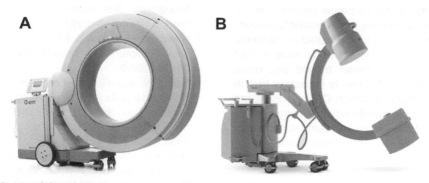

Fig. 4. The O-ARM (A) provides less exposure to the surgeon but more exposure to the patient than the C-ARM (B). ([A] *Courtesy of* Medtronic Inc., Minneapolis, MN and [B] *Courtesy of* Philips, Inc., Amsterdam, The Netherlands.)

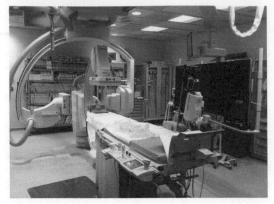

Fig. 5. Modern angiography suite.

and less radiation exposure. These technologies also might allow introduction of high-precision robotics into spinal surgery.

Lessons Learned from Interventional Neurosurgery

The main difference between interventional neurosurgery and minimally invasive spine surgery in terms of radiation exposure is probably that the former is performed in angiography suites designed specifically for this purpose, whereas the second is usually performed in regular ORs, most of which were built before the minimally invasive era. Whereas ORs sometimes barely provide enough space for the material to be moved around the room and have nonabsorbent walls, which can reflect radiation back into the OR, angiography suites are designed with the intention of having absorbent surfaces and enough space for shields to fit comfortably in the room. Further, angiography suites are designed with specific locations for the radiation source, the patient table, and the screens (**Fig. 5**). Another major advantage of angiography suites is ceiling-mounted shields, which are used between the radiation source and the surgeon to further decrease radiation exposure. This kind of shield is made available in modern ORs intended for radiation-based procedures. Another factor in the angiography suite is that personnel are usually better trained and more aware of radiation risks; this is especially true in low-volume centers, in which OR personnel are usually involved in multiple types of surgery. This issue can be addressed by improving staff training and, when feasible, increasing specialization.

SUMMARY

Radiation exposure is an increasing problem. Guidelines that help protect against radiation are well established, and the tools are readily available in most hospitals. However, limiting factors, such as making the tools lighter and more comfortable to wear and making the shielding more accessible, are likely to increase personnel compliance and improve protection. Reducing unnecessary exposure and decreasing unnecessary radiation as well as better staff education are probably the most important steps toward better radiation exposure prophylaxis.

REFERENCES

1. Smith ZA, Fessler RG. Paradigm changes in spine surgery: evolution of minimally invasive techniques. Nature reviews. Neurology 2012;8:443–50.
2. Rampersaud YR, Foley KT, Shen AC, et al. Radiation exposure to the spine surgeon during fluoroscopically assisted pedicle screw insertion. Spine 2000; 25:2637–45.
3. Davis H. Increasing rates of cervical and lumbar spine surgery in the United States, 1979-1990. Spine 1994;19:1117–22.
4. Schueler BA, Balter S, Miller DL. Radiation protection tools in interventional radiology. J Am Coll Radiol 2012;9:844–5.
5. Pitkanen MA, Hopewell JW. Effects of local single and fractionated X-ray doses on rat bone marrow blood flow and red blood cell volume. Strahlentherapie 1985;161:719–23.
6. Hamlet R, Heryet JC, Hopewell JW, et al. Late changes in pig skin after irradiation from beta-emitting sources of different energy. Br J Radiol Suppl 1986;19:51–4.
7. Parsons JT, Fitzgerald CR, Ian Hood C, et al. The effects of irradiation on the eye and optic nerve. Int J Radiat Oncol Biol Phys 1983;9:609–22.
8. United Nations Scientific Committee on the Effects of Atomic Radiation 2008 report: sources and effects of ionizing radiation. Classifications of types of radiation exposure 2008.
9. Rehani MM, Berry M. Radiation doses in computed tomography. The increasing doses of radiation need to be controlled. BMJ 2000;320:593–4.
10. Ghobadifar MA, Zarei S. Effect of collimation on radiation exposure and image quality. Korean J Pain 2013;26:307–8.
11. Baek SW, Ryu JS, Jung CH, et al. A randomized controlled trial about the levels of radiation exposure depends on the use of collimation C-ARM fluoroscopic-guided medial branch block. Korean J Pain 2013;26:148–53.
12. Rzeszotarski MS, Dixon RG, Heintz PH, et al. Radiation dose and safety in interventional radiology. Radiological Society of North America; 2012.
13. Schueler BA. Operator shielding: how and why. Tech Vasc Interv Radiol 2010;13:167–71.

14. Moore B, vanSonnenberg E, Casola G, et al. The relationship between back pain and lead apron use in radiologists. AJR Am J Roentgenol 1992;158:191–3.

15. Klein LW, Miller DL, Balter S, et al. Occupational health hazards in the interventional laboratory: time for a safer environment. Radiology 2009;250:538–44.

16. Nambiar S, Yeow JT. Polymer-composite materials for radiation protection. ACS Appl Mater Interfaces 2012;4:5717–26.

17. Yaffe MJ, Mawdsley GE, Lilley M, et al. Composite materials for X-ray protection. Health Phys 1991;60:661–4.

18. Miller DL, Vano E, Bartal G, et al. Occupational radiation protection in interventional radiology: a joint guideline of the Cardiovascular and Interventional Radiology Society of Europe and the Society of Interventional Radiology. J Vasc Interv Radiol 2010;21: 607–15.

19. King JN, Champlin AM, Kelsey CA, et al. Using a sterile disposable protective surgical drape for reduction of radiation exposure to interventionalists. AJR Am J Roentgenol 2002;178:153–7.

20. Worgul BV, Kundiyev YI, Sergiyenko NM, et al. Cataracts among Chernobyl clean-up workers: implications regarding permissible eye exposures. Radiat Res 2007;167:233–43.

21. Klein BE, Klein RE, Moss SE. Exposure to diagnostic X-rays and incident age-related eye disease. Ophthalmic Epidemiol 2000;7:61–5.

22. Klein BE, Klein R, Linton KL, et al. Diagnostic X-ray exposure and lens opacities: the Beaver Dam eye study. Am J Public Health 1993;83:588–90.

23. Moore WE, Ferguson G, Rohrmann C. Physical factors determining the utility of radiation safety glasses. Med Phys 1980;7:8–12.

24. Kuon E, Birkel J, Schmitt M, et al. Radiation exposure benefit of a lead cap in invasive cardiology. Heart 2003;89:1205–10.

25. Miller DL, Vano E, Bartal G, et al. Occupational radiation protection in interventional radiology: a joint guideline of the Cardiovascular and Interventional Radiology Society of Europe and the Society Of Interventional Radiology. Cardiovasc Intervent Radiol 2010;33:230–9.

26. Wagner LK, Mulhern OR. Radiation-attenuating surgical gloves: effects of scatter and secondary electron production. Radiology 1996;200:45–8.

27. Jones DP, Robertson PA, Lunt B, et al. Radiation exposure during fluoroscopically assisted pedicle screw insertion in the lumbar spine. Spine (Phila Pa 1976) 2000;25:1538–41.

28. Mulconrey DS. Fluoroscopic radiation exposure in spinal surgery: in vivo evaluation for operating room personnel. J Spinal Disord Tech 2013. [Epub ahead of print].

29. Kruger R, Faciszewski T. Radiation dose reduction to medical staff during vertebroplasty: a review of techniques and methods to mitigate occupational dose. Spine (Phila Pa 1976) 2003;28:1608–13.

30. Kallmes DF, O E, Roy SS, et al. Radiation dose to the operator during vertebroplasty: prospective comparison of the use of 1-cc syringes versus an injection device. AJNR Am J Neuroradiol 2003;24: 1257–60.

31. Harstall R, Heini PF, Mini RL, et al. Radiation exposure to the surgeon during fluoroscopically assisted percutaneous vertebroplasty: a prospective study. Spine (Phila Pa 1976) 2005;30:1893–8.

32. Synowitz M, Kiwit J. Surgeon's radiation exposure during percutaneous vertebroplasty. J Neurosurg Spine 2006;4:106–9.

33. Fitousi NT, Efstathopoulos EP, Delis HB, et al. Patient and staff dosimetry in vertebroplasty. Spine (Phila Pa 1976) 2006;31:E884–9 [discussion: E890].

34. Mroz TE, Yamashita T, Davros WJ, et al. Radiation exposure to the surgeon and the patient during kyphoplasty. J Spinal Disord Tech 2008;21: 96–100.

35. Schils F, Schoojans W, Struelens L. The surgeon's real dose exposure during balloon kyphoplasty procedure and evaluation of the cement delivery system: a prospective study. Eur Spine J 2013;22: 1758–64.

36. Ul Haque M, Shufflebarger HL, O'Brien M, et al. Radiation exposure during pedicle screw placement in adolescent idiopathic scoliosis: is fluoroscopy safe? Spine (Phila Pa 1976) 2006;31:2516–20.

37. Bindal RK, Glaze S, Ognoskie M, et al. Surgeon and patient radiation exposure in minimally invasive transforaminal lumbar interbody fusion. J Neurosurg Spine 2008;9:570–3.

38. Kim CW, Lee YP, Taylor W, et al. Use of navigation-assisted fluoroscopy to decrease radiation exposure during minimally invasive spine surgery. Spine J 2008;8:584–90.

39. Taher F, Hughes AP, Sama AA, et al. 2013 Young Investigator award winner: how safe is lateral lumbar interbody fusion for the surgeon? A prospective in vivo radiation exposure study. Spine (Phila Pa 1976) 2013;38:1386–92.

40. Mariscalco MW, Yamashita T, Steinmetz MP, et al. Radiation exposure to the surgeon during open lumbar microdiscectomy and minimally invasive microdiscectomy: a prospective, controlled trial. Spine (Phila Pa 1976) 2011;36:255–60.

41. Ahn Y, Kim CH, Lee JH, et al. Radiation exposure to the surgeon during percutaneous endoscopic lumbar discectomy: a prospective study. Spine (Phila Pa 1976) 2013;38:617–25.

42. Nottmeier EW, Pirris SM, Edwards S, et al. Operating room radiation exposure in cone beam computed tomography-based, image-guided spinal surgery. J Neurosurg Spine 2013;19:226–31.

43. Zhang J, Weir V, Fajardo L, et al. Dosimetric characterization of a cone-beam O-ARM imaging system. J Xray Sci Technol 2009;17:305–17.

44. Nottmeier EW, Bowman C, Nelson KL. Surgeon radiation exposure in cone beam computed tomography-based, image-guided spinal surgery. Int J Med Robot 2012;8:196–200.

45. Tabaraee E, Gibson AG, Karahalios DG, et al. Intraoperative cone beam computed tomography with navigation (O-ARM) versus conventional fluoroscopy (C-ARM): a cadaveric study comparing accuracy, efficiency, and safety for spinal instrumentation. Spine (Phila Pa 1976) 2013;38(22):1953–8.

46. Smith ZA, Sugimoto K, Lawton CD, et al. Incidence of lumbar spine pedicle breach following percutaneous screw fixation: a radiographic evaluation of 601 screws in 151 patients. J Spinal Disord Tech 2012. [Epub ahead of print].

47. Abdullah KG, Bishop FS, Lubelski D, et al. Radiation exposure to the spine surgeon in lumbar and thoracolumbar fusions with the use of an intraoperative computed tomographic 3-dimensional imaging system. Spine (Phila Pa 1976) 2012;37: E1074–8.

48. Moses ZB, Mayer RR, Strickland BA, et al. Neuronavigation in minimally invasive spine surgery. Neurosurg Focus 2013;35:E12.

Current Techniques in the Management of Cervical Myelopathy and Radiculopathy

Carter S. Gerard, MD*, John E. O'Toole, MD

KEYWORDS

- Minimally invasive • Posterior • Foraminotomy • Cervical

KEY POINTS

- Patients with radiculopathy caused by a lateralized osteophyte or disc herniation without cord compression, evidence of instability, or those for whom an anterior approach is contraindicated, are candidates for minimally invasive cervical discectomy or foraminotomy (MICD/F).
- Minimally invasive decompression of cervical stenosis (MIDCS) may be offered to patients who have less than 3 levels of disease, lack evidence of instability, and have normal cervical lordosis.
- In addition to equivalent efficacy, MICD/F and MIDCS offer the advantages of reduced blood loss, length of stay, postoperative pain, and muscle spasm; preservation of motion segments; and decreased risk of iatrogenic sagittal plan deformity.

INTRODUCTION

Several degenerative abnormalities of the cervical spine can be successfully treated with posterior decompressive techniques.[1–4] Although anterior cervical procedures represent a well-established treatment for cervical disc herniation, posterior cervical laminoforaminotomy consistently shows symptom improvement of 90% to 97%[3,5–8] for patients with foraminal stenosis or lateral disc herniation. Likewise, posterior decompression with either laminectomy or laminoplasty for patients with myelopathy from cervical stenosis shows clinical improvement in 62.5% to 83% of cases.[4,9,10] Posterior decompressive procedures avoid the complications associated with anterior approaches such as esophageal injury, recurrent laryngeal nerve paralysis, dysphagia, and adjacent-level disease after fusion.[11–14]

Although standard open approaches are effective, minimally invasive approaches have been developed to avoid the extensive subperiosteal stripping of paraspinal musculature that can result in significant postoperative pain, muscle spasm,

and dysfunction in 18% to 60% of patients.[4,11,15,16] Furthermore, preoperative loss of lordosis combined with long-segment decompression can contribute to the risk of sagittal plane deformity,[17–20] a known complication that often obliges fusion at the time of decompression. The use of a posterior fusion technique increases operative time, blood loss, surgical risk, and early postoperative pain, and potentially contributes to adjacent-level disease.

The principal tenet of minimal-access techniques is to reduce approach-related morbidity. To this end, the advent of muscle-splitting tubular retractor systems and associated instruments have allowed for the application of minimally invasive techniques to posterior cervical decompressive procedures.[16,21] Minimally invasive cervical discectomy/foraminotomy (MICD/F) was first described in a cadaver model, and has subsequently been shown to have clinical efficacy equal to that of open procedures in addition to having less blood loss, shorter hospital stay, and decreased postoperative pain.[7,22–27]

Department of Neurological Surgery, Rush University Medical Center, 1725 West Harrison Street, Professional Building Suite 855, Chicago, IL 60612, USA
* Corresponding author.
E-mail address: carter_gerard@rush.edu

Neurosurg Clin N Am 25 (2014) 261–270
http://dx.doi.org/10.1016/j.nec.2013.12.005

Whereas the goal of MICD/F is nerve-root decompression, minimally invasive decompression of cervical stenosis (MICDS) is performed with the aim of decompressing the spinal cord. MICDS is a familiar modification of minimally invasive techniques that have been applied extensively to the lumbar spine.[28] By preserving much of the normal osteoligamentous anatomy of the cervical spine, the MIDCS procedure reduces the risk of postlaminectomy kyphosis and avoids the need for prophylactic posterior fusion.[4,19,29] The use of minimally invasive laminoplasty has been reported with positive results, although investigators have encountered technical difficulties and prolonged operative times.[30,31]

PREOPERATIVE PLANNING

A preoperative radiographic evaluation follows a detailed history and physical examination, and should include magnetic resonance imaging (MRI) or postmyelographic computed tomography (CT), and anteroposterior (AP), lateral, and flexion/extension cervical radiographs. Preoperative electromyography (EMG) and nerve conduction studies may also assist in the neurologic localization of specific radiculopathy. Those patients with radicular symptoms that correlate with electrophysiologic and radiographic findings may be well suited for MICD/F, depending on the underlying pathologic profile. **Fig. 1**A shows a lateralized disc herniation without spinal cord compression on preoperative MRI scan. By contrast, **Fig. 1**B shows moderate cord and nerve-root compression arising from a herniated disc. The former would be an ideal candidate for MICD/F, whereas MICDS or an anterior approach would be safer and more effective in the latter. Regardless of the abnormality, whether a soft disc or an osteophyte,

it must be lateralized without significant canal stenosis to be amenable to MICD/F. MIDCS may be indicated for patients presenting with myelopathy or myeloradiculopathy caused by central spondylotic stenosis (eg, ligamentum flavum or facet hypertrophy). Those patients with moderate canal stenosis, normal cervical lordosis, primarily posterior disease, and without instability may be considered for MIDCS or traditional laminectomy or laminoplasty.[29,32,33]

EQUIPMENT

- Gardner-Wells tongs with traction or other head fixation device
- Microscope or endoscope (with compatible camera)
- Tubular retractor system
- Minimally invasive spinal instruments (including microcurettes and 1-mm and 2-mm rongeurs)
- High-speed drill
- Intraoperative fluoroscopy

PATIENT POSITIONING

General endotracheal anesthesia is induced with fiberoptic intubation utilized in patients with chronic spinal cord compression. If the patient is placed in the sitting position a precordial Doppler may be used to monitor for air embolism, although the risk of air embolism is very low. Foley catheterization is generally not needed. Routine perioperative antibiotics are administered, as is an intravenous corticosteroid at the surgeon's discretion. Paralytic agents are minimized after induction to allow for physical intraoperative feedback of nerve-root irritation. The patient is placed in Gardner-Wells tongs or Mayfield head holder, and placed prone on a Jackson table with the

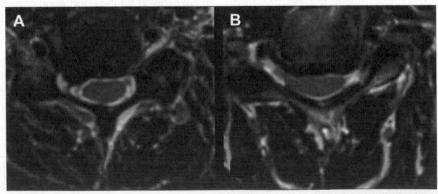

Fig. 1. Axial T2-weighted magnetic resonance imaging (MRI) scans of the cervical spine demonstrate (A) laterally herniated disc to the right with compression of the exiting nerve root and (B) a centrally located disc/osteophyte causing both spinal cord and nerve-root compression.

head gently flexed (**Fig. 2**). Alternatively, the patient may be placed in the sitting position. For the sitting position, the Mayfield 3-point head fixator is attached and the table progressively flexed to bring the patient into a semisitting position, such that head is flexed but not rotated and the posterior neck is perpendicular to the floor. Some prefer the sitting position because of the decreased blood pooling in the operative field and the gravity-dependent positioning of the shoulders for better lateral fluoroscopic images.[11,16] Regardless of the position, the legs, hands, and arms are well padded, particularly over the cubital tunnel, to prevent positional ulnar neuropathy. The fluoroscopic monitor is placed opposite the side of the approach so that the surgeon can look directly at the monitors while standing next to the patient and operating through the tubular retractor. The C-arm is placed beneath or anterior to the patient depending on available space. The neck is checked a final time to ensure the position allows adequate jugular venous drainage and airway patency.

SURGICAL APPROACH

This section outlines the technique for posterior MICD/F[5,11,16,21] and MIDCS.[19,30,32] The procedures described here use the METRx retractor (Medtronic Sofamor Danek, Memphis, TN); however, the principles are the same regardless of the retractor system used.

Before draping, an initial fluoroscopic image is acquired to confirm adequate visualization and to plan the initial entry point. The posterior neck is shaved, scrubbed, prepared, and draped in the usual manner. It is helpful to use adhesive lined drapes and/or an antibacterial adhesive layer such as Ioban (3M Health Care, St. Paul, MN) to maintain the orientation and position of the drapes during the procedure. Suction tubing, cautery lines, and the drill are typically draped over the

top or side of the field and secured against the drapes. The operative level(s) is once again confirmed on lateral fluoroscopy while a long Kirschner (K)-wire or Steinman pin is held over the lateral side of the patient's neck. For lower cervical levels (eg, C6–7, C7–T1) or in patients with high-riding shoulders in whom the operative level cannot be adequately visualized on lateral fluoroscopy despite maneuvers to push the shoulders down, both oblique and AP fluoroscopy can be used to localize the level and carefully dock as described below. A 2-cm longitudinal incision over the operative level is marked out approximately 1.5 cm off the midline on the operative side, and this is injected with local anesthesia. For 2-level procedures the incision should be placed midway between the targeted levels. For bilateral procedures, a midline skin incision can be used and the skin retracted to each side for independent dilations. After an initial stab incision, the K-wire is advanced slowly though the musculature under fluoroscopic guidance and docked at the inferomedial edge of the rostral lateral mass of the level of interest (**Fig. 3**). It is critical to engage bone and not to penetrate the interlaminar space where the laterally thinned ligamentum flavum may not protect against iatrogenic dural or spinal cord injury. At this point the incision is completed about 1 cm above and below the K-wire entry point, and the wire is removed. The axial forces that are applied during muscle dilation in the lumbar spine are more hazardous in the cervical spine. Therefore, the cervical fascia is incised equal to the length of the incision using monopolar cautery or scissors so that muscle dilation can proceed in a safe and controlled fashion. The K-wire is replaced under fluoroscopy again, and the tubular muscle dilators are serially inserted. Alternatively, a larger skin incision can be made and, once the fascia is incised, the muscle can be spread with Metzenbaum scissors and the first dilator then placed. This method avoids potential complications associated with the K-wire, and may be attractive for the novice practitioner. After dilation, the final 16-mm or 18-mm tubular METRx retractor is placed over the dilators and fixed into place over the laminofacet junction with a table-mounted flexible retractor arm, and the dilators are removed (see **Fig. 3**). The microscope is then brought into the operative field, or a 25° angled glass-rod endoscope is attached to a camera and then secured to the retractor system.

SURGICAL PROCEDURE

Monopolar cautery and pituitary rongeurs are used to clear the remaining soft tissue from the

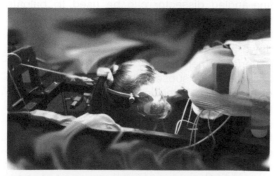

Fig. 2. Operative positioning of patient in Gardner-Wells tongs head fixation for MICD/F or MIDCS.

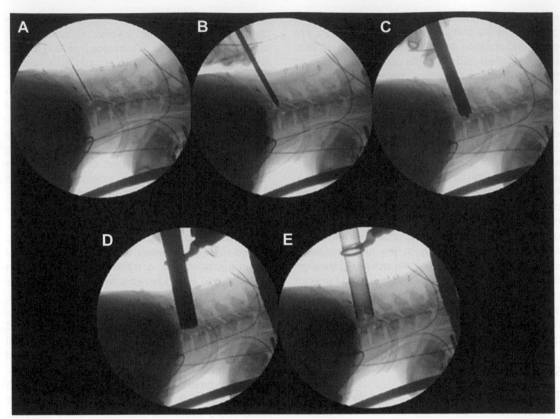

Fig. 3. Intraoperative lateral fluoroscopic images demonstrating the process of muscle dilation. (*A*) K-wire is docked on laminofacet junction over intervertebral foramen of interest (C6–7 in this case). (*B, C*) The first 2 muscle dilators are inserted serially. (*D*) Progression to largest dilator is complete. (*E*) An 18-mm tubular retractor is fixed into place and dilators are removed.

lateral mass and lamina of interest, taking care to start the dissection over solid bone laterally. A small up-angled curette is used to gently detach the ligamentum flavum from the undersurface of the inferior edge of the lamina, and a Kerrison punch with a small footplate is used to begin the laminotomy. At this point the MICD/F and MIDCS diverge in their course. The technique for MICD/F is described first, followed by that for MIDCS.

MICD/F Technique

The subsequent steps of this operation differ little from those of the open procedure. Depending on the degree of facet hypertrophy, the Kerrison punch may be used to complete most of the laminotomy and early foraminotomy, or the drill may be required early in the course of bone removal. The ligamentum flavum can be removed medially after the laminotomy to identify the lateral edge of the dura and proximal portion of the nerve root. The dorsal bony resection should follow

the nerve root into the foramen by removal of part of the medial facet. It is crucial to preserve at least 50% of the facet to maintain biomechanical integrity.[34,35] This amount of resection permits adequate exposure of the root in the foramen. At this point, the venous plexus overlying the nerve root should be carefully coagulated with low-power bipolar cautery and incised. With the root well visualized (**Fig. 4**), a fine-angled dissector can be used to palpate ventral to the nerve root for osteophytes or disc fragments. Should an osteophyte be present, a down-angled curette may be used to tamp the material further ventrally into the disc space or fragment it for subsequent removal. In the case of a soft disc herniation, a nerve hook may be passed ventrally and inferiorly to the root to gently tease the fragment away from the nerve for ultimate removal with a pituitary rongeur. In either case, additional drilling of the superomedial quadrant of the caudal pedicle allows greater access to the ventral abnormality and obviates the retraction of excessive nerve root superiorly.

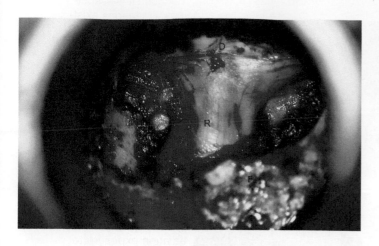

Fig. 4. After completion of the laminotomy and removal of less than 50% of the facet, the dura (D) is observed medially, while the nerve root (R) is seen laterally as it exits under the remaining facet (F). The top of the image is medial and the right is cranial.

The foramen is inspected one final time for any further signs of compression, and the field is irrigated with antibiotic-impregnated solution. Hemostasis is achieved with bipolar cautery, bone wax, and any of a variety of commercially available operative hemostatic agents. A methylprednisolone-soaked pledget may be placed over the root to reduce postoperative inflammation. Closure and postoperative care proceed as described below.

Summary of MICD/F

- The operative level is confirmed with fluoroscopy and K-wire or Steinman pin
- A 2-cm incision is made 1.5 cm off midline on the operative side, carrying the incision through the cervical fascia but avoiding muscle violation
- The K-wire or the initial dilator is advanced and docked at the inferomedial edge of the lateral mass of the level of interest
- The tubular muscle dilators are serially inserted
- The final 16-mm or 18-mm tubular retractor is placed over the dilators and fixed into place over the laminofacet junction
- A Kerrison punch or the drill is used to complete the laminoforaminotomy, preserving at least 50% of the facet
- The ligamentum flavum is removed medially to identify the lateral edge of the dura and proximal portion of the nerve root
- With the root well visualized (see **Fig. 4**), disc fragments or osteophytes may be addressed using a fine-angled dissector, nerve hook, or down-angled microcurette
- Hemostasis is achieved with bipolar cautery, bone wax, and operative hemostatic agents

- The tubular retractor is removed under direct observation
- The fascia and skin are closed with absorbable sutures and skin sealant

MICDS Technique

After completion of the ipsilateral laminotomy, the ligamentum flavum is left in place to protect the dura. The tubular retractor is then angled about 45° off the midline such that the microscope or endoscope is oriented to visualize the contralateral side. A plane between the ligament and undersurface of the spinous process is gently dissected with a fine curette. The undersurface of the spinous process and contralateral lamina are progressively drilled until reaching the contralateral facet. This initial decompression allows greater working space within which to remove hypertrophied ligament while avoiding downward pressure on the dura and spinal cord. Dissection and removal of the ligament with curettes and Kerrison rongeurs may now proceed safely. Any compressive elements of the contralateral facet or the superior edge of the caudal lamina may also be drilled off or removed with Kerrison rongeurs. After gently confirming decompression over to the contralateral foramen with a fine probe, the tube is returned to its original position to complete the ipsilateral removal of ligament and bone. This action should then reveal completely decompressed and pulsatile dura. If indicated, ipsilateral foraminotomy as already described may be performed at this time as well. The field is irrigated with antibiotic-impregnated solution and hemostasis is achieved with bipolar cautery, bone wax, and hemostatic agents. **Fig. 5** demonstrates a representative case of single-level C5-6 stenosis treated with MICDS.

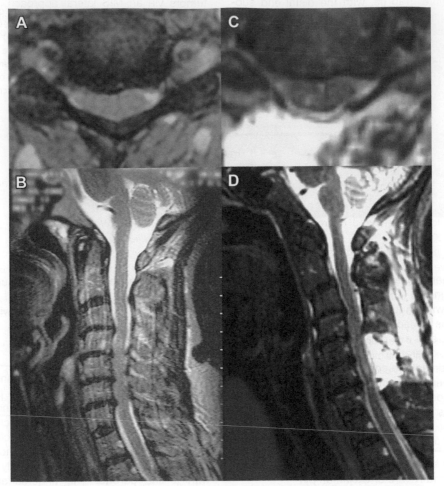

Fig. 5. A 69-year-old woman presented with chronic myelopathy from cervical stenosis and underwent a right-sided approach for C5-6 MIDCS. (*A*) Sagittal T2-weighted MRI demonstrates focal C5-6 spondylotic stenosis. (*B*) Axial T2-weighted MRI reveals severe focal compression at C5-6. (*C*) Postoperative axial T2-weighted MRI reveals decompression of the spinal cord. (*D*) Postoperative sagittal T2-weighted MRI shows the rostral-caudal extent of the decompression.

Summary of MICDS

- The operative level is confirmed with fluoroscopy and K-wire or Steinman pin
- A stab incision is made 2.0 to 2.5 cm off the midline on the operative side and carried through the cervical fascia
- The K-wire or initial dilator is advanced and docked at the inferomedial edge of the lateral mass of the level of interest
- The tubular muscle dilators are serially inserted
- The final 18-mm tubular retractor is placed over the dilators and fixed into place over the laminofacet junction
- The microscope is brought into the operative field, or a 25° angled glass-rod endoscope is attached to a camera and the retractor system

- A Kerrison punch or the drill is used to complete the hemilaminectomy
- The ligamentum flavum is exposed and left in place to protect the dura
- The tube is then angled about 45° off the midline to visualize the contralateral side
- The undersurface of the spinous process and contralateral lamina are progressively drilled until reaching the contralateral facet
- The contralateral ligament is removed using Kerrison rongeurs
- Compressive elements of the contralateral facet or the superior edge of the caudal are removed
- The contralateral foramen is inspected to confirm decompression
- The tube is returned to its original position to complete the ipsilateral removal of ligament and bone

- Hemostasis is achieved with bipolar cautery, bone wax, and operative hemostatic agents
- The tubular retractor is removed under direct observation
- The fascia and skin are closed with absorbable sutures and skin sealant

MANAGEMENT OF COMPLICATIONS

The reported complication rates after minimally invasive posterior cervical decompressive procedures range from 0% to 7%,[7,25–27,29,32,33] and are mostly attributable to durotomy. Direct suture repair of durotomy is challenging through the narrow-diameter tubes. Therefore, one technique for handling small defects is to simply cover the durotomy with muscle, fat, gelfoam, or dural substitute followed by fibrin glue or synthetic. Using this approach, overnight bed rest is usually sufficient to seal the defect. For larger dural tears that cannot be primarily closed, 2 to 3 days of lumbar cerebrospinal fluid (CSF) drainage may prevent a leak. Regardless, the lack of dead space and the small opening after minimally invasive surgery has reduced the rates of pseudomeningocele and CSF-cutaneous fistula to a minimal level.[36]

Potential neurologic complications include radicular injury from manipulation within the tight foramen, or direct mechanical spinal cord injury during dilation or decompression. Vertebral artery injury can be avoided by early detection of dark venous bleeding from the venous plexus surrounding the artery that may arise from accidental dilation lateral to the facet or during overly aggressive dissection laterally in the foramen. This type of bleeding can typically be controlled by packing with gelfoam or another hemostatic product. Postoperative surgical-site infection is exceedingly rare after minimally invasive posterior cervical procedures.[37] Although recurrent disease or postoperative instability are potential concerns, recent series have failed to show an increased risk.[24–27,29,32,33]

POSTOPERATIVE CARE

The tube is removed, and local anesthetic is injected into the fascia and muscles surrounding the incision. The wound is closed using 1 or 2 absorbable stitches for the fascia, 2 or 3 inverted stitches for the subcutaneous layer, and a running subcuticular stitch and Dermabond for the skin (**Fig. 6**). After awaking from general anesthesia, the patient is brought to the postanesthesia care unit and is mobilized as early as possible. No collar is necessary. If medically stable, patients are typically discharged home after 2 to 3 hours, although in some cases the authors have chosen to observe

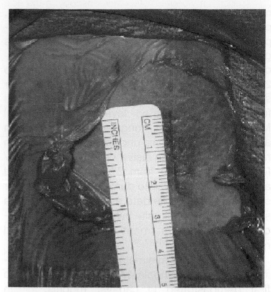

Fig. 6. MICD/F or MIDCS incision after closure is only 2 cm in length.

MIDCS patients overnight. Discharge medications generally include an opioid/acetaminophen combination pain reliever and a muscle relaxant. Nonsteroidal anti-inflammatory agents are also commonly used.

CLINICAL RESULTS IN THE LITERATURE

Recent series of MICD/F[7,11,16,24–27,38] have repeatedly demonstrated that efficacy is equivalent to that of open cases, but that blood loss, length of stay, and postoperative medication usage for pain are all reduced in MICD/F cases. Lidar and Salame[26] recently reported a series of 32 patients who underwent MICD/F. Mean operative time was 62 minutes, mean estimated blood loss 60 mL, and average hospital stay 1.5 days. All patients with motor deficits showed improvement after surgery. The mean Visual Analog Scale (VAS) for radicular pain decreased from 8 preoperatively to 4.8 immediately postoperatively, and finally to 0.75 at 12-month follow-up. The same series showed a decrease in mean preoperative VAS for neck pain from 6.75 to 5.75 immediately postoperatively and then to 0.9 at 12-month follow-up. The 36-item Short Form Questionnaire (SF-36) showed statistically significant improvements in all 8 domains; bodily pain index improved from 11 preoperatively to 80 ($P<.002$) at 6 months postoperatively while the physical functioning improved from 11 preoperatively to 86 ($P<.002$) at 6-month follow-up. Several investigators have reported excellent outcomes with multilevel foraminotomies.[6,27] Although neither of these series report an increased rate of instability or kyphosis, previous investigators have suggested that multiple levels of decompression or facetectomies greater than 50% may increase the risk for subsequent instability.[8,23,34] Recent series with up to 2 years of follow-up have not shown a need for subsequent anterior cervical discectomy and fusion at the operated level after successful MICD/F.[7,27] However, long-term rates of fusion at the index level remain unclear. The complication rates for minimally invasive cervical discectomy/foraminotomy range from 2% to 7%,[7,25–27] and are mostly attributable to durotomy without further sequelae. In total, the data establish MICD/F as a safe, effective, minimally invasive outpatient procedure for the treatment of isolated cervical radiculopathy.[11,16,24–27,38]

The feasibility of minimal-access multilevel laminectomy and laminoplasty techniques was also first demonstrated in cadaver models.[30,39] In separate studies, both techniques demonstrated a 43% expansion of the cross-sectional area of the spinal canal.[10,19,30] Clinical application of minimally invasive posterior cervical decompression for stenosis, however, has not been studied as extensively as MICD/F. The use of minimally invasive cervical laminoplasty has been reported in 4 patients. The investigators report the procedure to be technically safe, with a mean improvement of 1.25 points on the Nurick Scale postoperatively.[30] Benglis and colleagues[31] have also reported the technique to be safe but technically challenging, and requiring an operative time that is double that required for the open equivalent.

Clinical results of MIDCS were first published in 2005 by Yabuki and Kikuchi.[32] The results were favorable with no complications in the series of 10 patients. Four years later Minamide and colleagues[33] reported a series of 51 myelopathic patients who were treated with MIDCS. The results were consistent with the prior series, with the exception of an overall complication rate of 7%. The complications included durotomy, epidural hematoma, and C5 palsies. Finally, Dahdaleh and colleagues[29] recently published their series of 10 patients who underwent MICDS for cervical spondylotic myelopathy. This group treated an average of 2.2 levels of stenosis, reported a mean blood loss of 32.2 mL, and a mean hospital stay of 1.6 days. The mean Nurick Score fell from 1.6 preoperatively to 0.3 postoperatively. There were no significant changes in preoperative and postoperative Cobb angles. The patients had no complications, postoperative instability, or reoperation. The investigators comment that this technique is only suitable for a limited subset of patients: symptomatic patients with moderate

canal stenosis, normal cervical lordosis, primarily posterior disease, and without instability. During a 10-year period only 10 of the 256 patients treated for cervical spondylotic myelopathy were candidates for MIDCS. These results are similar to those reported in previous series, and support MIDCS as an effective technique for the treatment of symptomatic cervical stenosis for select patients.

SUMMARY

Posterior MICD/F and MIDCS offer decreased blood loss, reduced length of stay in hospital, reduced postoperative pain and muscle spasm, preservation of motion segments, and decreased risk of iatrogenic sagittal plane deformity, while offering equivalent efficacy in comparison with their traditional open counterparts.[7,22–27,29,32,33] These minimally invasive techniques are appealing for degenerative conditions of the cervical spine because they minimize both short-term and long-term operative morbidity while offering safe and efficacious decompression. Minimally invasive procedures for the cervical spine are likely to become commonplace as more practitioners adopt these established techniques.

REFERENCES

1. Aldrich F. Posterolateral microdiscectomy for cervical monoradiculopathy caused by posterolateral soft cervical disc sequestration. J Neurosurg 1990; 72(3):370–7. http://dx.doi.org/10.3171/jns.1990.72.3.0370.

2. Crandall PH, Batzdorf U. Cervical spondylotic myelopathy. J Neurosurg 1966;25(1):57–66. http://dx.doi.org/10.3171/jns.1966.25.1.0057.

3. Henderson CM, Hennessy RG, Shuey HM Jr, et al. Posterior-lateral foraminotomy as an exclusive operative technique for cervical radiculopathy: a review of 846 consecutively operated cases. Neurosurgery 1983;13(5):504–12.

4. Ratliff JK, Cooper PR. Cervical laminoplasty: a critical review. J Neurosurg 2003;98(Suppl 3):230–8.

5. Khoo L, Perez-Cruet M, Fessler R. Posterior cervical microendoscopic foraminotomy. In: Perez-Cruet M, Fessler R, editors. Outpatient spinal surgery. St Louis (MO): Quality Medical Publishing, Inc; 2006. p. 71–93.

6. Holly LT, Moftakhar P, Khoo LT, et al. Minimally invasive 2-level posterior cervical foraminotomy: preliminary clinical results. J Spinal Disord Tech 2007;20(1): 20–4. http://dx.doi.org/10.1097/01.bsd.0000211254.98002.80.

7. Ruetten S, Komp M, Merk H, et al. Full-endoscopic cervical posterior foraminotomy for the operation of

lateral disc herniations using 5.9-mm endoscopes: a prospective, randomized, controlled study. Spine 2008;33(9):940–8. http://dx.doi.org/10.1097/BRS. 0b013e31816c8b67.

8. Jagannathan J, Sherman JH, Szabo T, et al. The posterior cervical foraminotomy in the treatment of cervical disc/osteophyte disease: a single-surgeon experience with a minimum of 5 years' clinical and radiographic follow-up. J Neurosurg Spine 2009; 10(4):347–56. http://dx.doi.org/10.3171/2008.12. SPINE08576.

9. Kumar VG, Rea GL, Mervis LJ, et al. Cervical spondylotic myelopathy: functional and radiographic long-term outcome after laminectomy and posterior fusion. Neurosurgery 1999;44(4):771–7 [discussion: 777–8].

10. Wang MY, Shah S, Green BA. Clinical outcomes following cervical laminoplasty for 204 patients with cervical spondylotic myelopathy. Surg Neurol 2004; 62(6):487–92. http://dx.doi.org/10.1016/j.surneu. 2004.02.040 [discussion: 492–3].

11. Fessler RG, Khoo LT. Minimally invasive cervical microendoscopic foraminotomy: an initial clinical experience. Neurosurgery 2002;51(Suppl 5):S37–45.

12. Hilibrand AS, Robbins M. Adjacent segment degeneration and adjacent segment disease: the consequences of spinal fusion? Spine J 2004;4(Suppl 6): 190S–4S. http://dx.doi.org/10.1016/j.spinee.2004. 07.007.

13. Ishihara H, Kanamori M, Kawaguchi Y, et al. Adjacent segment disease after anterior cervical interbody fusion. Spine J 2004;4(6):624–8. http://dx.doi. org/10.1016/j.spinee.2004.04.011.

14. Xia XP, Chen HL, Cheng HB. Prevalence of adjacent segment degeneration after spine surgery: a systematic review and meta-analysis. Spine 2013;38(7):597–608. http://dx.doi.org/10.1097/BRS. 0b013e318273a2ea.

15. Hosono N, Yonenobu K, Ono K. Neck and shoulder pain after laminoplasty. A noticeable complication. Spine 1996;21(17):1969–73.

16. Siddiqui A, Yonemura K. Posterior cervical microendoscopic diskectomy and laminoforaminotomy. In: Kim D, Fessler R, Regan J, editors. Endoscopic spine surgery and instrumentation: percutaneous procedures. New York: Thieme; 2005. p. 66–73.

17. Albert TJ, Vacarro A. Postlaminectomy kyphosis. Spine 1998;23(24):2738–45.

18. Kaptain GJ, Simmons NE, Replogle RE, et al. Incidence and outcome of kyphotic deformity following laminectomy for cervical spondylotic myelopathy. J Neurosurg 2000;93(Suppl 2):199–204.

19. Perez-Cruet M, Samartzis D, Fessler R. Microendoscopic cervical laminectomy. In: Perez-Cruet M, Khoo L, Fessler R, editors. An anatomic approach to minimally invasive spine surgery. St Louis (MO): Quality Medical Publishing, Inc; 2006. p. 16.11–7.

20. Yonenobu K, Okada K, Fuji T, et al. Causes of neurologic deterioration following surgical treatment of cervical myelopathy. Spine 1986;11(8): 818–23.

21. Khoo L, Bresnahan L, Fessler R. Cervical endoscopic foraminotomy. In: Fessler R, Sekhar L, editors. Atlas of neurosurgical techniques: spine and peripheral nerves, vol. 1. New York: Thieme; 2006. p. 785–92.

22. Burke TG, Caputy A. Microendoscopic posterior cervical foraminotomy: a cadaveric model and clinical application for cervical radiculopathy. J Neurosurg 2000;93(Suppl 1):126–9.

23. Roh SW, Kim DH, Cardoso AC, et al. Endoscopic foraminotomy using MED system in cadaveric specimens. Spine 2000;25(2):260–4.

24. Kim KT, Kim YB. Comparison between open procedure and tubular retractor assisted procedure for cervical radiculopathy: results of a randomized controlled study. J Korean Med Sci 2009;24(4):649. http://dx.doi.org/10.3346/jkms.2009.24.4.649.

25. Winder MJ, Thomas KC. Minimally invasive versus open approach for cervical laminoforaminotomy. Can J Neurol Sci 2011;38(2):262–7.

26. Lidar Z, Salame K. Minimally invasive posterior cervical discectomy for cervical radiculopathy: technique and clinical results. J Spinal Disord Tech 2011;24(8):521–4. http://dx.doi.org/10.1097/BSD. 0b013e31820679e3.

27. Lawton CD, Smith ZA, Lam SK, et al. Clinical outcomes of microendoscopic foraminotomy and decompression in the cervical spine. World Neurosurg 2012. http://dx.doi.org/10.1016/j.wneu.2012. 12.008.

28. Khoo LT, Fessler RG. Microendoscopic decompressive laminotomy for the treatment of lumbar stenosis. Neurosurgery 2002;51(Suppl 5):S146–54.

29. Dahdaleh NS, Wong AP, Smith ZA, et al. Microendoscopic decompression for cervical spondylotic myelopathy. Neurosurg Focus 2013;35(1):E8. http://dx.doi.org/10.3171/2013.3.FOCUS135.

30. Perez-Cruet M, Wang M, Samartzis D. Microendoscopic cervical laminectomy and laminoplasty. In: Kim D, Fessler R, Regan J, editors. Endoscopic spine surgery and instrumentation: percutaneous procedures. New York: Thieme; 2005. p. 74–87.

31. Benglis DM, Guest JD, Wang MY. Clinical feasibility of minimally invasive cervical laminoplasty. Neurosurg Focus 2008;25(2):E3. http://dx.doi.org/10. 3171/FOC/2008/25/8/E3.

32. Yabuki S, Kikuchi S. Endoscopic partial laminectomy for cervical myelopathy. J Neurosurg Spine 2005; 2(2):170–4. http://dx.doi.org/10.3171/spi.2005.2.2. 0170.

33. Minamide A, Yoshida M, Yamada H, et al. Clinical outcomes of microendoscopic decompression surgery for cervical myelopathy. Eur Spine J 2009;

19(3):487–93. http://dx.doi.org/10.1007/s00586-009-1233-0.

34. Raynor RB, Pugh J, Shapiro I. Cervical facetectomy and its effect on spine strength. J Neurosurg 1985;63(2): 278–82. http://dx.doi.org/10.3171/jns.1985.63.2.0278.

35. Zdeblick TA, Zou D, Warden KE, et al. Cervical stability after foraminotomy. A biomechanical in vitro analysis. J Bone Joint Surg Am 1992;74(1):22–7.

36. Ruban D, O'Toole JE. Management of incidental durotomy in minimally invasive spine surgery. Neurosurg Focus 2011;31(4):E15. http://dx.doi.org/10.3171/2011.7.FOCUS11122.

37. O'Toole JE, Eichholz KM, Fessler RG. Surgical site infection rates after minimally invasive spinal surgery. J Neurosurg Spine 2009;11(4):471–6. http://dx.doi.org/10.3171/2009.5.SPINE08633.

38. Adamson TE. Microendoscopic posterior cervical laminoforaminotomy for unilateral radiculopathy: results of a new technique in 100 cases. J Neurosurg 2001;95(Suppl 1):51–7.

39. Wang MY, Green BA, Coscarella E, et al. Minimally invasive cervical expansile laminoplasty: an initial cadaveric study. Neurosurgery 2003;52(2):370–3 [discussion: 373].

Minimally Invasive Treatment of Thoracic Disc Herniations

Laura A. Snyder, MD[a],*, Zachary A. Smith, MD[b],
Nader S. Dahdaleh, MD[b], Richard G. Fessler, MD, PhD[c]

KEYWORDS

- Thoracic disc • Minimally invasive • Disc herniation • Microendoscopic discectomy
- Microscopic discectomy • Costrotransversectomy • Lateral extracavitary approach

KEY POINTS

- Although thoracic disc herniations can be a challenging pathologic abnormality, they can be treated minimally invasively as multiple techniques have been developed.
- The microendoscopic and microscopic discectomy can be performed for soft, lateral, and smaller thoracic disc herniations using skills with which most minimally invasive surgeons are already comfortable.
- The mini-open lateral approach may be better used for large, calcified central disc herniations.

INTRODUCTION

Thoracic disc herniations present significant challenges for the spine surgeon in their diagnosis as well as in their treatment. As only one in one million people will present with a clinically significant thoracic disc herniation, most spine surgeons are less experienced in treating this disease process.[1] Knowledge of thoracic spinal anatomy is critical for the safe application of surgical techniques for thoracic disc treatment. This article addresses the nuances of evaluation, surgical planning, and treatment of thoracic disease pathologic abnormalities. Furthermore, it highlights the expanding role of minimally invasive techniques in the treatment of this challenging pathologic abnormality.

PREOPERATIVE EVALUATION

Challenges in thoracic disc herniation include identifying the source of the patients' symptoms. The symptom that commonly brings these patients to a spine surgeon's attention is unilateral radicular pain, or pain radiating from the upper or middle back to the chest. Numbness or strange sensations in similar radicular distributions are also possible, but many patients will complain of strange sensations or shooting, electric shocklike pains into the legs or abdomen that do not necessarily follow classic radicular patterns. Furthermore, patients may also complain of difficulty ambulating, feeling off balance, and feeling that their legs are heavy. On examination, patients may or may not demonstrate symptoms of myelopathy. Lower extremity reflexes may be hyperreflexic, and Babinski testing may demonstrate upgoing toes. Patients can have difficulty with tandem gait or with toe proprioception. When patients do demonstrate weakness on examination, often it is a generalized weakness of the legs or decompensation of the leg muscles due to decreased use. Rarely is one leg weaker than the other, and this may or may not correlate with which side the offending thoracic disc herniation abuts the spinal cord.

Often patients may have very vague complaints and a nonlocalizing examination that surgeons must sort through. A detailed history and examination are pertinent because many patients with

[a] Department of Neurological Surgery, Barrow Neurological Institute, St. Joseph's Hospital and Medical Center, 350 W. Thomas Rd., Phoenix, AZ, 85013, USA; [b] Department of Neurological Surgery, Northwestern University, Feinberg School of Medicine, 676 N St. Clair, Suite 2210, Chicago, IL, 60611, USA; [c] Department of Neurological Surgery, Rush University Medical Center, 1725 W. Harrison St., Suite 855, Chicago, IL, 60612, USA
* Corresponding author.
E-mail address: laura.snyder@bnaneuro.net

Neurosurg Clin N Am 25 (2014) 271–277
http://dx.doi.org/10.1016/j.nec.2013.12.006

signs and symptoms from a thoracic disc may present with multiple thoracic disc herniations on magnetic resonance imaging (MRI). In many cases, a cervical spine MRI is warranted to rule out potential cervical disease contributing to myelopathy. Symptomatic patients without evidence of cord compression should be given a trial of conservative therapy for 4 to 6 weeks, including physical therapy, nonsteroidal anti-inflammatory drugs, and oral or epidural steroids. Symptomatic patients with evidence of cord compression should be considered surgical candidates and conservative therapy is not warranted in these patients.

SURGICAL PLANNING

For all techniques, preventing intraoperative injury starts before incision. The preoperative MRI should include imaging that allows the surgeon to determine the correct herniated thoracic disc level counting from C2 down or from the sacrum up. Intraoperatively, it is usually easier to count the thoracic level upward from the sacrum or using the ribs as a reference because the shoulders can obstruct the view of the cervical and upper thoracic spine. Thus, all patients should have preoperative chest anteroposterior and lateral radiographs as well as lumbar anteroposterior and lateral radiographs for intraoperative reference, in case a patient should have transitional lumbar vertebrae or an extra rib. To assist with intraoperative localization, some surgeons prefer that interventional radiology place a preoperative fiducial at the correct thoracic level, although this requires that the surgeon trust the radiologist.[2] Furthermore, preoperative somatosensory evoked potentials and motor evoked potentials should be obtained on positioning to monitor any changes with dissection intraoperatively.

Once the offending level is verified, surgeons have a few options in deciding surgical treatment. A midline open laminectomy is never recommended, because even mild retraction or manipulation of the thoracic cord can lead to significant postoperative deficits.[3-8] Soft, lateral disc herniations have been traditionally accessed via a unilateral transpedicular approach or costotransversectomy on the side to which the disc is eccentric.[9-15] Because of the stabilization of the rib on the other side and the rest of the rib cage, disruption of the facet at the level of the thoracic disc often does not require surgical stabilization of the level.[15-17] Many of the currently described minimally invasive techniques for thoracic disc herniations are best used for treatment of these soft, lateral discs.[18-21]

For central disc herniations or calcified disc herniations, traditional thoracotomy with an anterolateral transpleural or lateral extracavitary technique has been used to remove the thoracic disc safely without retraction of the thoracic cord or accidental injury to the surrounding great vessels.[5,22] Calcification may be present in anywhere from 30% to 70% of thoracic disc herniations.[23] Thus, a computed tomographic scan of the thoracic spine should be considered as part of preoperative planning to help determine the proper approach. As thoracic pedicle anatomy can be variable, a computed tomographic scan also allows for pedicle evaluation in case stabilization or fusion is determined to be necessary. Although there are minimally invasive techniques for central disc herniations and calcified discs, it must be noted that even with these advancements, depending on the experience of a given surgeon, a calcified disc or a large central disc may still often be more safely and properly treated with an open approach.[24-27]

SURGICAL TECHNIQUE
Thoracoscopic Disc Removal

In the early 1990s, thoracic surgeons had identified video-assisted thoracoscopic surgery (VATS) for lung lesions as a way to improve pulmonary function and decrease pain over thoracotomy. In 1993, Mack and colleagues[28] reported a reliable way to access the thoracic spine using VATS.[29,30] In 1994, Horowitz and colleagues[31] described the use of VATS for thoracic discectomy, which was expanded on by Caputy in 1995.[32] Multiple series followed that identified VATS as a less morbid approach than thoracotomy to perform thoracic disc resection from an anterior approach.[33-37] A series by Rosenthal and Dickman[36] in 1998 evaluated the thoracoscopic approach and demonstrated that it had less morbidity than costotransversectomy as well, with less neurologic deficits and less intercostal neuralgia. More recent series have continued to demonstrate efficacy in these techniques because disc removal is sufficient and improvement in outcomes is long-term.[38-40]

In this technique, the patient is placed in the lateral decubitus position, and the surgeons stand on the patient's ventral side. Three port sites are usually planned with fluoroscopy localization of the operating level, one port site for thoracoscopic visualization and two port sites for entry of working instruments. A Kelly clamp is used to enter the pleural space after incision at one of the port sites, and the pleura is taken down away from the chest cavity. The patient is turned slightly ventrally to have the collapsed lung fall away from the thoracic spine. The pleura over the desired disc level is removed; the segmental vessels are coagulated, and then the rib head is drilled away at this level. The pedicle is removed at this level to see normal thecal sac. A portion of the vertebral bodies above and below the offending disc space is also removed so that disc fragments can be pulled into this space anteriorly and removed. Although placement of a graft in this space has been described, as well as thoracoscopic fusion, most often this is not required.[41,42] A chest tube is left in one of the port sites and the lung is reinflated.

Unfortunately, the thoracoscopic technique has a steep learning curve. The long instruments wielded using 2-dimensional visualization can make this a significantly difficult technique and one that many residents are not exposed to in training. There are anesthetic risks with collapsing the lung, and patients must be watched closely postoperatively with the chest tube in place, especially if intraoperatively there was a cerebral spinal fluid leak or an intradural disc herniation.[5,24]

Endoscopic Disc Removal

Use of the endoscope in combination with smaller posterolateral exposures has also been described for the treatment of thoracic disc herniations. Stillerman and colleagues[43,44] described a transfacet, pedicle-sparing approach. A 4-cm opening was used to expose and partially remove the medial facet complex and then a discectomy was performed. In some cases, an open endoscope was used to aid completion of the discectomy.

Jho[45,46] in 1998 described a transpedicular minimally invasive technique of thoracic disc resection by a combination of a tubular retractor, the operating microscope, and a 70° microscope. In this technique, a 2-cm paramedian incision at the facet joint of the involved disc level was used to place a tubular 1.5-cm retractor. The operating microscope was used to drill away the facet and a portion of the pedicle. The 70° endoscope allowed visualization of the ventral side of the thoracic cord, and the herniated disc fragments could be pushed into and removed through a cavity created in the intervertebral space.

This technique provided less incisions and less morbidity than the thoracoscopic technique. It also came from a transpedicular approach and posterolateral anatomy with which more spine surgeons were comfortable than that seen through the thoracoscopic technique. However, not many spine surgeons adopted the technique because visualization through the 70° endoscope could be confusing.

Microendoscopic and Microscopic Discectomy

In 2004, Perez-Cruet and colleagues[20] described microendoscopic thoracic discectomy. Their report described results in 7 patients with 9 thoracic discs removed by use of a 30° microendoscope. A incision was made 3 to 4 cm from midline and tubular dilators were centered at the superior aspect of the caudal transverse process at the level of the herniated disc. The microendoscope was passed through and fixated to the final tubular retractor. The medial portion of the facet complex could be removed with a high-speed drill, and then the pedicle could be removed over the disc space. Once the lateral edge of the dura could be identified, annular incision and disc removal could be performed.

Issacs and colleagues[47] evaluated this same approach in 9 cadavers. Their results demonstrated that a sufficient amount of the thoracic disc herniation could be removed with average facet removal of 35.5%. As a large portion of the facet remained in place and a large majority of the functioning disc was left in place, no fusion was required. Eichholz and colleagues[48] found this technique to have smaller incisions and less tissue disruption than the traditional lateral extracavitary approach for thoracic disc herniation in their report in 2006.

The authors use the approach described by Perez-Cruet and Issacs for soft, lateral, and smaller central discs (**Figs. 1–3**). A K-wire is not

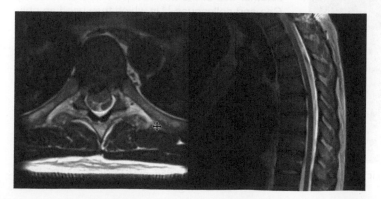

Fig. 1. Thoracic herniated disc treated by microendoscopic discectomy.

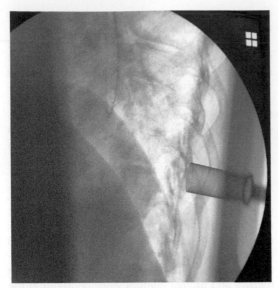

Fig. 2. Tube docking site for microendoscopic and microscopic discectomy.

used to start the retractor dilation because of potential thoracic cord injury, and the fascia is opened using a bovie to place the smallest dilator. Due to the angulation of the facets in the thoracic spine, occasionally more muscle needs to be removed than after initial dilation in the lumbar spine. The usual complications of open surgery due to extensive tissue resection, bone removal, and entrance into the thorax are avoided. Starting at 3 to 4 cm laterally, angulation of the tubular retractor and angulation of the 30° endoscope allow medial visualization of the dural sac without spinal cord manipulation. Using this technique, the senior author (R.G.F.) has never had a patient requiring intraoperative fusion or

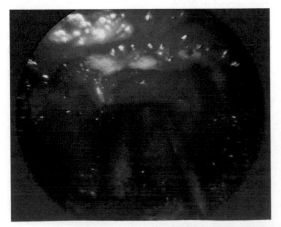

Fig. 3. Intraoperative view of thoracic microendoscopic discectomy.

fusion at a later date. As described by Issacs, stability is maintained by leaving the functioning disc in place as well as most of the facet.

Lidar and colleagues[49] described a similar technique as Perez-Cruet and colleagues and Issacs and colleagues, but they used a 15° endoscope and rib head resection as necessary. All 10 of their patients had significantly decreased Visual Analog Scale and returned to work with American Spinal Cord Injury Association (ASIA) scale improvements. Smith and colleagues[50] reported 16 patients in which thoracic microendoscopic discectomy was performed on 18 thoracic disc herniations. Of these patients, 13 patients had excellent outcomes. No complications occurred, and no cases required conversion to open technique. It must be noted that calcified discs were excluded from the thoracic microendoscopic technique in their study. Operative time ranged from 88 to 252 minutes per level (mean, 153 minutes per level). Mean blood loss was 69 mL, and mean hospital stay was 21 hours.

The microendoscopic technique requires a learning curve, and it may take surgeons time to adjust to the 2-dimensional visualization. However, the skills that are required are similar to those that minimally invasive spine surgeons have become comfortable with while performing microendoscopic lumbar discectomies. The instruments are not quite as long as those used in thoracoscopic procedures and are thus not as difficult to wield.

Although the medial visualization of the dura may not be quite as good as with a 30° or 15° endoscope, surgeons who are comfortable performing tubular minimally invasive lumbar microdiscectomies using a microscope may still have good outcomes using the microscope rather than endoscope. Regev and colleagues[21] reported their series of 12 patients in which they used a similar tubular docking and drilling technique as well as the microscope for thoracic microdiscectomy. All 12 patients improved and had no complications. Another use of the microscope was described by Cho and colleagues,[18] in which they used an oblique parasagittal docking site, lateral to the facet joint and between the transverse processes. Initial incision was 5 to 6 cm from the spinous process. They drilled through the lateral facets to approach the disc herniation, and they too demonstrated good outcomes in 5 patients.

Khoo and colleagues[51] described 13 patients who had minimally invasive microscopically assisted lateral extracavitary approaches. Tubular retractors were docked along the rib angle toward the transverse process and pedicle of the body inferior to the target level of the herniation. For improved visualization using the microscope, the patient was rotated away from the surgeon such that the working portal was almost orthogonal to the floor. Posterolateral disc herniations were directly visualized and removed, but in the cases of central herniations, a working cavity was created in and around the disc space. A Woodson elevator or down-pushing back-angled curettes could then be used to push the herniated fragments into the working cavity for safe removal, allowing for improved resection of calcified discs.

Khoo's report also involved introducing an interbody cage into this working cavity, after the intervertebral space had been sufficiently cleared and packed with bone graft. In most cases, they used a straight carbon fiber synthetic cage of 7- to 9-mm height. Their use of an interbody fusion was in response to biomechanical and clinical studies indicating that thoracic discectomies can cause vertebral motion and rotation, making the spine more susceptible to delayed deformity, progressive axial pain, and pathologic fracture.[52–55] In the senior author's experience (R.G.F.), fusion should not be required unless a significant amount of the functioning disc or the vertebral bodies above and below have been violated to remove the herniated portion of the disc, as may occur with large calcified central disc herniations.

Mini-Open Lateral Approach

In attempts to improve resection of central, calcified thoracic discs, some surgeons have experimented with mini-open lateral techniques. This technique was first described by Deviren and colleagues in 2008[56] and was expanded on by Dakwar and colleagues[57] and Uribe and colleagues.[26,58] Patients are placed in a true lateral position and a 2- to 3-cm incision is made between the ribs, taking a portion of the ribs if necessary. Blunt dissection between the pleura and the rib is performed as far as possible toward the rib head. The initial dilator is passed posteriorly in the thoracic cavity along the ribs to the intersection of the rib head and spine at the desired level. Further dilation proceeds until a larger expandable retractor can be locked into place. The final pleura overlying the lateral spine is removed, and the rib head and a portion of the pedicle are drilled away to expose the disc space. The disc can be well visualized and removed with standard techniques. Wedge osteotomies can be performed on the posterior aspect of the vertebral bodies as necessary, and especially if the disc is calcified, so that it can be pulled away from the dura into the cavity. A chest tube can be left in place or an

underwater red-rubber catheter Valsalva technique for thoracic cavity air expulsion can be performed.

Multiple other centers and studies have adopted a permutation of this technique for treatment of herniated discs. In 2011, Kasliwal and Deutsche[24] described their mini-open lateral approach for 7 patients. Three patients improved one point on the Nurita scale, all patients with radicular pain improved, and there were no complications nor conversions to open procedures. Uribe and colleagues[26] described 60 patients in which a lateral mini-open approach was used to treat 75 symptomatic discs at 5 institutions. They included calcified discs in their series. Excellent or good overall outcomes occurred in 80%; fair or unchanged outcomes occurred in 15%, and poor outcomes occurred in 5%. Myelopathy, radiculopathy, axial back pain, and bladder and/or bowel dysfunction improved in 83.3%, 87.0%, 91.1%, and 87.5% of cases, respectively. Four major complications occurred (6.7%): pneumonia in 1 patient (1.7%); extrapleural free air in 1 patient (1.7%); new lower-extremity weakness in 1 patient (1.7%); and wound infection in posterior instrumentation in 1 patient (1.7%). Because of the multiple centers involved, this study demonstrated the reproducibility of this approach with good results.

Because the exposure and technique are similar to that used in the extreme lateral lumbar interbody fusions, many spine surgeons can feel more comfortable with the mini-open lateral approach over other minimally invasive techniques. As opposed to the thoracoscopic or endoscopic techniques, the microscope provides 3-dimensional imaging and familiar hand-eye coordination skills for most spine surgeons. Although the learning curve is less than that with the thoracoscopic approaches, it still requires developing comfort with longer instruments due to the long operating corridor. This corridor makes controlling complications and bleeding more difficult, and thus, surgeons operating using this technique must be prepared to convert to an open thoracotomy. However, it is worth learning this minimally invasive technique because it is one that can be used to treat large central and calcified discs. There is significantly less muscle and tissue trauma than open techniques, and as opposed to the posterolateral endoscopic technique described by Perez-Cruet and Issacs,[20,47] there is improved anterior visualization of the disc space.

SUMMARY

Thoracic disc herniations have always posed significant challenges to spine surgeons. Because the thoracic cord will not tolerate retraction, access to the disc without disruption of important surrounding structures remains difficult. With increasing use and development of minimally invasive techniques, spine surgeons now reliably remove offending thoracic disc herniations safely with less morbidity than traditional techniques. Adoption of minimally invasive techniques for thoracic disc resection can lead to reduced operative time, less blood loss, and quicker patient recovery.

REFERENCES

1. Jeckey D, Devlin VJ. Thoracic Disc Herniation. In: Devlin VJ, editor. Spine Secrets. Philadelphia: Hanley & Belfus; 2003. p. 264–6.

2. Upadhyaya CD, Wu JC, Chin CT, et al. Avoidance of wrong-level thoracic spine surgery: intraoperative localization with preoperative percutaneous fiducial screw placement. J Neurosurg Spine 2012;16(3):280–4.

3. Carson J, Gumpert J, Jefferson A. Diagnosis and treatment of thoracic intervertebral disc protrusions. J Neurol Neurosurg Psychiatry 1971;34(1):68–77.

4. Knecht CD. Results of surgical treatment for thoracolumbar disc protrusion. J Small Anim Pract 1972; 13(8):449–53.

5. Maiman DJ, Larson SJ, Luck E, et al. Lateral extracavitary approach to the spine for thoracic disc herniation: report of 23 cases. Neurosurgery 1984;14(2):178–82.

6. Lesoin F, Rousseaux M, Autricque A, et al. Thoracic disc herniations: evolution in the approach and indications. Acta Neurochir (Wien) 1986;80(1–2):30–4.

7. Russell T. Thoracic intervertebral disc protrusion: experience of 67 cases and review of the literature. Br J Neurosurg 1989;3(2):153–60.

8. Dietze DD Jr, Fessler RG. Thoracic disc herniations. Neurosurg Clin N Am 1993;4(1):75–90.

9. Lesoin F, Jomin M. Posterolateral approach to thoracic disk herniations through transversoarthropediculectomy. Surg Neurol 1985;23(4):375–9.

10. Rossitti S. The extreme lateral approach to thoracic disc herniations: technique and preliminary results. Neurochirurgia (Stuttg) 1993;36(5):161–3.

11. Garrido E. Modified costotransversectomy: a surgical approach to ventrally placed lesions in the thoracic spinal canal. Surg Neurol 1980;13(2): 109–13.

12. el-Kalliny M, Tew JM Jr, van Loveren H, et al. Surgical approaches to thoracic disc herniations. Acta Neurochir (Wien) 1991;111(1–2):22–32.

13. Simpson JM, Silveri CP, Simeone FA, et al. Thoracic disc herniation. Re-evaluation of the posterior approach using a modified costotransversectomy. Spine (Phila Pa 1976) 1993;18(13):1872–7.

14. Hamburger C. Modification of costotransversectomy to approach ventrally located intraspinal lesions. Preliminary report. Acta Neurochir (Wien) 1995;136(1–2):12–5.

15. Levi N, Gjerris F, Dons K. Thoracic disc herniation. Unilateral transpedicular approach in 35 consecutive patients. J Neurosurg Sci 1999;43(1):37–42 [discussion: 42–3].

16. Le Roux PD, Haglund MM, Harris AB. Thoracic disc disease: experience with the transpedicular approach in twenty consecutive patients. Neurosurgery 1993;33(1):58–66.

17. Bilsky MH. Transpedicular approach for thoracic disc herniations. Neurosurg Focus 2000;9(4):e3.

18. Cho JY, Lee SH, Jang SH, et al. Oblique paraspinal approach for thoracic disc herniations using tubular retractor with robotic holder: a technical note. Eur Spine J 2012;21(12):2620–5.

19. Sheikh H, Samartzis D, Perez-Cruet MJ. Techniques for the operative management of thoracic disc herniation: minimally invasive thoracic microdiscectomy. Orthop Clin North Am 2007;38(3): 351–61 [abstract vi].

20. Perez-Cruet MJ, Kim BS, Sandhu F, et al. Thoracic microendoscopic discectomy. J Neurosurg Spine 2004;1(1):58–63.

21. Regev GJ, Salame K, Behrbalk E, et al. Minimally invasive transforaminal, thoracic microscopic discectomy: technical report and preliminary results and complications. Spine J 2012;12(7):570–6.

22. Chen TC. Surgical outcome for thoracic disc surgery in the postlaminectomy era. Neurosurg Focus 2000;9(4):e12.

23. Burkett CJ, Greenberg MS. Cervical and thoracic spine degenerative disease. In: Baaj AA, Mummaneni PV, Uribe JS, et al, editors. Handbook of spine surgery. New York: Thieme Medical Publishers; 2012.

24. Kasliwal MK, Deutsch H. Minimally invasive retropleural approach for central thoracic disc herniation. Minim Invasive Neurosurg 2011;54(4):167–71.

25. Borm W, Bazner U, Konig RW, et al. Surgical treatment of thoracic disc herniations via tailored posterior approaches. Eur Spine J 2011;20(10):1684–90.

26. Uribe JS, Smith WD, Pimenta L, et al. Minimally invasive lateral approach for symptomatic thoracic disc herniation: initial multicenter clinical experience. J Neurosurg Spine 2012;16(3):264–79.

27. Russo A, Balamurali G, Nowicki R, et al. Anterior thoracic foraminotomy through mini-thoracotomy for the treatment of giant thoracic disc herniations. Eur Spine J 2012;21(Suppl 2):S212–20.

28. Mack MJ, Regan JJ, McAfee PC, et al. Video-assisted thoracic surgery for the anterior approach to the thoracic spine. Ann Thorac Surg 1995;59(5):1100–6.

29. Landreneau RJ, Mack MJ, Hazelrigg SR, et al. Video-assisted thoracic surgery: basic technical

concepts and intercostal approach strategies. Ann Thorac Surg 1992;54(4):800–7.

30. Lewis RJ, Caccavale RJ, Sisler GE. Special report: video-endoscopic thoracic surgery. N J Med 1991; 88(7):473–5.

31. Horowitz MB, Moossy JJ, Julian T, et al. Thoracic discectomy using video assisted thoracoscopy. Spine (Phila Pa 1976) 1994;19(9):1082–6.

32. Caputy A, Starr J, Riedel C. Video-assisted endoscopic spinal surgery: thoracoscopic discectomy. Acta Neurochir (Wien) 1995;134(3–4):196–9.

33. McAfee PC, Regan JR, Zdeblick T, et al. The incidence of complications in endoscopic anterior thoracolumbar spinal reconstructive surgery. A prospective multicenter study comprising the first 100 consecutive cases. Spine (Phila Pa 1976) 1995;20(14):1624–32.

34. Dickman CA, Mican CA. Multilevel anterior thoracic discectomies and anterior interbody fusion using a microsurgical thoracoscopic approach. Case report. J Neurosurg 1996;84(1):104–9.

35. Visocchi M, Masferrer R, Sonntag VK, et al. Thoracoscopic approaches to the thoracic spine. Acta Neurochir (Wien) 1998;140(8):737–43 [discussion: 743–4].

36. Rosenthal D, Dickman CA. Thoracoscopic microsurgical excision of herniated thoracic discs. J Neurosurg 1998;89(2):224–35.

37. Burke TG, Caputy AJ. Treatment of thoracic disc herniation: evolution toward the minimally invasive thoracoscopic technique. Neurosurg Focus 2000; 9(4):e9.

38. Anand N, Regan JJ. Video-assisted thoracoscopic surgery for thoracic disc disease: classification and outcome study of 100 consecutive cases with a 2-year minimum follow-up period. Spine (Phila Pa 1976) 2002;27(8):871–9.

39. Sasani M, Fahir Ozer A, Oktenoglu T, et al. Thoracoscopic surgery for thoracic disc herniation. J Neurosurg Sci 2011;55(4):391–5.

40. Oskouian RJ Jr, Johnson JP, Regan JJ. Thoracoscopic microdiscectomy. Neurosurgery 2002; 50(1):103–9.

41. Dickman CA, Mican CA. Multilevel anterior thoracic discectomies and anterior interbody fusion by using a microsurgical thoracoscopic approach. Case report. Neurosurg Focus 1999;7(5):e3.

42. Hott JS, Feiz-Erfan I, Kenny K, et al. Surgical management of giant herniated thoracic discs: analysis of 20 cases. J Neurosurg Spine 2005;3(3):191–7.

43. Stillerman CB, Chen TC, Day JD, et al. The transfacet pedicle-sparing approach for thoracic disc removal: cadaveric morphometric analysis and preliminary clinical experience. J Neurosurg 1995; 83(6):971–6.

44. Stillerman CB, Chen TC, Couldwell WT, et al. Experience in the surgical management of 82 symptomatic herniated thoracic discs and review of the literature. J Neurosurg 1998;88(4):623–33.

45. Jho HD. Endoscopic microscopic transpedicular thoracic discectomy. Technical note. J Neurosurg 1997;87(1):125–9.

46. Jho HD. Endoscopic transpedicular thoracic discectomy. J Neurosurg 1999;91(Suppl 2):151–6.

47. Isaacs RE, Podichetty VK, Sandhu FA, et al. Thoracic microendoscopic discectomy: a human cadaver study. Spine (Phila Pa 1976) 2005; 30(10):1226–31.

48. Eichholz KM, O'Toole JE, Fessler RG. Thoracic microendoscopic discectomy. Neurosurg Clin N Am 2006;17(4):441–6.

49. Lidar Z, Lifshutz J, Bhattacharjee S, et al. Minimally invasive, extracavitary approach for thoracic disc herniation: technical report and preliminary results. Spine J 2006;6(2):157–63.

50. Smith JS, Eichholz KM, Shafizadeh S, et al. Minimally invasive thoracic microendoscopic diskectomy: surgical technique and case series. World Neurosurg 2013;80(3-4):421–7.

51. Khoo LT, Smith ZA, Asgarzadie F, et al. Minimally invasive extracavitary approach for thoracic discectomy and interbody fusion: 1-year clinical and radiographic outcomes in 13 patients compared with a cohort of traditional anterior transthoracic approaches. J Neurosurg Spine 2011;14(2):250–60.

52. Broc GG, Crawford NR, Sonntag VK, et al. Biomechanical effects of transthoracic microdiscectomy. Spine (Phila Pa 1976) 1997;22(6):605–12.

53. Otani K, Yoshida M, Fujii E, et al. Thoracic disc herniation. Surgical treatment in 23 patients. Spine (Phila Pa 1976) 1988;13(11):1262–7.

54. Korovessis PG, Stamatakis MV, Baikousis A, et al. Transthoracic disc excision with interbody fusion. 12 patients with symptomatic disc herniation followed for 2-8 years. Acta Orthop Scand Suppl 1997;275:12–6.

55. Currier BL, Eismont FJ, Green BA. Transthoracic disc excision and fusion for herniated thoracic discs. Spine (Phila Pa 1976) 1994;19(3):323–8.

56. Deviren V, Pekmezci M, Tay B. Thoracic disc herniation: extreme lateral approach. In: Goodrich AJ, editor. eXtreme lateral interbody fusion (XLIF). 6th edition. St Louis (MO): Quality Medical Publishing, Inc; 2008. p. 241–59.

57. Dakwar E, Cardona RF, Smith DA, et al. Early outcomes and safety of the minimally invasive, lateral retroperitoneal transpsoas approach for adult degenerative scoliosis. Neurosurg Focus 2010; 28(3):E8.

58. Uribe JS, Dakwar E, Le TV, et al. Minimally invasive surgery treatment for thoracic spine tumor removal: a mini-open, lateral approach. Spine (Phila Pa 1976) 2010;35(Suppl 26):S347–54.

Minimally Invasive Transforaminal Lumbar Interbody Fusion (MI-TLIF)

Surgical Technique, Long-Term 4-year Prospective Outcomes, and Complications Compared with an Open TLIF Cohort

Albert P. Wong, MD[a], Zachary A. Smith, MD[a],
James A. Stadler III, MD[a], Xue Yu Hu, MD[b], Jia Zhi Yan, MD[c],
Xin Feng Li, MD[d], Ji Hyun Lee, PA-C[e], Larry T. Khoo, MD[e,*]

KEYWORDS

- TLIF • Transforaminal lumbar interbody fusion • Minimally invasive surgery
- Minimally invasive spine • Spine surgery outcomes • TLIF complications

KEY POINTS

- Minimally invasive transforaminal lumbar interbody fusion (MI-TLIF) can decompress central and foraminal stenosis from a unilateral or bilateral approach.
- MI-TLIF permits 3-column arthrodesis from a single posterior incision.
- MI-TLIF techniques can be used to effectively reduce spondylolisthesis, increase disc height, and restore segmental lordosis.
- MI-TLIF has better perioperative outcomes and similar long-term outcomes when compared with open TLIF, with trends toward improvement in cost and functional outcomes in the minimally invasive cohort.
- Operative complications associated with MI-TLIF are similar to those of open TLIF, with some caveats: cerebrospinal fluid leak, infection, neurologic deficit, malpositioned instrumentation, and Kirschner-wire fracture.

INTRODUCTION

Degenerative disease of the lumbar spine can present with low back pain, radiating pain or paresthesias down the lower extremities, weakness of the legs, impaired ambulation, or bladder and bowel incontinence. Radicular symptoms in the lower extremities can be treated by a foraminotomy, discectomy, or laminectomy for the corresponding abnormality. However, these surgical techniques

Sources of Support: None.

[a] Department of Neurological Surgery, Northwestern University Feinberg School of Medicine, 676 St. Clair, Suite 2210, Chicago, IL 60611, USA; [b] Department of Orthopaedics, Xijing Hospital, The Fourth Military Medical University, 127 Changle West Road, Xi'an, Shaanxi 710032, China; [c] Department of Orthopaedics, Beijing Tiantan Hospital, The Capital Medical University, Beijing 100050, People's Republic of China; [d] Department of Orthopaedic Surgery, Renji Hospital, Shanghai Jiaotong University School of Medicine, Shanghai 200127, People's Republic of China; [e] The Spine Clinic of Los Angeles, Good Samaritan Hospital, University of Southern California, 1245 Wilshire Blvd, Suite 717, Los Angeles, CA 90117, USA
* Corresponding author. The Spine Clinic of Los Angeles, 1245 Wilshire Boulevard, Suite #717, Los Angeles, CA 90017.
E-mail address: lkhoo@laspineclinic.com

neurosurgery.theclinics.com

have limited success in the treatment of low back pain that originates from the discoligamentous complex, facet joint-mediated pain, malalignment of the spinal column, or spinal instability.

Traditionally, structural causes of low back pain have been treated successfully with spinal fusion, which can be accomplished with a posterolateral fusion, posterior interbody fusion (PLIF), direct lateral interbody fusion (DLIF), or anterior lumbar interbody fusion (ALIF). The transforaminal lumbar interbody fusion (TLIF) approach was pioneered by Harms and Rolinger[1] in 1982, with great success. The TLIF technique permits decompression of both central and foraminal stenosis as well as 3-column arthrodesis through a single posterior approach.

The traditional open TLIF requires a long, midline incision with dissection of the posterior tension band and bilateral paraspinal soft tissue for surgical exposure. Excellent clinical and radiographic outcomes have been reported with open TLIF for patients with lumbar degenerative disease and lumbar spondylolisthesis. The authors initially described minimally invasive unilateral and bilateral laminectomies and facetectomies in early 2000, demonstrating the technique, efficacy, and long-term utility over the last decade.[2] In 2002, this less invasive approach to lumbar decompression was combined with tubular discectomy, interbody arthrodesis, cage placement, and percutaneous pedicle screw instrumentation, to constitute one of the earliest descriptions and case series of minimally invasive PLIF.[3] Subsequently, minimally invasive approaches have been applied successfully to the traditional TLIF technique. Minimally invasive transforaminal lumbar interbody fusion (MI-TLIF) has demonstrated improved perioperative outcomes similar to those achieved with open TLIF regarding surgical blood loss, operative time, length of hospital stay, and overall fusion rates. Nonetheless, the MI-TLIF approach has perioperative complications inherent to the emerging surgical technique: cerebrospinal fluid (CSF) leak, wrong-level surgery, Kirschner (K)-wire or Jamshidi needle fracture, pedicle screw breach, increased radiation exposure, and increased rates of pseudarthrosis. The surgical technique, long-term outcomes, and complications of MI-TLIF are reviewed in this article.

SURGICAL TECHNIQUE
Positioning

The patient is intubated under general anesthesia and is placed prone onto a radiolucent operating table. For optimal lordotic sagittal balance, an open Jackson frame is the preferred choice. A Wilson frame may be used to improve access to the intervertebral disc space for decompression, but may lead to decreased postoperative lumbar lordosis. Somatosensory evoked potentials (SSEPs) and continuous electromyographic potentials (cEMG) are continuously monitored throughout the surgery. Triggered electromyographic potentials (tEMG) can be used to optionally test the needle, tap, and screw during pedicle cannulation. Under anterior-posterior (AP) fluoroscopic guidance, the midline over the spinous processes is outlined with a skin marker and 2 paramedian lines are drawn approximately 1 to 2 cm lateral to the lateral borders of the pedicles, as seen on the fluoroscopic image (**Fig. 1**A). The skin incisions are preliminarily swabbed with betadine. At this point, #18-gauge spinal needles are passed through the incisions bilaterally down to the pedicle entry points at the junction of the transverse process and the pedicle under AP fluoroscopy. Approximately 5 mL of 0.25% Marcaine with 1:200,000 epinephrine are then used to inject the cylinder of soft tissue from these entry points, through the muscles and the skin itself, to reduce bleeding and postoperative pain (see **Fig. 1**A). The patient is then prepped and draped in standard sterile fashion. With lateral fluoroscopy, the initial tubular dilator is used to further localize and confirm the surgical level (L4–L5) (see **Fig. 1**B).

Incision and Localization

The paramedian skin marks are incised with a scalpel about 3 cm long through the dermis, subcutaneous tissue, and fascia. Blunt dissection with fingers can be used to split the plane further and to bilaterally palpate the transverse process–facet junctions of the superior and inferior levels. AP and lateral fluoroscopy is then adjusted to the proper Ferguson angle to ensure a level view of the superior endplates of the operative level vertebrae (see **Fig. 1**B, C).

Ipsilateral Percutaneous Placement of Pedicle Screws and Rods

Under AP fluoroscopic guidance, two #11 Jamshidi needles are inserted through the incisions, again down to the level of the pedicle entry points of the superior vertebral level at approximately the 3 o'clock and 9 o'clock positions of the pedicle (**Fig. 2**A). Each needle is then advanced approximately 2 cm through the incisions, taking care to not pass beyond the medial border of the circular pedicle projection on AP fluoroscopy to the corresponding 9 o'clock and 3 o'clock positions (see

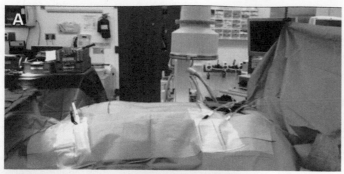

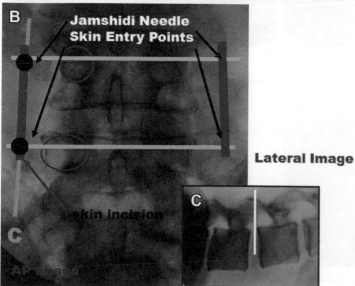

Fig. 1. (*A*) The patient is placed in the prone position on a radiolucent table, on top of a radiolucent Jackson or Wilson frame. (*B, C*) Paramedian skin incisions 3 cm in length are drawn paramedian and 1 to 2 cm lateral to the pedicles. Similarly, horizontal skin lines are drawn under anteroposterior (AP) fluoroscopy to allow for preinjection and localization of the operative level.

Fig. 2B). Pedicle entry points should be placed more lateral and inferior along the pedicle such as to ensure that the screw head stays well away from the facet complex, to avoid adjacent facet impingement. At this depth in most patients, the needles typically end in the posterior third of the vertebral bodies on lateral fluoroscopy (see Fig. 2C). At this point, vertebral body bone marrow aspiration can be performed after pedicle cannulation, with the osteoprogenitor cellular concentrate then admixed into an appropriate matrix to be combined with bone to be saved from the decompression. K-wires are placed and the cannulated Jamshidi needles are removed. A tap is placed over the K-wire to create a working channel, followed by placement of the percutaneous screw. The process of tapping should be monitored with fluoroscopic guidance (see Fig. 2D). tEMG stimulation of the tap and/or screw can be used at this point with plastic insulation sleeves to ensure that impedance is higher than 11 to 12 mA. Initially, minimally invasive pedicle screws with sleeve extenders are placed only contralateral to the side

of the planned lamino-facetectomy decompression (ie, right-sided screws for a left-sided TLIF) (Fig. 3A). Triangulating bicortical screw placement is recommended when reduction of listhesis is desired, to improve screw pullout strength and minimize the chance of correction loss. The same sequence of targeting, cannulation, K-wire placement, stimulation, tapping, and screw placement is then repeated for the inferior level (see Fig. 3C, D).

Using the original contralateral incision, an appropriately sized rod is placed with a 90° handle, and passed underneath the fascia and through the polyaxial pedicle screw heads. Set screws are then placed through the pedicle screw extenders to secure the rod in place. For cases of mobile spondylolisthesis, the reduction mechanisms of several commercially available MI spinal (MIS) screw systems will often be used at this point to partially or completely reduce the listhesis (see Fig. 3E). In cases where there is a more rigid slip and/or the presence of osteoporosis, aggressive reduction should be avoided at this point pending

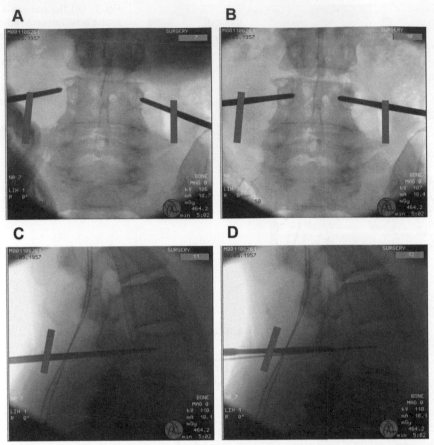

Fig. 2. (*A*) After opening the paramedian incision, #11 Jamshidi targeting needles are simultaneously placed at the pedicle screw entry points at the junction of the transverse process and facet joints under AP fluoroscopic guidance. (*B*) The needles are advanced 2 cm through the pedicles from 3 to 9 o'clock and 9 to 3 o'clock, respectively, to the medial border of the pedicles. (*C*) A lateral image is obtained to confirm the typical posterior third position of the needles at this point. (*D*) Kirschner (K)-wires are then exchanged through the Jamshidi needles and appropriately sized taps used to prepare the pedicles bilaterally.

additional release of the facet joints during decompression. The ipsilateral K-wires are then angled away from the incisions and stapled to the surgical drape to provide access for the decompression portal (see **Fig. 3**F; **Fig. 4**C).

Bony Decompression

A K-wire is placed onto the ipsilateral facet joint. Lateral fluoroscopy is used to confirm the correct surgical level and angle for surgical approach to the disc space. Sequential muscle-splitting tubular dilators are placed until the final static tubular or expandable retractor is locked into place with the flexible retractor arm between the K-wires (see **Fig. 4**A–C). Bipolar cautery is first used to circumferentially coagulate the soft-tissue vasculature around the edges of the tubular retractor. Monopolar electrocautery is then used to remove the soft tissue overlying the facet joint and the lamina. An

up-angled curette is used to define the sublaminar plane (see **Fig. 4**D; **Fig. 5**A). The lateral border of the facet, with particular focus on the pars interarticularis, is identified. A hemilaminotomy is performed with Kerrison rongeurs up to the rostral pedicle and down to the caudal pedicle. The remainder of the facet joint may be resected with rongeurs, osteotomes, or a pneumatic drill bit (see **Fig. 5**A, B). Hemostasis is achieved with bone wax and thrombin-soaked gelfoam.

Exposure of the Thecal Sac and Disc Space

The ligamentum flavum is carefully resected to expose the underlying thecal sac. The thecal sac is decompressed from the central canal laterally until the traversing nerve root is clearly identified. Facet joint and ligament resection should be performed as far lateral as possible to provide an optimal angle of approach for the discectomy

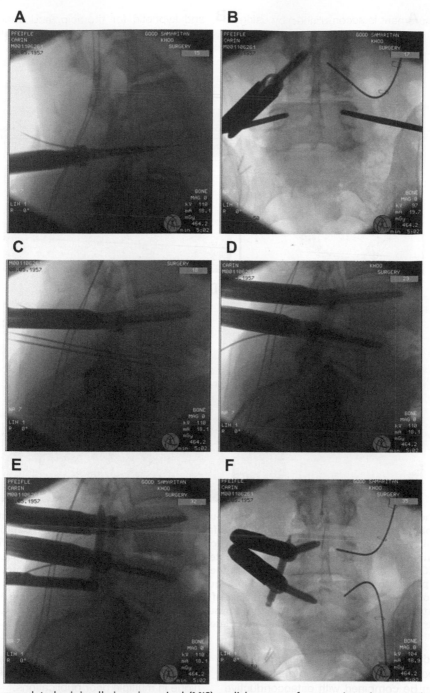

Fig. 3. (*A*) A cannulated minimally invasive spinal (MIS) pedicle screw of appropriate size to optimally achieve near-bicortical triangulating position is placed over the K-wire contralateral to the side of the intended decompression and TLIF. (*B*) The inferior level is then targeted under AP fluoroscopy with the #11 Jamshidi needles. (*C*) K-wires are again exchanged for the Jamshidi needles under lateral fluoroscopy to confirm their depth into the vertebral body. (*D*) Another contralateral MIS pedicle screw with extension sleeve is placed over the K-wire at the inferior vertebral body. (*E*) Using an angled MIS rod inserter, the rod is threaded down the extension sleeves of the contralateral MIS screws and temporarily locked loosely in place. Partial reduction via the MIS screw sleeves of any listhesis present can sometimes be achieved at this juncture in mobile segments. (*F*) AP fluoroscopy demonstrates for a left-sided MI-TLIF the typical placement at this point of the right contralateral MIS screws and rod in place, with the ipsilateral K-wires bent out of the way and stapled to the surgical field drapes to allow for the ipsilateral left MIS portal access to begin the decompression.

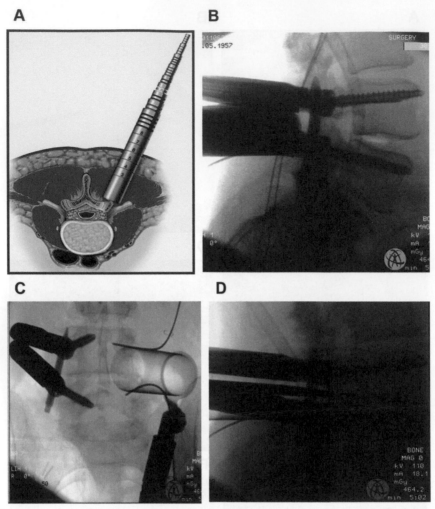

Fig. 4. (*A*) The tubular system of dilators is passed through the left paramedian incision to separate the muscle fibers in an oblique TLIF trajectory down to the target facet complex of the operative level. Depth markings on the dilators allow for portal diameter and length selection at this point. (*B*) Lateral fluoroscopy demonstrates the ipsilateral series of dilators pointed toward the disc space to facilitate interbody discectomy and subsequent cage placement. (*C*) The working portal is seen between the K-wires on the left side on AP fluoroscopy, providing appropriate pedicle-to-pedicle exposure for the subsequent left L4-5 hemilaminectomy, total facetectomy, and discectomy to follow. (*D*) Once the soft tissue is clear of the facet complex through the working MIS portal, an angled curette can be passed underneath either the superior articulating process or the pars to confirm the correct plane of dissection at the target level under lateral fluoroscopic guidance.

and interbody fusion (see **Fig. 5**C). Autograft from the bony decompression is saved for fusion material, and can be combined with osteoconductive material and vertebral body bone marrow aspiration obtained earlier during pedicle cannulation. Typically, 5 mL of local bone graft, 10 mL of extender matrix, and 4 mL of concentrated aspirate can be combined to yield 15 to 20 mL of composite graft material per level. In cases where there is severe bilateral central recess and foraminal stenosis, the working portal is angled such that decompression can be carried underneath the spinous process to achieve a contralateral

laminectomy, facetectomy, and foraminotomy. The authors have previously described this technique in multiple prior publications.[2]

Discectomy, Correction, and Interbody Fusion

The disc is incised with a long-handled scalpel, and the discectomy is performed with a combination of curettes and pituitary rongeurs. If necessary, a nerve-root retractor is placed medially to gently retract the traversing nerve root and thecal sac to expose the underlying disc (see **Fig. 5**C). Meticulous removal of the cartilaginous endplates

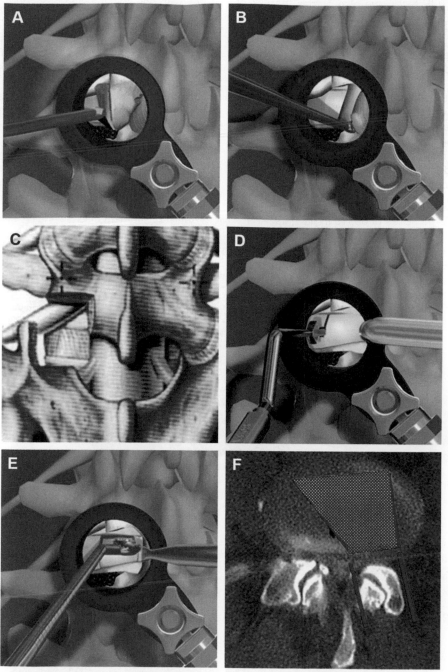

Fig. 5. (*A*) Once the soft tissue is clear of the facet complex through the working MIS portal, an angled curette can be passed underneath either the superior articulating process or the pars to confirm the correct plane of dissection at the target level to orient the surgeon. (*B*) A high-speed drill and/or osteotomes combined with Kerrison rongeurs is then used to progressively complete a total facetectomy and hemilaminectomy of the ipsilateral level. (*C*) Schematic demonstrating the typical amount of bone removed during an ipsilateral TLIF laminectomy and facetectomy. Additional laminectomy can be completed to further decompress the central thecal sac and provide more bone autograft fusion material if desired. (*D*) A Love nerve-root retractor is used to gently displace the thecal sac to expose the target disc space, which is incised with an extended #11 blade to begin the annulotomy for discectomy and interbody preparation. (*E*) An extended period of time is spent with straight and angled curettes, endplate shavers, and rasps to ensure that a near total discectomy and denuding of the cartilaginous endplate is completed and to optimize the chance of solid bony interbody fusion. (*F*) Schematic of the computed tomography myelogram demonstrates the typical goal of the funnel-shaped interbody preparation that should be achieved in a typical unilateral MI-TLIF discectomy approach.

will ensure the largest surface area available for bony fusion (see **Fig. 5**D). With meticulous use of angled instruments, approximately 60% to 80% of the disc space can be effectively prepared for arthrodesis through a unilateral approach (see **Fig. 5**E).

Sequentially larger disc space shavers are used to assist with the discectomy and preparation of the endplates for fusion. Blunt interbody dilators can also be used to progressively distract severely collapsed disc spaces, to restore the intervertebral height and facilitate the insertion of interbody discectomy tools (**Fig. 6**A). Particular attention should be paid to avoid using blunt dilators to distract the soft central area of the vertebral endplate, where inadvertent bony cavitation can occur. The dilator should be advanced cautiously such that distraction occurs primarily along the central far anterior ring hypophysis, where the endplate strength is maximal (see **Fig. 6**A). During interbody paddle distraction, the contralateral screws can also be simultaneously distracted and the rod temporarily locked to maintain the increased interbody height to facilitate optimal cage height placement. Furthermore, several MIS pedicle screw systems have reduction threads or mechanisms to also reduce the spondylolisthesis at this moment, as the distraction typically mobilizes and releases

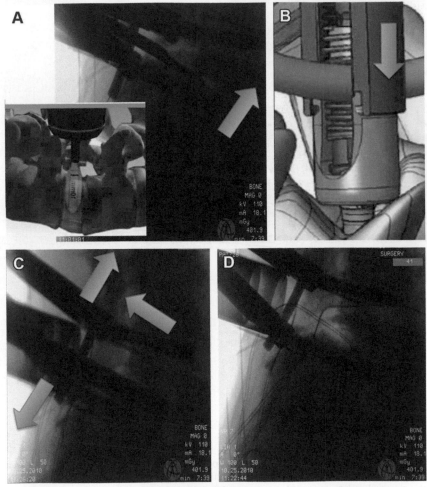

Fig. 6. (A) Lateral fluoroscopic image demonstrates the ipsilateral placement of a paddle interbody distractor through the working portal to begin the steps needed for progressive restoration of intervertebral disc height. (B) Diagrammatic representation shows the threaded reduction sleeves available on several MIS pedicle screw systems to allow for reduction of spondylolisthetic segments via the contralaterally placed screws in combination with simultaneous ipsilateral paddle distraction. (C) Lateral fluoroscopy demonstrates the height restoration and reduction of the operative segment in comparison with A, by simultaneously distracting ipsilaterally with the blunt interbody paddle distractor and reducing the contralateral MIS pedicle screw-rods via the reduction threads in the screw extension sleeves. (D) Lateral fluoroscopy demonstrates the restored, albeit nonlordotic, intervertebral space with full reduction of the grade-2 listhesis and collapse seen in A. Arrows (A–C) are used to show force vectors and movement for distraction and reduction.

the segment (see **Fig. 6**B). This combined maneuver of ipsilateral interbody paddle height elevation, and contralateral screw distraction with reduction as needed, has been highly effective at correcting the slip and lordosis in most grade 2 and lower spondylolisthesis cases treated by the authors (see **Fig. 6**C, D). The interbody cage and the disc space are then packed with 15 mL of the previously mentioned composite bone graft (**Fig. 7**A). Bone morphogenetic protein (BMP) may also be used with caution to ensure that the bioactive material remains anterior in the disc space, and that the annulotomy is well sealed at the end with Tisseel (Baxter Biosurgery, Deerfield, IL) and gelfoam to avoid unwanted leakage with subsequent radiculitis, seromas, and possible delayed heterotopic bone formation. In this series of 198 patients (144 MI-TLIF, 54 open TLIF) reported here, the authors did not use BMP in any of the primary surgeries. The cage is placed into the prepared disc space under AP and lateral fluoroscopic guidance to ensure that the graft is near the center as well as

resting fully on the anterior ring hypophysis, to minimize the risk of delayed subsidence through the softer, center portion of the vertebral endplates (see **Fig. 7**A–C). Hemostasis is achieved with Surgifoam (Ethicon, a Johnson & Johnson Company, New Brunswick, NJ) and bipolar cautery of the epidural veins and soft tissue followed by antibiotic irrigation. A piece of gelfoam is placed within the annulotomy and sealed with Tisseel if desired to prevent leakage of bone marrow and bioactive materials from the interbody space. The ipsilateral working portal is then carefully removed to avoid inadvertent removal of the ipsilateral K-wires within the pedicles.

The previously stapled ipsilateral K-wires are then released, and the pedicle screws with their extender sleeves are placed over them and threaded into the vertebral bodies. An ipsilateral rod is then introduced as was performed with the contralateral screws previously (**Fig. 8**A). When both rods are secured, bilateral compression is applied to the construct, before final locking of

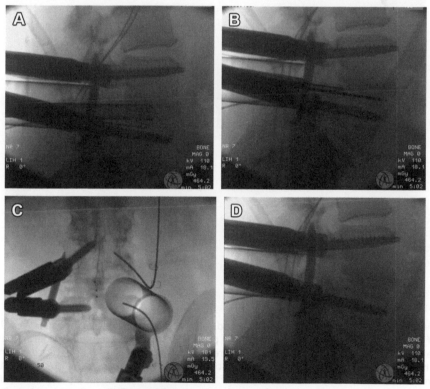

Fig. 7. (*A*) A funnel is used to pack the restored interbody space with approximately 15 mL of composite graft material obtained from bone saved from the decompression, transpedicular vertebral body bone marrow aspirate, and synthetic bone matrix extenders. (*B*) An expandable 15° polyetheretherketone (PEEK) prosthetic intervertebral cage is inserted at 7 mm height and expanded to a final height of 15 mm under lateral fluoroscopic control to ensure that there is good contact with the strong load-bearing anterior ring hypophysis of the inferior endplate. (*C*) AP fluoroscopy is used to ensure proper medial placement to avoid inducing a coronal tilt and to ensure maximal hypophyseal contact with anterior ring. (*D*) Final cage position is then confirmed again after final expansion of the PEEK cage.

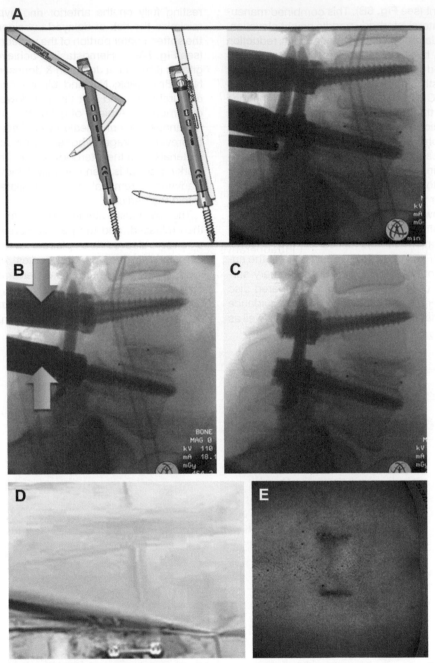

Fig. 8. (*A*) The pivoting, rotational movement of the rod inserter is demonstrated as the rod is then threaded after placement of the ipsilateral MIS pedicle screws over the previously stapled K-wires. (*B, C*) Lateral fluoroscopy demonstrates the important simultaneously bilateral compression of the MIS extension sleeves to maximize segment lordosis around the PEEK cage and to optimize overall postoperative sagittal balance. (*D*) Schematic AP representation of the final construct superimposed on a diagram of the spinal column shows ideal placement of the screws and TLIF oblique PEEK cage. (*E*) The typical skin incisions of a 1-level and 2-level TLIF are demonstrated after closure, re-injection with 0.25% Marcaine with 1:200,000 epinephrine, and Dermabond sealant. Note the untouched nature of the central musculoligamentous tension complex. *Arrows* (*B*) demonstrate compressive force applied on construct.

the set screws to maximize segmental lordosis and improve overall sagittal balance (see **Fig. 8**B). AP and lateral radiographs are used to confirm appropriate final placement of bilateral

screws and rods (see **Fig. 8**C, D). Either a small handheld retractor or tubular portal is then placed down through the contralateral incision between the MIS pedicle extension sleeves. In this fashion, the contralateral facet and transverse processes can be decorticated and irrigated, with the remaining 5 to 8 mL of composite bone graft used to pack the bony posterolateral gutter. The MIS pedicle screw extension sleeves and the contralateral retractor are then all removed, leaving the final construct in place (see **Fig. 8**C, D). The wounds are irrigated and closed with a combination of absorbable sutures and a skin adhesive for an optimal cosmetic closure. At this point, reinjection of local anesthetic (ie, 0.25% Marcaine with 1:200,000 epinephrine) into the skin and underlying muscle will help decrease postoperative pain.

RESULTS: OUTCOMES OF MI-TLIF VERSUS OPEN TLIF
Demographics

From a single working group of surgeons, the authors prospectively studied 144 single-level and 2-level MI-TLIF lumbar surgical procedures. As a control, 54 open TLIF procedures using the classic open TLIF techniques from the same institution were also prospectively followed. Surgical parameters, hospitalization data, radiographic data, and standardized clinical outcome measures were followed over a 4-year period with a mean follow-up of 45 months (**Table 1**). Demographics for both groups demonstrated a similar mean age (60 years old) and a male to female ratio (45:55). The clinical diagnoses were similar in both groups: spondylolisthesis ± tilt with stenosis (46%), postlaminectomy instability with stenosis (25%), and degenerative disc disease with stenosis (19%). The distribution of surgical levels was also similar, although there were more L5-S1 levels treated in the MI-TLIF group because the surgeons in the open TLIF group often preferred ALIF treatment for simple degenerative disease and stenosis at L5-S1 (see **Table 1**).

Perioperative Data

Although the authors first described minimally invasive interbody fusion, cage placement, decompression, and instrumentation in early 2002, this series of 144 MI-TLIF procedures represent surgical cases (years 2006–2008) that were well past the initial learning curve of the first 100 MI-TLIF procedures earlier from 2002 to 2004. As a result, the MI-TLIF group had shorter surgical times (2.05 hours) than the open group (3.75 hours) ($P<.001$), as less time is taken up by opening, closure, and instrumentation. This finding stands in contrast to results of some of the other comparative MI-TLIF and open TLIF studies from the earlier portion of other working groups' learning curves. The more than 3-fold decrease in blood loss of 115 mL versus 485 mL in the MI-TLIF group also accounted for decreased time spent obtaining hemostasis as well as an optimized clinical workflow ($P<.01$). Postoperatively, this resulted also in a 5-fold decreased rate of postoperative transfusion in the MI-TLIF group (2.1% vs 11.1%, $P<.001$). An overall trend of lower postoperative pain and disability in the first few weeks (Visual Analog Scale [VAS] Back, 3 months: 26 vs 38; Oswestry Disability Index [ODI]: 39 vs 45; $P = .01$) also resulted in a 37% decrease in the length of stay (LOS) (2.75 days vs 4.40 days, $P<.01$) in the MI-TLIF group (see **Table 1**). Inpatient institutional cost data reflected this improvement in length of surgery, blood loss, transfusion, infection, and LOS, with $3554 savings seen per level in the MI-TLIF group during a separate subcohort retrospective analysis of patients' costs in 68 single-level fusions (34 MI-TLIF vs open TLIF: $19,925 vs $23,479; $P<.01$) (**Table 2**). MI-TLIF procedures, however, are associated with significantly increased radiation exposure to the patient, surgeon, and operating room personnel. This feature was observed in a 2.5-fold increase in milliSieverts (mSv) per level for the MI-TLIF group of 1.90 mSv versus 0.75 mSv for the open TLIF group ($P<.01$).

Radiographic and Fusion Outcomes

Fusion success was measured by dynamic flexion-extension lumbar radiographs in conjunction with a computed tomography (CT) scan obtained within the 16- to 24-month postoperative window (mean: 19.2 months). Both groups showed statistically similar fusion rates of 92.5% (MI-TLIF) and 93.5% (open TLIF), which is similar to that in the published literature of MI-TLIF series (see **Table 2**; **Table 3**). In this series of 198 patients (144 MI-TLIF, 54 open), the authors did not use BMP in any of the primary surgeries, as they had previously encountered a significant incidence of delayed heterotopic foraminal and recess bone formation, causing recurrent radiculopathy, at a mean of 21 months following the primary MI-TLIF procedure. Segmental correction of lordosis (5.65° vs 4.10°) and percentage of subsidence (11.75% vs 11.8%) were statistically equivalent for both groups, as was the incidence of surgery for pseudarthrosis revision (2.1% vs 1.9%, $P<.01$).

Clinical Standardized Outcomes

During the 6- to 24-month postoperative period, clinical standardized outcome measures (ODI, VAS Back, VAS Leg) were statistically similar for both study cohorts (**Fig. 9**A, see **Table 2**). However, there was a statistically superior ($P<.01$) VAS Back (26 vs 38) and VAS Leg (26 vs 19),

Table 1
Aggregated perioperative data, outcomes, and complications for MI-TLIF (144) versus open TLIF (54)

Variable	Present Series of MI-TLIF	Control Series of Open TLIF
Demographics		
No. of patients (levels)	144 (79 1-level, 55 2-level)	54 (35 1-level, 21 2-level)
Mean age (y)	61	58
Males/females	61/83	25/29
Follow-up, mo (range)	45 (34–60)	46 (33–58)
L5/S1, L4/5, L3/4, L2/3 (%)	45, 43, 9, 3	39, 52, 7, 2
Perioperative Data		
Mean operating room time per level (h)	2.05	3.75
Mean blood loss (mL)	**115**	**485**
Radiation exposure (mSv/level)	**1.90**	**0.75**
Average length of stay (d)	**2.75**	**4.40**
Radiographic Outcomes		
CT-Based fusion rate (18–24 mo) (%)	92.5	93.5
Lordotic change (degrees per level)	5.65	4.10
Subsidence (3–6 mo; 6–12 mo) (%)	9.25, 2.5	8.80, 3
Revision for pseudarthrosis	2.1% (3)	1.9% (2)
Complications and Revisions	% (no. of patients)	% (no. of patients)
Immediate postoperative radiculitis/deficit	5.7% (8)	5.6% (3)
Delayed postoperative radiculitis/deficit (>48 h)	2.8 (4)	3.7 (2)
Cerebrospinal fluid leaks	3.5 (5)	3.7 (2)
Vascular or abdominal injury	0.7 (1)	0.0 (0))
Persistent stenosis and symptoms	4.9 (7)	5.5 (3)
Screw misplacement requiring revision	1.4 (2)	3.7 (2)
Cage misplacement/migration and revision	0.7 (1)	1.9 (1)
Need for postoperative transfusion	**2.1 (3)**	**11.1 (6)**
Respiratory infections	**2.1 (3)**	**9.3 (5)**
Urinary tract infections	**2.1 (3)**	**7.4 (4)**
Wound infections (superficial)	4.2 (6)	12.9 (7)
Deep infections (needing surgery)	**0.0 (0)**	**5.6 (3)**
Postoperative diagnosed hematoma	**2.1 (3)**	**9.3 (5)**
Symptomatic deep vein thrombosis	**1.4 (2)**	**5.1 (4)**
Overall reoperation rate (4 y)	**8.3 (12)**	**20.4 (12)**
Repeat decompression	1.4 (2)	0.0 (0)
Revision for hardware issues	2.1 (3)	3.7 (2)
Vascular or abdominal repair	0.7 (1)	0.0 (0)
Infections/hematoma drainage	**0.0 (0)**	**5.6 (3)**
Pseudarthrosis	2.1 (3)	1.9 (2)
New adjacent-level degeneration	**2.1 (3)**	**7.4 (4)**

Values achieving statistical significance (P≤01) are highlighted in bold.

Table 2
Aggregated outcomes for MI-TLIF studies compared with the present series (n = 198 with 144 MI-TLIF)

Variable	Literature Review	Present Series of MI-TLIF	Control Series of Open TLIF
Total studies	28		
N	1291	144	54
Follow-up, mo (range)	12–72	45 (34–60)	46 (33–58)
Visual Analog Scale (VAS) Back Pain			
Studies included	17		
No. of patients (levels)	721	144 (79 1-level, 55 2-level)	54 (35 1-level, 21 2-level)
Preoperative score (mean)	6.68	6.37	6.72
Postoperative score (mean)	1.92	1.05 (1 y), 2.25 (4 y)	1.70 (1 y), 3.95 (4 y)
Change (mean)	4.76	5.32 (1 y), 4.12 (4 y)	5.02 (1 y), 2.77 (4 y)
Percentage improvement (mean)	71.2	83 (1 y), **65 (4 y)**	75 (1 y), **42 (4 y)**
VAS Leg Pain			
Studies included	13		
No. of patients (levels)	556	144 (79 1-level, 55 2-level)	54 (35 1-level, 21 2-level)
Preoperative score (mean)	7.06	8.90	8.82
Postoperative score (mean)	1.72	1.15 (1 y), 1.43 (4 y)	1.30 (1 y), 2.22 (4 y)
Change (mean)	5.34	7.75 (1 y), 7.47 (4 y)	7.52 (1 y), 6.60 (4 y)
Percentage improvement (mean)	75.7	87 (1 y), 83 (4 y)	85 (1 y), 75 (4 y)
Oswestry Disability Index			
Studies included	24		
No. of patients (levels)	1072	144 (79 1-level, 55 2-level)	54 (35 1-level, 21 2-level)
Preoperative score (mean)	48.9	52.8	51.2
Postoperative score (mean)	19.4	18 (1 y), 26 (4 y)	21 (1 y), 33 (4 y)
Change (mean)	29.5	34.8 (1 y), 26.8 (4 y)	30.2 (1 y), 18.2 (4 y)
Percentage improvement (mean)	60.3	66 (1 y), **51 (4 y)**	59 (1 y), **36 (4 y)**
Fusion Rate			
Studies included	24		
No. of patients (levels)	1132	144 (79 1-level, 55 2-level)	54 (35 1-level, 21 2-level)
Fusion percentage (mean)	93.5	92.5	93.5
Systems Cost			
No. of patients (levels)		34 (34 1-level)	34 (34 1-level)
Hospital surgery/admission costs (US$)		**19,925**	23,479

Variables achieving statistical significance (P≤01) are highlighted in bold.

with resultant decreased narcotic requirements, seen in the MI-TLIF group (see **Fig. 9**B). The difference in ODI score only demonstrated a trend (P<.05) toward less pain, but did not reach statistical significance at 3 months (ODI 39 vs 45) (see **Fig. 9**A). Overall at 1 year, there was no difference in the VAS Leg pain scores, with a mean improvement of 85% and 87% seen for both groups. There was again a trend for better sustained VAS Leg pain improvement at 4 years (MI-TLIF 83%, vs open TLIF 75%), but this was not statistically significant. The same equivalence was seen at 1 year for VAS Back pain scores (1.05/83% improvement for MI-TLIF vs 1.70/75% improvement for open TLIF) (see **Fig. 9**B, see **Table 2**). Of particular note, however, was the statistically significant trend at 3 years and significance at 4 years of better VAS Back pain scores for the less invasive cohort (2.25/65% improvement for MI-TLIF vs 3.95/42% improvement for open TLIF; P<.01).

Table 3
Summary of MI-TLIF outcome literature

Authors,[Ref.] Year	Design	n (MI Subset)	Follow-Up	Significant Results and Comment
Adogwa et al,[4] 2011[a,b]	RS	30 (15)	2 y	Cohort comparison of MI-TLIF and open TLIF MI-TLIF showed shorter LOS, duration of narcotic use, and time to return to work Similar VAS, ODI, EQ-5D score improvements at 2 y between groups
Archavlis & Carvi,[5] 2013[a,b,c]	RS	49 (24)	26 mo	Cohort comparison of MI-TLIF and open TLIF Similar LOS, VAS, ODI, walking distance at 2 y between groups 92% with bony fusion, similar between groups
Beringer & Mobasser,[6] 2006	RS	8	6 mo	Assessment of unilateral percutaneous pedicle screws with MI-TLIF Bony fusion in all patients at 6 mo
Deutsch & Musacchio,[7] 2006	RS	20	6–12 mo	Assessment of unilateral percutaneous pedicle screws with MI-TLIF 85% of patients with >20-point reduction in ODI Significant reduction in ODI and pain scores 55% with bony fusion at 6 mo
Dhall et al,[8] 2008[c]	RS	42 (21)	>2 y	Cohort comparison of MI-TLIF and open TLIF MI-TLIF showed shorter LOS Similar improvement in Prolo scores between groups 1 patient with pseudarthrosis in MI-TLIF group, none in open TLIF group
Jang & Lee,[9] 2005	RS	23	13–28 mo	Assessment of ipsilateral pedicle screws and contralateral facet screw with MI-TLIF Significant improvement in pain scores, ODI 22/24 of operated levels showed bony fusion 21/23 patients satisfied with outcomes
Kasliwal & Deutsch,[10] 2012[a,b,c]	RS	40	12–62 mo	Assessment of local bony shavings as autograft 65% of patients with >20-point reduction in ODI and >50% reduction in VAS scores 93% of patients with some improvement of ODI and VAS 68% with bony fusion at 1 y
Kim et al,[11] 2009[a,b,c]	RS	94 (46)	30 mo	Cohort comparison of MI-TLIF and ALIF with percutaneous pedicle screws Similar improvements in VAS and ODI scores between groups 92% with bony fusion after MI-TLIF, similar to ALIF Improved disc height, listhesis, and segmental lordosis with MI-TLIF; ALIF with more increases in disc height, segmental lordosis, and whole lumbar lordosis
Kim et al,[12] 2012[a,b,c]	RS	44	68 mo	Assessment of long-term outcome for MI-TLIF Significant improvements in VAS and ODI scores 80% patient satisfaction rate 98% with bony fusion

Study	Design	N	Follow-up	Summary
Kim et al,[13] 2011[a,b,c]	RS	56	32 mo	Assessment of clinical and radiological outcomes following MI-TLIF 93% of patients with good or excellent clinical outcomes Disc height and whole lumbar lordosis significantly improved 95% with bony fusion
Lau et al,[14] 2013	RS	16	17 mo	Assessment of MI-TLIF for spondylolisthesis in normal weight and obese cohorts Similar improvements in VAS and ODI between groups
Lee et al,[15] 2010[a,b,c]	RS	20	18 mo	Assessment of clinical and radiological outcomes following MI-TLIF Significant improvements in VAS and ODI scores, and in spinal canal cross-sectional area 92% with bony fusion
Lee et al,[16] 2008[b,c]	RS	27	39 mo	Assessment of MI-TLIF in elderly patients Significant improvements in VAS and ODI scores 89% with ≥ 2 point VAS, $\geq 25\%$ ODI, $\geq 50\%$ patient satisfaction score improvements with no major complications 72% subjective patient satisfaction rate Significant increases in segmental lordosis and sacral tilt 78% with bony fusion
Lee et al,[17] 2012[a,b,c]	PC	144 (72)	2 y	Cohort comparison of MI-TLIF and open TLIF MI-TLIF group used less morphine, ambulated sooner, and had shorter LOS Similar improvement in VAS, SF36, ODI, NASS scores between groups 97% with bony fusion in MI-TLIF group, similar to open group
Luo et al,[18] 2012[b,c]	RS	16	18 mo	Assessment of MI-TLIF with computer-aided fluoroscopic navigation and EMG Significant improvements in VAS and ODI
Min & Yoo,[19] 2013[a,b,c]	RS	127	25 mo	Assessment of single- and multilevel MI-TLIF Similar improvement in VAS and ODI between groups Changes in disc height, segmental lordosis, and whole lumbar lordosis similar between groups 90% with bony fusion, similar between groups
Park & Foley,[20] 2008[a,b,c]	RS	40	35 mo	Assessment of MI-TLIF with reduction of spondylolisthesis Significant improvements in VAS and ODI scores Mean translational reduction of 76% Bony fusion noted in all patients
Park et al,[21] 2011[a,b,c]	RS	66	36 mo	Comparison of MI-TLIF for spondylotic spondylolisthesis, degenerative spondylolisthesis, and degenerative segmental instability Similar improvements in VAS, ODI, and functional scores between groups 77% with bony fusion, similar between groups
Parker et al,[22] 2013[b,c]	RS	100 (50)	2 y	Cost-effectiveness analysis between MI-TLIF and open TLIF Shorter LOS and time to return to work in MI-TLIF group Similar improvements in VAS, ODI, SF12, Zung depression, and EQ-5D scores between groups Similar gains in QALYs between groups MI-TLIF group had significantly lower 2-y total cost

(continued on next page)

Table 3
(continued)

Authors,[Ref.] Year	Design	n (MI Subset)	Follow-Up	Significant Results and Comment
Peng et al,[23] 2009[a,b,c]	PC	58 (29)	2 y	Cohort comparison of MI-TLIF and open TLIF MI-TLIF group showed reduced morphine use and LOS Similar improvements in VAS, ODI, SF36, and NASS scores between groups 100% with bony fusion in both groups
Rodriguez-Vela et al,[24] 2013[a,b]	PC	41 (21)	36–54 mo	Randomized comparison of MI-TLIF and open TLIF Similar improvements in VAS, ODI, SF26, and NASS scores between groups
Rosen et al,[25] 2008	RS	110	15 mo	Correlation of obesity and body habitus to clinical outcomes Linear regression showed no correlation between BMI or weight and SF36 scores or perioperative outcomes
Rouben et al,[26] 2011[b,c]	RS	169	49 mo	Assessment of clinical outcomes following MI-TLIF 80% showed >20% improvement in ODI, mean improvement 41% Significant improvements in VAS 1- and 2-level fusions improved similarly 96% with bony fusion at 1 y
Scheufler et al,[27] 2007[c]	RS	53	16 mo	Comparison of MI-TLIF with institutional reference cohort of mini-open TLIF MI-TLIF showed better early postoperative pain scores and Roland-Morris pain scores at follow-up, compared with mini-open TLIF group Similar improvements in AAOS questionnaire scores between groups at follow-up 87% of patients rated outcome as good or excellent, none reported poor 94% with bony fusion at 16 mo
Schizas et al,[28] 2009[b,c]	RS	36 (18)	22 mo	Cohort comparison of MI-TLIF and open TLIF MI-TLIF group showed shorter LOS Similar improvement in VAS and ODI between groups
Schwender et al,[29] 2005[b,c]	RS	49	23 mo	Assessment of clinical and radiographic outcomes after MI-TLIF Significant improvements in VAS and ODI, narcotic use discontinued 2–4 wk postoperatively All patients showed bony fusion at last follow-up
Shunwu et al,[30] 2010[b]	PC	62 (32)	24–42 mo	Cohort comparison of MI-TLIF and open TLIF MI-TLIF group showed better perioperative outcomes, including LOS MI-TLIF group had more improvement in VAS and ODI scores than open group
Sonmez et al,[31] 2013[a,b,c]	PC	20	2 y	Comparison of unilateral and bilateral pedicle screws in MI-TLIF Similar improvements in VAS and ODI between groups 8/10 with bony fusion in unilateral group at 2 y, compared with 9/10 in bilateral group

Study	Type	N	Follow-up	Findings
Tsahtsarlis & Wood,[32] 2012	RS	34	6 mo	Assessment of clinical and radiographic outcomes after MI-TLIF / Significant improvements in ODI / 97% with bony fusion at 6 mo
Villavicencio et al,[33] 2010[c]	RS	139 (76)	38 mo	Cohort comparison of MI-TLIF and open TLIF / MI-TLIF group had shorter LOS than open group / Similar improvements in VAS, ODI, MacNab, and patient satisfaction scores between groups
Villavicencio et al,[34] 2012	RS	52 (32)	25 mo	Comparison of same-day discharge and <24 h admission for MI-TLIF and open TLIF / Similar perioperative outcomes, improvements in VAS, and patient satisfaction scores / 96% with bony fusion at follow-up
Wang et al,[35] 2011	RCT	79 (41)	33 mo	Randomized comparison of MI-TLIF and open TLIF / MI-TLIF group with shorter postoperative recovery time / Early postoperative ODI with more improvement in MI-TLIF group compared with open group / Similar improvements in VAS and late ODI between groups / Less sacrospinalis injury in MI-TLIF group, based on MRI and EMG
Wang et al,[36] 2010[a,b,c]	PC	85 (42)	26 mo	Cohort comparison of single-level MI-TLIF and open TLIF for low-grade spondylolisthesis / MI-TLIF group with better perioperative outcomes, including LOS / Similar improvements in VAS and ODI between groups / 41/42 fusion rate in MI-TLIF group, compared with 42/43 in open group
Wang et al,[37] 2011[a,b,c]	PC	52 (25)	28 mo	Cohort comparison of MI-TLIF and open TLIF for patients with prior open discectomy / Similar improvements in VAS and ODI between groups / 24/25 fusion rate in MI-TLIF group, compared with 26/27 in open group
Wang et al,[38] 2012[a,b,c]	PC	81 (42)	36 mo	Cohort comparison of MI-TLIF and open TLIF for patients in overweight or obese patients / Similar improvements in VAS and ODI between groups / 41/42 fusion rate in MI-TLIF group, compared with 38/39 in open group
Wu et al,[39] 2012	RS	151	10 mo	Cohort comparison of patients <65 y and >65 y old following MI-TLIF / Younger patients showed a shorter LOS / Similar improvements in VAS and ODI between groups / 88% with bony fusion, no significant differences between groups
Xue et al,[40] 2012	RCT	80	25 mo	Randomized comparison of unilateral pedicles screws with MI-TLIF and open TLIF / Similar improvements in VAS, ODI, and Prolo scores between groups / 34/37 fusion rate in unilateral MI-TLIF group, compared with 41/43 in bilateral open group
Zairi et al,[41] 2013	RS	100 (40)	2 y	Cohort comparison of MI-TLIF and open TLIF / Similar improvements in VAS and ODI between groups / 98% with bony fusion at 1 y

Abbreviations: AAOS, American Academy of Orthopedic Surgeons; BMI, body mass index; EMG, electromyography; EQ-5D, EuroQol 5D Health Questionnaire; LOS, length of stay; MRI, magnetic resonance imaging; NASS, North American Spine Society; ODI, Oswestry Disability Index; PC, prospective cohort; QALY, quality-adjusted life year; RCT, randomized controlled trial; RS, retrospective; SF, Short-Form 12-, 26-, 36-item questionnaire; VAS, Visual Analog Scale.

[a] Study included in back and/or leg VAS analysis.
[b] Study included in ODI analysis.
[c] Study included in fusion rate analysis.

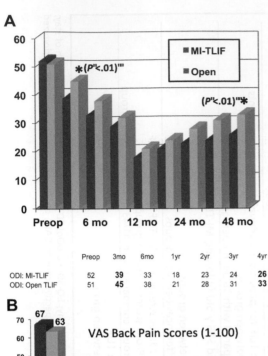

A

	Preop	3mo	6mo	1yr	2yr	3yr	4yr
ODI: MI-TLIF	52	**39**	33	18	23	24	**26**
ODI: Open TLIF	51	**45**	38	21	28	31	**33**

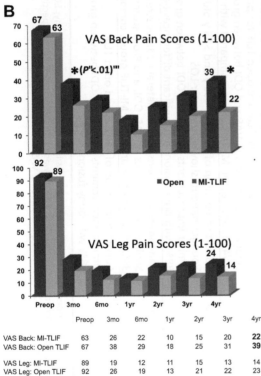

B

	Preop	3mo	6mo	1yr	2yr	3yr	4yr
VAS Back: MI-TLIF	63	26	22	10	15	20	**22**
VAS Back: Open TLIF	67	38	29	18	25	31	**39**
VAS Leg: MI-TLIF	89	19	12	11	15	13	14
VAS Leg: Open TLIF	92	26	19	13	21	22	23

Fig. 9. (*A*) Four-year comparative Oswestry Disability Index Score outcomes. (*B*) Outcomes of 4-year comparative Back and Leg Pain Visual Analog Scale scores. * Designates a *P*<.05.

This difference was underscored and affirmed by the statistical difference in the ODI score as well, with a 15% overall better ODI score in the MI-TLIF group at 4 years (26 ODI MI-TLIF, 33 ODI open TLIF; *P*<.01). These overall differences are demonstrated graphically in **Fig. 9**A, B with

statistically different segments highlighted with an asterisk on the graphs, and in bold within the data tables. When compared with literature values from the review below and **Table 3**, the overall VAS Leg, VAS Back, and ODI scores seen in the present study of MI-TLIF patients tracks well with the summarized published control data (see **Table 2**).

Complications

The overall incidence of complications at the time of surgery are summarized in **Table 1**, and demonstrate statistical equivalence (*P*>.01) with regard to postoperative new neurologic deficits/radiculitis (7.8% MI-TLIF, 9.3% open TLIF), CSF leaks (3.5% vs 3.7%), persistent radicular compressive symptoms (4.9% vs 5.5%), and hardware replacement requiring revision (2.1% vs 5.6%). There was one case of anterior injury of the ileum during interbody disc preparation requiring laparotomy for surgical repair that occurred in a case of revision MI-TLIF seen early on in the cohort. Overall, however, the blood loss was much lower in the MI-TLIF group, as noted earlier (115 mL vs 485 mL) with a 4-fold lower risk of postoperative transfusion seen in the less invasive cohort (2.1% vs 11.1%; *P*<.01). On analysis of the postoperative complications observed, there was a striking superiority seen in MI-TLIF for all measures. There was a 3- to 4-fold increase in systemic respiratory (2.1% and 9.3%) and urinary infections (2.1% vs 7.4%) in the MI-TLIF group (*P*<.001). This difference is attributed to the overall earlier mobilization and ambulation, decreased postoperative pain, and shorter LOS seen in the MI-TLIF group. Accordingly, the incidence of hematoma and deep vein thrombosis is also much higher in the open TLIF group (2.1% vs 9.3%; 1.4% vs 5.4%), likely for the same reasons (*P*<.001).

The most important difference between the two groups is seen in the overall wound infection rate. As MI-TLIF is accepted now as having less tissue trauma, blood loss, need for drainage, and a smaller potential dead space, it comes as no surprise that there is 3-fold increase in superficial wound infection in the open TLIF group (12.9% vs 4.2%). More striking, however, is the 5-fold increase in the number of deep wound infections requiring wound revision, irrigation, and debridement seen in the open TLIF group (5.6% vs 0%) (*P*<.001). Each of these secondary surgical costs for infection led to total additional costs of $83,755 for the 3 cases seen in the open TLIF group, as they occurred within 5 weeks of the original surgery. Distributing these additional costs, the mean cost of the open TLIF group thus rises to $25,000 per surgery, thereby resulting in a mean 1-year difference of approximately $5105 per patient. For the 144 patients treated with MI-TLIF, this could represent a cost saving of $735,123 at 1 year to the institution. In addition to the individual patient benefits already discussed.

LITERATURE REVIEW

The literature documents improvement in functional outcomes for patients with degenerative disc disease, recurrent disc herniation, spondylolysis, or spondylolisthesis treated by TLIF.[1,42–44] The traditional open technique provides excellent 3-column bony fusion and decompression of neurologic elements from a single, posterior midline incision. The posterior approach to a 3-column arthrodesis avoids potential injury to anterior or retroperitoneal structures.[45–47] By removing the facet joint, a posterolateral approach via TLIF permits direct access to the disc space for interbody fusion, minimizing retraction or injury to the thecal sac and nerve roots.[43,44,48–50] However, the benefits of 3-column fusion from a posterior midline open TLIF are diminished by numerous factors: extensive soft-tissue dissection required for a posterolateral approach, increased operative blood loss, necessity for blood transfusions, increased postoperative pain, and extended recovery time.[51–54]

MI-TLIF is performed through a paramedian incision, preserving the posterior tension band and attachments of the paraspinal musculature. Muscle-splitting tubes are used to minimize soft-tissue trauma, resulting in decreased operative blood loss, diminished postoperative pain, and a quicker recovery time.[2,3,20,25,29,55–61] The perioperative benefits of minimally invasive approaches to the lumbar spine are well documented in the literature.

Similarly, clinical and radiographic outcomes of MI-TLIF have shown excellent results comparable with those of open TLIF (see **Table 1**). Numerous studies, mostly retrospective in nature, have consistently demonstrated statistical similarity of long-term improvement in VAS scores, ODI scores, and bony fusion rates between groups, with durability of clinical improvement over several years.[5,8,17,22–24,28,33,35–38,41,62] The perioperative outcomes of MI-TLIF appear to be better than those for open TLIF; studies have generally showed a decrease in length of hospital stay, intraoperative blood loss, and perioperative narcotic use.[4,8,17,22,23,28,30,33,36] Of significance, MI-TLIF is cost-effective in comparison with open TLIF.[22]

Aggregated data from multiple studies allows better understanding of the reported long-term outcomes of MI-TLIF (see **Table 1**, column 1).

Studies were systematically searched for back and/or leg VAS scores, ODI scores, and fusion rates, the most commonly reported outcome measures for MI-TLIF. The available data were included if documented for a follow-up of at least 1 year. Collectively, the data demonstrated robust outcomes of MI-TLIF. On average, VAS scores for back and leg pain improved 4.76 and 5.34 points, or 71.2% and 75.7%, respectively. ODI decreased 29.5 points on average, an improvement of 60.3%. Overall bony fusion rate was calculated at 93.5%. As summarized earlier, the authors' data from the 144 MI-TLIF patients demonstrate similar outcomes for the VAS Back, VAS Leg, and ODI scores at 1 and 2 years. As this report represents one of the largest and longest follow-up MI-TLIF series published to date, these benefits have also been demonstrated to be maintained over 4 years. Moreover, statistical superiority of the MI-TLIF technique with regard to back pain was also observed in the 4-year ODI (26 vs 33) and VAS Back (2.25 vs 3.95) scores. Although the exact causes of this observation require further study, the authors believe that the overall decreased tissue trauma and iatrogenic biomechanical destabilization associated with open TLIF exposures may play a significant role in this finding. This notion is indeed supported by the overall increased reoperation rate in the open TLIF group (20.4% vs 8.3% MI-TLIF). These data are partially accounted for by the 5.6% incidence of delayed postoperative wound revisions and debridements for infection/seromas, which clearly would be associated with more tissue trauma, paraspinal muscle injury/atrophy, and worsened long-term scarring of the posterior musculoligamentous complex. Finally, the 7.4% versus 2.1% incidence of reoperation seen in the open TLIF group for symptomatic adjacent segment degeneration ($P = .01$) would also seem to hint at the biomechanically less invasive nature of the MI-TLIF approach.

Complications from MI-TLIF are similar to those of open TLIF (injury to the nerve root, durotomy, wound infection), with some added caveats (see **Tables 2** and **3**; **Table 4**). An injury to the nerve roots may lead to a dermatomal or myotomal loss of function. Fracture of the K-wire during percutaneous pedicle screw placement may lead to a foreign body that is difficult to remove. A postoperative hematoma may result in progressive pain in the back or lower extremity, weakness, or bladder and bowel dysfunction requiring emergent exploration and evacuation. A wound infection may present with expanding erythema around the incision site, swelling, fluctuance, tenderness, drainage from the wound, or systemic signs of

Table 4
Summary of MI-TLIF complications in the literature

Authors,[Ref.] Year	n	Complications	Rate
Adogwa et al,[4] 2011	15	None	
Archavlis and Carvi,[5] 2013	24	2 contralateral radiculopathy 2 revision surgery 1 durotomy 1 malpositioned screw (reoperation) 1 pseudarthrosis 1 ASD	29%
Deutsch and Musacchio,[7] 2006	20	2 durotomy 1 radiculopathy (reoperation to adjust L5 pedicle screw)	
Dhall et al,[8] 2008	21	2 transient L5 sensory loss 1 malpositioned screw (reoperation) 1 cage migration (reoperation) 1 pseudarthrosis	
Isaacs et al,[58] 2005	20	1 transient leukopenia (due to perioperative antibiotic)	
Kim et al,[11] 2009	46	1 nerve-root injury (screw misplacement) 1 UTI 1 wound dehiscence	
Lau et al,[63] 2011	10	1 wound infection 1 pseudarthrosis 1 ventricular tachycardia and subfascial infection (reoperation) 1 instrumentation not connected (reoperation)	40%

Lau et al,[14] 2013	16	Normal Weight
		  1 durotomy
		Obese
		  1 transient radiculopathy
			Normal
			1/7 (14.3%)
			Obese
			1/9 (11.1%)

Lee et al,[16] 2008	27	1 drug eruption 1 UTI	7.4%

Lee and Fessler,[64] 2012	84	3 Major
		  1 CHF
		  1 respiratory distress
		  1 bowel injury
		17 Minor
		  5 urinary retention
		  3 durotomy
		  2 arrhythmias
		  1 leg dysesthesia
		  1 corneal abrasion
		  1 *Clostridium difficile* infection
		  1 neuromonitoring issue
		  1 UTI
		  1 transient hypoxia
		  1 pneumonia
			Young
			8/49 (16.33%)
			Elderly
			7/35 (20%)

Lee et al,[17] 2012	72	1 Major
		  1 malpositioned screw (reoperation)
		2 Minor
		  1 durotomy
		  1 pneumonia
		4 Technical
		  4 cage migrations (asymptomatic)	

(continued on next page)

Table 4
(*continued*)

Authors,[Ref.] Year	n	Complications	Rate
Luo et al,[18] 2012	16	None	0%
Park et al,[21] 2011	66	15 nonunion 2 adjacent segment disease (reoperation) 1 deep wound infection (reoperation)	18/66 (27.3%)
Peng et al,[23] 2009	29	2 iliac crest bone graft site infection	2/29 (6.9%)

Rosen et al,[25] 2008	107	Normal
		  2 urinary retention
		  1 LE weakness
		  1 durotomy
		  1 wound infection
		  1 CHF exacerbation
		  1 HTN
		  1 hypotension
		  1 ileus
		Overweight
		  3 delirium
		  3 postop. radiculopathy
		  1 durotomy
		  1 urinary retention
		  1 HTN
		  1 hypotension
		Obese
		  2 delirium
		  2 postop. radiculopathy
		  1 positioning injury
		  1 urinary retention
			Normal
			9/38
			
			Overweight
			10/34
			
			Obese
			6/35

Schizas et al,[28] 2009	18	3 nonunion/pseudarthrosis 1 durotomy 1 brachial plexus injury (transient) 1 L5 root paresis (transient)	

Schwender et al,[29] 2005	49	2 malpositioned screw (reoperation)
		2 new radiculopathy (reoperation)
		  1 graft dislodgment
		  1 contralateral neuroforaminal stenosis	

Selznick et al,[65] 2009	31	Primary Surgery
		  1 durotomy
		  1 intraoperative pedicle fracture
		Revision Surgery
		  3 CSF leak
		  1 screw malposition
		  1 seizure (due to AVM)
			Primary
			2/17
			
			Revision
			5/14

Shunwu et al,[30] 2010	32	2 malpositioned screw 3 superficial wound infection 1 ileus >3 d	
Tsahtsarlis and Wood,[32] 2012	34	2 malpositioned screw 1 PE 1 neurologic symptom (transient unilateral L5 nerve-root pain)	

(*continued on next page*)

Table 4
(continued)

Authors,[Ref.] Year	n	Complications	Rate

Villavicencio et al,[33] 2010	76	14 Major
		   5 neurologic deficit >3 mo
		   4 malpositioned screw (reoperation)
		   3 malpositioned allograft (reoperation)
		   1 infection
		   1 conversion to open
		10 Minor
		   3 neurologic deficit <3 mo
		   3 malpositioned screw
		   2 hematoma
		   1 durotomy
		   1 anemia
			Major
			18.4%
			
			Minor
			13.2%

Villavicencio et al,[66] 2006	73	6 Major
		   3 neurologic deficit >3 mo
		   2 infection
		   1 malpositioned screw (reoperation)
		16 Minor
		   8 malpositioned screw (no reoperation)
		   5 neurologic deficit <3 mo
		   3 hematomas
			Major
			8.2%
			
			Minor
			21.9%

Wang et al,[36] 2010	42	2 radiculopathy
		   1 graft dislodgement
		   1 epidural hematoma
		2 durotomy
		1 nonunion	

Wang et al,[37] 2011	25	3 durotomy 1 nonunion	
Wang et al,[38] 2012	43	4 durotomy 2 superficial wound infection 1 nonunion	9.5%

Wu et al,[39] 2012	151	7 Major
		   6 malpositioned screw
		   1 neurologic deficit (foot drop)
		9 Minor
		   7 durotomy without CSF leak
		   1 urinary retention
		   1 pneumonia
			16/151
			10.6%

Abbreviations: ASD, adjacent segment disease; AVM, arteriovenous malformation; CHF, congestive heart failure; CSF, cerebrospinal fluid; HTN, hypertension; LE, lower extremity; PE, pulmonary embolism; UTI, urinary tract infection.

an infection (fever, tachycardia, leukocytosis, or progressively elevated inflammatory markers). CSF leakage may present with postoperative postural headaches, active leakage of clear fluid from the incision site, high output of clear fluid from a surgical drain, or expanding pseudomeningocele on postoperative imaging. In most cases, MI-TLIF approaches with CSF leaks are successfully treated with flat bed rest for 24 hours. If the CSF leak persists, options include placement of a lumbar drain, radiology placement of a blood patch, or operative exploration for primary repair.

When compared with the published literature, complications reviewed herein, and **Table 4**, the incidence and type of complications seen in the present series are very similar, with the same benefits in wound infection, transfusion, and hematoma. As this series is again one of the longest in duration, the authors are also one of the first to observe the increased incidence of adjacent-level revision surgery (7.4% vs 2.1%) at 4 years seen in the open TLIF group. Again, it is likely that this phenomenon is due to the biomechanically less destabilizing nature of the MI-TLIF approach, although additional study will be needed with larger multicenter trials to further understand this observation. Of the risks of MI-TLIF, perhaps the most serious is the greater than 2-fold increase in the amount of radiation exposure per procedure (1.90 mSv vs 0.75 mSv). Thus it is essential for surgeons and operating room personnel to wear complete protective gear including aprons, thyroid shields, eyewear, and lead gloves to minimize radiation exposure. Stepping away from the fluoroscopic beam and judicious use of low-exposure "spot" shots are also important in this regard. For the 144 cases discussed here the cumulative radiation exposure was 273.6 mSv over a 34-month period, which is associated with a 2.7% increased lifetime risk of cancer. Additional improvements in the MI-TLIF workflow as well as the incorporation of guidance and virtual imaging technologies are clearly needed to reduce this radiation risk to both patients and clinicians.

SUMMARY

The present series of 144 MI-TLIF patients prospectively compared with 54 open TLIF patients demonstrates statistically significant benefits in operating room time, blood loss, primary infection rates, secondary medical complications, LOS, transfusion need, hospital costs, short-term and long-term pain outcomes, and short-term and long-term ODI scores. With the decreased muscle trauma and likely decreased iatrogenic instability from MI-TLIF approaches, a trend is also observed toward decreased adjacent-level reoperation at 4 years. A review of the literature clearly demonstrates that MI-TLIF can be performed safely, with excellent long-term outcomes. Published series of MI-TLIF demonstrate decreased operative blood loss, shorter duration of hospitalization, and similar long-term clinical outcomes when compared with open TLIF. The data from the present series match closely with published series in this regard. For these reasons, the authors believe that adoption of MI-TLIF will continue to grow as the evidence of its superiority continues to grow in the evidence-based outcomes literature. However, the steep surgical learning curve and the increased radiation exposure associated with MI-TLIF procedures will still need to be addressed as a greater number of surgeons continue to adopt them into their daily spinal surgical practice.

ACKNOWLEDGMENTS

The authors would like to thank Ms Kim Catbagan, Ms Almace Ignacio, Mrs Kristine Khoo, and Mrs Lorena Castillo, without whose assistance in collecting standardized outcome data, VAS scores, clinical follow-up data, and follow-up radiographic images/measurements this study would simply not have been achievable.

REFERENCES

1. Harms J, Rolinger H. A one-stage procedure in operative treatment of spondylolistheses: dorsal traction-reposition and anterior fusion (author's transl). Z Orthop Ihre Grenzgeb 1982;120:343–7.
2. Asgarzadie F, Khoo LT. Minimally invasive operative management for lumbar spinal stenosis: overview of early and long-term outcomes. Orthop Clin North Am 2007;38:387–99 [abstract vi–vii].
3. Khoo L, Palmer S, Laich D, et al. Percutaneous posterior lumbar interbody fusion: a cadaveric pre-clinical study and preliminary case series. Neurosurgery 2002;51(Suppl 5):200–10.
4. Adogwa O, Parker SL, Bydon A, et al. Comparative effectiveness of minimally invasive versus open transforaminal lumbar interbody fusion: 2-year assessment of narcotic use, return to work, disability, and quality of life. J Spinal Disord Tech 2011;24:479–84.
5. Archavlis E, Carvi YN. Comparison of minimally invasive fusion and instrumentation versus open surgery for severe stenotic spondylolisthesis with high-grade facet joint osteoarthritis. Eur Spine J 2013;22(8):1731–40.
6. Beringer WF, Mobasser JP. Unilateral pedicle screw instrumentation for minimally invasive transforaminal lumbar interbody fusion. Neurosurg Focus 2006;20:E4.
7. Deutsch H, Musacchio MJ Jr. Minimally invasive transforaminal lumbar interbody fusion with unilateral pedicle screw fixation. Neurosurg Focus 2006;20:E10.
8. Dhall SS, Wang MY, Mummaneni PV. Clinical and radiographic comparison of mini-open transforaminal lumbar interbody fusion with open transforaminal lumbar interbody fusion in 42 patients with long-term follow-up. J Neurosurg Spine 2008;9:560–5.
9. Jang JS, Lee SH. Minimally invasive transforaminal lumbar interbody fusion with ipsilateral pedicle screw and contralateral facet screw fixation. J Neurosurg Spine 2005;3:218–23.
10. Kasliwal MK, Deutsch H. Clinical and radiographic outcomes using local bone shavings as autograft in minimally invasive transforaminal lumbar interbody fusion. World Neurosurg 2012;78:185–90.
11. Kim JS, Kang BU, Lee SH, et al. Mini-transforaminal lumbar interbody fusion versus anterior lumbar interbody fusion augmented by percutaneous pedicle screw fixation: a comparison of surgical outcomes in adult low-grade isthmic spondylolisthesis. J Spinal Disord Tech 2009;22:114–21.

12. Kim JS, Jung B, Lee SH. Instrumented minimally invasive spinal-transforaminal lumbar interbody fusion (MIS-TLIF); minimum 5-years follow-up with clinical and radiologic outcomes. J Spinal Disord Tech 2012. [Epub ahead of print].

13. Kim MC, Chung HT, Kim DJ, et al. The clinical and radiological outcomes of minimally invasive transforaminal lumbar interbody single level fusion. Asian Spine J 2011;5:111–6.

14. Lau D, Ziewacz J, Park P. Minimally invasive transforaminal lumbar interbody fusion for spondylolisthesis in patients with significant obesity. J Clin Neurosci 2013;20:80–3.

15. Lee CK, Park JY, Zhang HY. Minimally invasive transforaminal lumbar interbody fusion using a single interbody cage and a tubular retraction system: technical tips, and perioperative radiologic and clinical outcomes. J Korean Neurosurg Soc 2010; 48:219–24.

16. Lee DY, Jung TG, Lee SH. Single-level instrumented mini-open transforaminal lumbar interbody fusion in elderly patients. J Neurosurg Spine 2008; 9:137–44.

17. Lee KH, Yue WM, Yeo W, et al. Clinical and radiological outcomes of open versus minimally invasive transforaminal lumbar interbody fusion. Eur Spine J 2012;21:2265–70.

18. Luo W, Zhang F, Liu T, et al. Minimally invasive transforaminal lumbar interbody fusion aided with computer-assisted spinal navigation system combined with electromyography monitoring. Chin Med J (Engl) 2012;125:3947–51.

19. Min SH, Yoo JS. The clinical and radiological outcomes of multilevel minimally invasive transforaminal lumbar interbody fusion. Eur Spine J 2013;22: 1164–72.

20. Park P, Foley KT. Minimally invasive transforaminal lumbar interbody fusion with reduction of spondylolisthesis: technique and outcomes after a minimum of 2 years' follow-up. Neurosurg Focus 2008;25:E16.

21. Park Y, Ha JW, Lee YT, et al. Surgical outcomes of minimally invasive transforaminal lumbar interbody fusion for the treatment of spondylolisthesis and degenerative segmental instability. Asian Spine J 2011;5:228–36.

22. Parker SL, Mendenhall SK, Shau DN, et al. Minimally invasive versus open transforaminal lumbar interbody fusion (TLIF) for degenerative spondylolisthesis: comparative effectiveness and cost-utility analysis. World Neurosurg 2013. [Epub ahead of print].

23. Peng CW, Yue WM, Poh SY, et al. Clinical and radiological outcomes of minimally invasive versus open transforaminal lumbar interbody fusion. Spine (Phila Pa 1976) 2009;34:1385–9.

24. Rodriguez-Vela J, Lobo-Escolar A, Joven E, et al. Clinical outcomes of minimally invasive versus open approach for one-level transforaminal lumbar interbody fusion at the 3- to 4-year follow-up. Eur Spine J 2013;22(12):2857–63.

25. Rosen DS, Ferguson SD, Ogden AT, et al. Obesity and self-reported outcome after minimally invasive lumbar spinal fusion surgery. Neurosurgery 2008; 63:956–60 [discussion: 60].

26. Rouben D, Casnellie M, Ferguson M. Long-term durability of minimal invasive posterior transforaminal lumbar interbody fusion: a clinical and radiographic follow-up. J Spinal Disord Tech 2011;24: 288–96.

27. Scheufler KM, Dohmen H, Vougioukas VI. Percutaneous transforaminal lumbar interbody fusion for the treatment of degenerative lumbar instability. Neurosurgery 2007;60:203–12 [discussion: 12–3].

28. Schizas C, Tzinieris N, Tsiridis E, et al. Minimally invasive versus open transforaminal lumbar interbody fusion: evaluating initial experience. Int Orthop 2009;33:1683–8.

29. Schwender JD, Holly LT, Rouben DP, et al. Minimally invasive transforaminal lumbar interbody fusion (TLIF): technical feasibility and initial results. J Spinal Disord Tech 2005;18(Suppl):S1–6.

30. Shunwu F, Xing Z, Fengdong Z, et al. Minimally invasive transforaminal lumbar interbody fusion for the treatment of degenerative lumbar diseases. Spine (Phila Pa 1976) 2010;35:1615–20.

31. Sonmez E, Coven I, Sahinturk F, et al. Unilateral percutaneous pedicle screw instrumentation with Minimally Invasive TLIF for the treatment of recurrent lumbar disk disease: 2 years follow-up. Turk Neurosurg 2013;23:372–8.

32. Tsahtsarlis A, Wood M. Minimally invasive transforaminal lumber interbody fusion and degenerative lumbar spine disease. Eur Spine J 2012;21:2300–5.

33. Villavicencio AT, Burneikiene S, Roeca CM, et al. Minimally invasive versus open transforaminal lumbar interbody fusion. Surg Neurol Int 2010; 1:12.

34. Villavicencio AT, Nelson EL, Mason A, et al. Preliminary results on feasibility of outpatient instrumented transforaminal lumbar interbody fusion. J Spinal Disord Tech 2012;26(6):298–304.

35. Wang HL, Lu FZ, Jiang JY, et al. Minimally invasive lumbar interbody fusion via MAST Quadrant retractor versus open surgery: a prospective randomized clinical trial. Chin Med J (Engl) 2011; 124:3868–74.

36. Wang J, Zhou Y, Zhang ZF, et al. Comparison of one-level minimally invasive and open transforaminal lumbar interbody fusion in degenerative and isthmic spondylolisthesis grades 1 and 2. Eur Spine J 2010;19:1780–4.

37. Wang J, Zhou Y, Zhang ZF, et al. Minimally invasive or open transforaminal lumbar interbody fusion as revision surgery for patients previously treated by

open discectomy and decompression of the lumbar spine. Eur Spine J 2011;20:623–8.

38. Wang J, Zhou Y, Feng Zhang Z, et al. Comparison of clinical outcome in overweight or obese patients after minimally invasive versus open transforaminal lumbar interbody fusion. J Spinal Disord Tech 2012. [Epub ahead of print].

39. Wu WJ, Liang Y, Zhang XK, et al. Complications and clinical outcomes of minimally invasive transforaminal lumbar interbody fusion for the treatment of one- or two-level degenerative disc diseases of the lumbar spine in patients older than 65 years. Chin Med J (Engl) 2012;125:2505–10.

40. Xue H, Tu Y, Cai M. Comparison of unilateral versus bilateral instrumented transforaminal lumbar interbody fusion in degenerative lumbar diseases. Spine J 2012;12:209–15.

41. Zairi F, Arikat A, Allaoui M, et al. Transforaminal lumbar interbody fusion: comparison between open and mini-open approaches with two years follow-up. J Neurol Surg A Cent Eur Neurosurg 2013;74:131–5.

42. Houten JK, Post NH, Dryer JW, et al. Clinical and radiographically/neuroimaging documented outcome in transforaminal lumbar interbody fusion. Neurosurg Focus 2006;20:E8.

43. Moskowitz A. Transforaminal lumbar interbody fusion. Orthop Clin North Am 2002;33:359–66.

44. Rosenberg WS, Mummaneni PV. Transforaminal lumbar interbody fusion: technique, complications, and early results. Neurosurgery 2001;48:569–74 [discussion: 74–5].

45. Faciszewski T, Winter RB, Lonstein JE, et al. The surgical and medical perioperative complications of anterior spinal fusion surgery in the thoracic and lumbar spine in adults. A review of 1223 procedures. Spine (Phila Pa 1976) 1995;20:1592–9.

46. McDonnell MF, Glassman SD, Dimar JR 2nd, et al. Perioperative complications of anterior procedures on the spine. J Bone Joint Surg Am 1996;78:839–47.

47. Rajaraman V, Vingan R, Roth P, et al. Visceral and vascular complications resulting from anterior lumbar interbody fusion. J Neurosurg 1999; 91:60–4.

48. Brantigan JW, Steffee AD, Lewis ML, et al. Lumbar interbody fusion using the Brantigan I/F cage for posterior lumbar interbody fusion and the variable pedicle screw placement system: two-year results from a Food and Drug Administration investigational device exemption clinical trial. Spine (Phila Pa 1976) 2000;25:1437–46.

49. Brantigan JW, Neidre A, Toohey JS. The Lumbar I/F Cage for posterior lumbar interbody fusion with the variable screw placement system: 10-year results of a Food and Drug Administration clinical trial. Spine J 2004;4:681–8.

50. Wetzel FT, LaRocca H. The failed posterior lumbar interbody fusion. Spine (Phila Pa 1976) 1991;16: 839–45.

51. Gejo R, Matsui H, Kawaguchi Y, et al. Serial changes in trunk muscle performance after posterior lumbar surgery. Spine (Phila Pa 1976) 1999;24: 1023–8.

52. Rantanen J, Hurme M, Falck B, et al. The lumbar multifidus muscle five years after surgery for a lumbar intervertebral disc herniation. Spine (Phila Pa 1976) 1993;18:568–74.

53. Sihvonen T, Herno A, Paljarvi L, et al. Local denervation atrophy of paraspinal muscles in postoperative failed back syndrome. Spine (Phila Pa 1976) 1993;18:575–81.

54. Styf JR, Willen J. The effects of external compression by three different retractors on pressure in the erector spine muscles during and after posterior lumbar spine surgery in humans. Spine (Phila Pa 1976) 1998;23:354–8.

55. Fessler RG, O'Toole JE, Eichholz KM, et al. The development of minimally invasive spine surgery. Neurosurg Clin N Am 2006;17:401–9.

56. Foley KT, Holly LT, Schwender JD. Minimally invasive lumbar fusion. Spine (Phila Pa 1976) 2003; 28:S26–35.

57. Holly LT, Schwender JD, Rouben DP, et al. Minimally invasive transforaminal lumbar interbody fusion: indications, technique, and complications. Neurosurg Focus 2006;20:E6.

58. Isaacs RE, Podichetty VK, Santiago P, et al. Minimally invasive microendoscopy-assisted transforaminal lumbar interbody fusion with instrumentation. J Neurosurg Spine 2005;3:98–105.

59. Lawton CD, Smith ZA, Barnawi A, et al. The surgical technique of minimally invasive transforaminal lumbar interbody fusion. J Neurosurg Sci 2011; 55:259–64.

60. Shih P, Wong AP, Smith TR, et al. Complications of open compared to minimally invasive lumbar spine decompression. J Clin Neurosci 2011;18:1360–4.

61. Wong AP, Smith ZA, Lall RR, et al. The microendoscopic decompression of lumbar stenosis: a review of the current literature and clinical results. Minim Invasive Surg 2012;2012:325095.

62. Habib A, Smith ZA, Lawton CD, et al. Minimally invasive transforaminal lumbar interbody fusion: a perspective on current evidence and clinical knowledge. Minim Invasive Surg 2012;2012: 657342.

63. Lau D, Lee JG, Han SJ, et al. Complications and perioperative factors associated with learning the technique of minimally invasive transforaminal lumbar interbody fusion (TLIF). J Clin Neurosci 2011; 18:624–7.

64. Lee P, Fessler RG. Perioperative and postoperative complications of single-level minimally invasive

transforaminal lumbar interbody fusion in elderly adults. J Clin Neurosci 2012;19:111–4.

65. Selznick LA, Shamji MF, Isaacs RE. Minimally invasive interbody fusion for revision lumbar surgery: technical feasibility and safety. J Spinal Disord Tech 2009;22:207–13.

66. Villavicencio AT, Burneikiene S, Bulsara KR, et al. Perioperative complications in transforaminal lumbar interbody fusion versus anterior-posterior reconstruction for lumbar disc degeneration and instability. J Spinal Disord Tech 2006;19:92–7.

Minimally Invasive Extracavitary Transpedicular Corpectomy for the Management of Spinal Tumors

Rajiv Saigal, MD, PhD[a], Rishi Wadhwa, MD[a],
Praveen V. Mummaneni, MD[b], Dean Chou, MD[b],*

KEYWORDS

- Minimally invasive spine surgery • Spine metastasis • Spinal tumors • Extracavitary
- Transpedicular corpectomy • Epidural spinal cord compression

KEY POINTS

- For patients with metastatic epidural spinal cord compression, circumferential surgical decompression combined with adjuvant radiotherapy leads to improved ambulation and may improve urinary continence, pain, Frankel scores, and overall survival.
- To achieve circumferential decompression and maintain or restore spinal stability, tumor resection and reconstruction of the anterior spinal column is often required.
- Compared with combined anteroposterior approaches, transpedicular corpectomy has a lower complication rate, lower estimated blood loss, and shorter operative time, and showed improved American Spinal Injury Association scores.
- Typically, minimally invasive cases involve use of tubular retractors at the corpectomy level, but this may inhibit complete vertebral body resection and makes expandable cage placement more difficult, and therefore many surgeons opt for a mini-open approach.
- Compared with open transpedicular corpectomy, minimally invasive spine surgery and mini-open approaches also lead to effective neurologic improvement and pain alleviation, with a trend toward reduced operative times, blood loss, and complication rates.

 Video of Mini-Open Transpedicular Corpectomy T12 Metastatic Renal Cell Cancer accompanies this article at http://www.neurosurgery.theclinics.com/

INTRODUCTION: NATURE OF THE PROBLEM

Spinal metastasis is a large and growing clinical problem. As cancer survivors live longer because of improved adjuvant therapies, the burden of spinal metastasis is expected to increase.[1–3] Estimates of metastatic epidural spinal cord compression cases range from 8400 to 25,000 annually in the United States, with approximately 76,000

Disclosures: None (Dr R. Saigal & Dr R. Wadhwa); Royalties: DePuy Spine, Quality Medical Publishing, Thieme Publishers, Honoraria: Globus, Stock: Spinicity (Dr P.V. Mummaneni); Consultant: Globus, Honoraria: Depuy, Orthofix (Dr D. Chou).

[a] Department of Neurological Surgery, University of California, San Francisco, 505 Parnassus Avenue, San Francisco, CA 94143-0112, USA; [b] Department of Neurological Surgery, UCSF Spine Center, University of California, San Francisco, 505 Parnassus Avenue, San Francisco, CA 94143-0112, USA
* Corresponding author. Department of Neurological Surgery, University of California, San Francisco, 505 Parnassus Avenue, Box 0112, San Francisco, CA 94143-0112.
E-mail address: ChouD@neurosurg.ucsf.edu

Neurosurg Clin N Am 25 (2014) 305–315
http://dx.doi.org/10.1016/j.nec.2013.12.008

hospitalizations from 1998 to 2006.[4–6] Among patients dying of cancer, 3.4% are hospitalized annually because of spinal metastasis, with mean hospitalization charges of $61,655 in 2006.[4] A much higher number, between 30% and 90% of deceased patients with cancer, have been found to harbor spinal metastasis in cadaver studies.[7] Older studies showed that breast, lung, and prostate cancers were the most common sources, in descending order.[8–10] However, a more modern study using the Nationwide Inpatient Sample (NIS) showed a rearranging in relative prevalence: lung cancer (24.9%), prostate cancer (16.2%), multiple myeloma (11.1%), lymphoma (8.7%), breast cancer (6.9%), renal cell carcinoma (3.5%), and colorectal carcinoma (2.1%).[4] Pain and neurologic dysfunction are the most common presenting findings,[2] and appropriate clinical treatment is critically important.

Palliative surgical decompression for spinal metastatic lesions was once a controversial topic. Early data on surgical intervention showed mixed results, likely because of inadequate decompression with laminectomy alone.[11–13] As surgical treatment advanced to include circumferential decompression, results improved.[7] In 2005, the landmark Patchell study showed definitively that surgical decompression with adjuvant radiation leads to functional neurologic improvement for patients with metastatic epidural spinal cord compression and neurologic deficits.[3] Although the primary outcome was ambulation (84% of the cohort with surgery plus radiation vs 57% of the cohort with radiation alone), improvement was also seen in the secondary outcome measures of urinary continence, pain, Frankel scores, and overall survival. A recent retrospective study even showed a trend toward increased survival with repeat surgery for recurrent spinal metastasis (19.6 vs 12.8 months; $P = .085$).[14]

The thoracic spine receives 70% of spinal metastases, followed by 20% for the lumbar spine and 10% for the cervical; the vertebral body is the most common site.[15] For patients with spinal instability from a pathologic vertebral body fracture but without neurologic deficit, vertebral augmentation may be a viable treatment option.[16] For others with neurologic deficit from epidural spinal cord compression, corpectomy is often necessary. Early techniques of corpectomy and anterior column reconstruction involved anterior approaches through the thoracic cavity.[17] Since then, extracavitary approaches have grown in popularity because of their more streamlined approach and decreased morbidity. Extracavitary transpedicular corpectomy with expandable cage placement allows for circumferential decompression and anterior column reconstruction from a posterior approach.

Posterior transpedicular corpectomies can be completed from an open, mini-open, or minimally invasive approach. Percutaneous pedicle screw placement has been associated with decreased multifidus atrophy, decreased blood loss, and comparable clinical outcomes relative to open screw placement.[18,19] Small series on minimally invasive[20] or mini-open[21] approaches for decompression of metastatic epidural lesions have shown promising early results. A systematic review of minimally invasive spine surgery approaches in the management of metastatic spine disease found effective neurologic improvement and pain alleviation, and trends toward reduced operative times, blood loss, and complication rates relative to traditional open approaches.[2] As one such example, this article reviews mini-open extracavitary transpedicular corpectomy for management of these complex metastatic lesions.

PREOPERATIVE PLANNING

Considerable preoperative planning is required before undertaking a minimally invasive transpedicular corpectomy for spinal metastasis. Discussion with a medical and radiation oncologist is necessary to determine propriety for surgery. Multiple complementary imaging modalities aid surgical planning. Use of neuromonitoring and discussion with anesthesia regarding perfusion goals enhances patient safety.

Oncologic Consultation

For patients with new diagnoses of spinal metastasis, consultation with both a medical oncologist and a radiation oncologist is suggested. Patchell criteria for spinal decompression include nonmedical primary tumors and expected survival of at least 3 months.[3] The medical oncologist can ensure completion of staging to estimate survival. The medical oncologist can additionally comment on cancer-related or medically related comorbidities that may preclude surgery. For example, many patients with cancer have immunosuppression and/or poor nutritional status that diminish the chances of successful postoperative recovery.[7] If the burden of illness is too high or expected survival is less than 3 months, the patient is likely a poor candidate for surgical intervention.

A radiation oncologist may also be consulted to assess the radiosensitivity of the lesion. Metastatic spine lesions from radiosensitive leukemia, lymphomas, germ-cell tumors, and multiple myeloma are usually better treated with radiation alone. If deemed appropriate for surgery, there is still a role for discussion and planning of adjuvant postoperative radiation. Traditionally, postoperative radiation consisted of conventional external-beam radiotherapy delivered in 10 fractions of 3 Gy each.[3] However, stereotactic radiosurgery is an emerging therapy with improved local control. Many tumors that are traditionally considered radioresistant do actually respond to stereotactic radiosurgery, and in some of these cases surgery may not be necessary.[22] These examples include renal cell carcinoma and colon cancer.[22] The radiation oncologist can be helpful in discussing the optimal extent of intended surgical resection. Nonetheless, cases of acute neurologic deficit and/or instability generally require surgical intervention.

Imaging

Radiograph, computed tomography (CT), and magnetic resonance imaging (MRI) provide complementary information and should all be part of the preoperative planning when possible. If the spine is sufficiently stable and the patient can tolerate upright radiographs (sitting or preferably standing), sagittal balance can be assessed under weight-bearing conditions. These imaging modalities can often reveal significant abnormalities not obvious on a supine examination. CT is best for evaluating bone quality and extent of tumor invasion. The number of levels requiring vertebrectomy and reconstruction can then be determined. Additionally, measurements of adjacent pedicle size are useful in the planning of implanted hardware. MRI is best for visualizing the neural elements and assessing the exact locations of spinal cord or nerve compression. Gadolinium-enhanced MRI sequences precisely define the tumor anatomy and may reveal subtle findings not readily visible on CT. **Fig. 1** shows preoperative imaging in a case example involving a 56-year-old man with metastatic melanoma to T10.

Angiography/Embolization

Preoperative angiography is generally not required but should be considered for vascular tumors. Angiography can define the tumor vasculature and influence the surgical approach. In particular, identification of the segmental level and side of the artery of Adamkiewicz helps the surgeon avoid compromise of this important segmental feeder.[23,24] For vascular tumors such as renal cell and thyroid carcinoma, preoperative embolization of important feeding vessels can decrease intraoperative blood loss. However, risk of intraoperative blood loss must be weighed against risk

of neurologic deficit from preoperative embolization, as high as 25% in some series.[17]

Neuromonitoring

Use of real-time neuromonitoring is a helpful adjunct for the surgeon performing a transpedicular corpectomy. Somatosensory-evoked potentials (SSEP), motor-evoked potentials (MEP), and electromyographic signals can provide the surgeon with immediate feedback throughout the case. The mechanism of transpedicular vertebral body resection often destabilizes the spine, and the authors typically use temporary rod placement to protect against unplanned translation of the spinal column. Any spinal translation could stretch or kink the cord and may result in MEP or SSEP changes. Similarly, any downward pressure on the cord during surgery could cause injury. If alerted by MEP or SSEP changes, the surgeon may pause surgery, make technical adjustments, and/or request an increased mean arterial pressure (MAP) to aid in cord perfusion.

Use of Approach Surgeon

An approach surgeon is not needed for the posterior mini-open transpedicular carpectomy, which is a major advantage over open anterior thoracoabdominal or open lateral approaches.

Anesthetic Concerns

Open discussion with anesthesia before incision is helpful to protect neural function. It is important to remember that the most common indication for spinal tumor surgery is epidural spinal cord compression. The compressed spinal cord is already in a compromised position. Further hemodynamic insults with episodes of hypotension may add risk of spinal cord injury. A clear MAP goal can be discussed with the anesthesiologist and maintained for the duration of the case. A common goal is to maintain MAP greater than 85 mm Hg.[25] If any episodes of hypotension occur during the case, a surgical pause can allow the anesthesiologist to correct the MAP before resuming surgery.

Intraoperative Imaging

The surgeon must choose between intraoperative plain films, fluoroscopy, and/or CT scan to localize the level of interest. Sometimes the pathologic level is easy to visualize because of fracture, loss of vertebral body height, and/or pathologic angulation. However, the thoracic spine is notoriously difficult to visualize, especially in obese patients. The authors recommend localization in the

A Sagittal T1 post-contrast

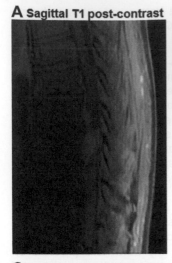

B Axial T1 post-contrast at T10

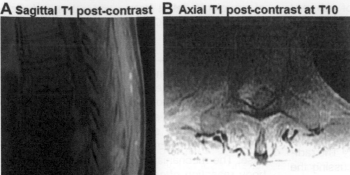

C Axial CT scan at T10

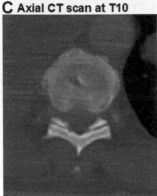

D PET scan

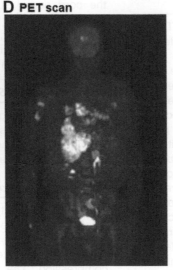

Fig. 1. Preoperative imaging in a 56-year-old man with metastatic melanoma to T10. (*A*) Sagittal T1 with gadolinium enhancement shows the metastatic lesion causes epidural spinal cord compression. (*B*) Axial T1 contrast image at T10 shows that the epidural compression was primarily right-sided. (*C*) Axial computed tomography scan, bone window, at T10. Some loss of bone density is seen in the vertebral body, but the metastatic lesion itself is not well visualized. (*D*) Positron emission tomography whole-body scan shows metastatic disease involving the skeleton, lungs, mediastinum and hila, and adrenal glands.

thoracic spine with anteroposterior views identifying the C7-T1 junction. It is critical to understand that the T1 rib is broad, round, and extremely close to the T2 rib. However, rib counting on intraoperative radiographs can be challenging. For patients with a large body habitus, an abnormal number of ribs, or transitional lumbar vertebrae, or for those harboring small metastatic lesions, preoperative CT-guided fiducial screw placement decreases localization time and radiation exposure and helps avoid wrong-level surgery.[26]

SURGICAL APPROACH
Preparation and Patient Positioning

After general anesthesia is induced, the patient is placed prone on the operating room table. A Jackson table is favored because of its radiolucence. This feature is particularly important if an

anteroposterior radiograph is used for localization. All pressure points are padded. The authors tuck the arms for thoracic spine abnormalities. A preoperative radiograph is taken to localize the level. The patient's skin is sterilely prepped and surgical drapes are applied with sufficient space to span the planned upper and lower instrumented vertebrae and to allow for localization.

Surgical Procedure

Although multiple percutaneous stab incisions are a viable option, the authors prefer a single midline skin incision but separate fascial incisions. In their experience (and also the experience of Dr Rick Fessler and Dr Michael Wang), the single midline incision leads to better postoperative cosmesis.[27,28] Hemostasis is obtained with monopolar electrocautery. The dissection is then performed in the extrafascial plane to minimize disruption of the fascia and the underlying soft tissues.

Intraoperative radiography is used to confirm the intended surgical levels. Using a posterior pedicle screw fixation system, the authors then place minimally invasive pedicle screws at least 2 and often 3 levels above and below the intended corpectomy level. This procedure is generally performed with fluoroscopic guidance. Image-guided screw placement is also an option that may minimize radiation exposure to the surgeon and operating room staff. For fluoroscopic guidance, Jamshidi needles are first introduced into the pedicles. From an anteroposterior view, the lateral aspect or midpoint of the pedicle is targeted. The Jamshidi is first gently docked in the cortical bone with a mallet. A lateral image is then taken to ensure a trajectory parallel to the pedicle. After correcting the trajectory, anteroposterior imaging should be used during the first 15 to 20 mm of Jamshidi advancement, taking care not to breach the medial pedicle border and risk entry into the spinal canal. After reaching this depth with no medial breach, the Jamshidi should be advanced a few millimeters further into the vertebral body under lateral fluoroscopy. A Kirschner wire (K-wire) is then gently placed through the center of the Jamshidi needle into the vertebral body. Once the K-wire is docked a few centimeters into the vertebral body, the Jamshidi is carefully and slowly removed. The K-wire should be held in place with a needle driver or hemostat while removing the Jamshidi to prevent inadvertent K-wire removal, which would necessitate restarting the procedure.

Once the Jamshidi is removed and the K-wire is retained at a suitable depth, a cannulated tap and then a cannulated screw is placed over the K-wire. Frequent lateral imaging is a critical safety mechanism during screw advancement. Friction from the cannulated screw can easily carry the K-wire anteriorly through the front of the vertebral body during screw advancement. This important pitfall must be avoided to prevent injury to the aorta, pleura, and other vital structures ventral to the vertebral body. Through bobbing the K-wire up and down by a few millimeters during the placement of the screw, the surgeon can avoid the problem of the K-wire being forced anteriorly during screw placement. Once the cannulated screw is advanced through the pedicle and into the vertebral body, the K-wire can be safely removed. The screw can then be advanced to the final desired depth. The same procedure is then repeated to place the remaining pedicle screws. **Fig. 2** illustrates the technique for minimally invasive pedicle screw placement.

After placement of all screws, a decompressive laminectomy is performed at the pathologic levels. **Fig. 3**A shows the fascial opening at this level. The laminectomy is performed widely to include removal of the transverse processes. Even in the absence of dorsal compression or mass, a laminectomy is still performed to access the spine and achieve circumferential decompression in case the tumor recurs at the index level. The inferior portion of the superior adjacent lamina and the superior portion of the inferior adjacent lamina are also removed to allow for further decompression of the spinal canal. The ligamentum flavum is fully removed. Thoracic nerve roots may be ligated if they are surrounded by tumor, but often only unilateral ligation is necessary. Because of the possibility of ischemic injury, the nerve root may be clipped first with a temporary clip or ligature, and then the surgeon can wait 5 to 15 minutes to monitor MEP and SSEP signals. If the signals are stable, then the nerve root may be sacrificed without too much worry that this will inhibit spinal cord perfusion and function. During this waiting period, the authors proceed with ipsilateral pedicle removal using rongeurs and a high-speed drill. The remaining pedicle is removed. The intervertebral discs surrounding the corpectomy level should be identified and the correct level corroborated again with lateral radiographic imaging.

The transpedicular corpectomy is then completed using a combination of high-speed burr, curettes, and osteotomes to remove all of the bone at the pathologic levels. Multiple specimens of metastatic tumor are sent to the pathology laboratory for diagnosis. To prevent spine translation, an ipsilateral temporary rod is placed after completion of corpectomy on one side. Once the spine is stabilized, the remaining vertebral body is removed from the contralateral side. After all bone is removed, great care is taken to remove the posterior longitudinal ligament (PLL). The PLL should be carefully dissected off of the ventral dura because it is often filled with tumor, and leaving the PLL can lead to immediate recurrence. Once dissected, a safe plane is maintained with a Woodson dissector and the PLL is cut rostrally and caudally with a 15 blade, then removed. The discs bordering the corpectomy are removed and the endplates are prepared with a rasp.

To create a pathway for cage placement, the rib head must be mobilized. The rib head can be resected altogether, but that necessitates pleural dissection and risks pneumothorax.[27] Alternatively, a less-invasive option is to preserve the rib head while drilling open a hinge with a matchstick bur. The hinge is drilled approximately 3 cm

A Surgeon's view

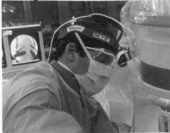

B Jamshidi needle placement

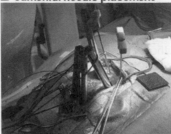

C Lateral C-arm x-ray during Jamshidi placement

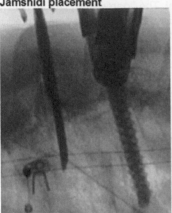

D AP x-ray. K-wire remains after right Jamshidi is removed

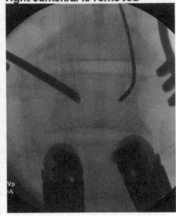

E Cannulated pedicle screw is advanced under x-ray guidance

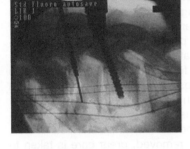

Fig. 2. Minimally invasive pedicle screw placement. (*A*) Surgeon's view. The C-arm is shown at top right, positioned for anteroposterior (AP) imaging. The fluoroscopy monitor is shown at top left. (*B*) Jamshidi needles (*upper right*) are placed at the next level while caudal screw heads are retracted and kept together with a band (*bottom left*). (*C*) Lateral C-arm radiograph during Jamshidi placement. Jamshidi is seen at left in the image. The implanted pedicle screw for the adjacent caudal level is seen at right. (*D*) Anteroposterior radiograph after K-wire placement on the right. A Jamshidi needle is seen on the left. Previously placed pedicle screws are seen at the adjacent caudal level (*bottom of image*). (*E*) Lateral C-arm radiograph shows advancing cannulated pedicle screw over guiding K-wire.

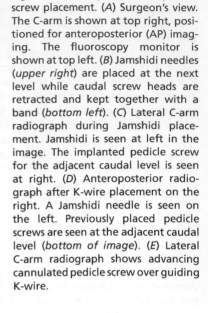

A Fascial opening for corpectomy

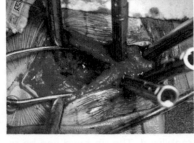

B Expandable cage placement, intra-op x-ray

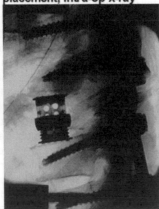

Fig. 3. Expandable cage placement. (*A*) Fascia is opened and retracted at the corpectomy level. (*B*) Lateral intraoperative radiograph shows cage placement after expansion.

lateral to the costovertebral junction. The rib head can then swing inwards in a "trapdoor" fashion, allowing space for cage placement.[27] The pleura remains intact deep to the rib and no pleural dissection is needed. An expandable cage is selected and packed with autograft and/or allograft material. The cage is advanced lateral to the spinal cord while pushing laterally on the rib head. The cage is medialized once it is safely past the spinal cord. Once in the desired position, the cage is expanded to make contact with the surrounding endplates. Anteroposterior and lateral radiographs verify correct placement of the cage. If necessary, the cage can be contracted, adjusted, and reexpanded. Additional graft material can be placed around the cage to increase the likelihood of arthrodesis.

After verification of final cage placement (see **Fig. 3**B), the final rods are placed and set screws are positioned and tightened. One or two crosslinks are placed. The entire wound is irrigated with several liters of antibiotic or iodine-based irrigation. Two large-bore drains are left in the epidural space to prevent epidural hematoma. Highlights from the surgical procedure are shown in the supplemental Video 1.

IMMEDIATE POSTOPERATIVE CARE

Patients are usually monitored in the intensive care unit for one night with hourly neurologic checks. Patients are given intravenous electrolyte fluid replacement until they are awake and recovered sufficiently to tolerate oral intake. Pain is controlled through a patient-controlled analgesic device delivering morphine or hydromorphone; oral narcotics; or muscle relaxants as needed. Sequential compressive devices are used in patients who are supine.

REHABILITATION AND RECOVERY

Patients are usually transferred to the surgical ward on postoperative day one. Physical and occupational therapy begin on the same day to mobilize the patient. Activity orders include getting out of bed to chair with meals and ambulation with assistance 3 times per day. Deep venous thrombosis prophylaxis with subcutaneous heparin commences at 48 hours postoperatively. Patients typically undergo postoperative anteroposterior and lateral radiographs to fully visualize the implanted hardware. If the patient is able to tolerate standing anteroposterior and lateral 36-inch-long cassette radiographs, these are also completed to assess alignment with weight-bearing. The authors typically do not use any external orthoses

in these patients. **Fig. 4** shows postoperative imaging for the example case of a 56-year-old man with metastatic melanoma to T10, status post mini-open T10 transpedicular corpectomy/expandable cage placement, and T8-T12 posterior spinal fusion with instrumentation.

CLINICAL RESULTS IN THE LITERATURE

Open thoracotomy is a viable approach to the thoracic spine, with risks including hemothorax, chylothorax, pleural effusion, atelectasis, and pulmonary contusion.[29,30] Although this approach offers clear ventral visualization of the metastatic vertebral body, complication rates hover around 11.0% to 11.5%.[29,31] In an initial technical note of 8 mini-open transpedicular corpectomy cases from 2008 to 2009, the authors found a mean estimated blood loss of 1250 mL and a low complication rate.[21] No statistical difference was seen between open and mini-open cases for these parameters, but this was only a technical note, not results from a large series. One mini-open wound infection was seen in a patient with multiple percutaneous stab incisions, but no infections were seen in the 7 cases of a single midline incision. No epidural hematomas were seen, which compared favorably with a 25% hematoma rate in a matched cohort of open transpedicular corpectomy. For the mini-open cases, 1 of 8 required reoperation for inferior screw pullout, but this case had only 1 instrumented level above and below the corpectomy.[21] The current standard is for at least 2 and often 3 levels of instrumentation rostral and caudal to the corpectomy level. Many patients with cancer will have poor bone density associated with their disease, and more levels of instrumentation are needed for adequate biomechanical strength.

Although the approach described here is mini-open, other minimally invasive options use a tubular retractor at the corpectomy level.[32] Kim and colleagues[32] tested a minimally invasive technique in 6 cadavers and then demonstrated utility in 4 clinical cases. In the clinical cases, they reported an average estimated blood loss of 495 mL, a mean operating time of 5.8 hours, a 4.7-day average length of stay, and neurologic improvement in the 3 patients with preoperative symptoms. However, they used a unilateral tubular retractor at the corpectomy level, which prevented complete resection of the vertebral body on the contralateral side.

Mummaneni,[33] and later Lall and colleagues,[30] reviewed the 4 major approaches to the ventral thoracic spinal canal: transthoracic, retropleural, costotransversectomy, and transpedicular (shown

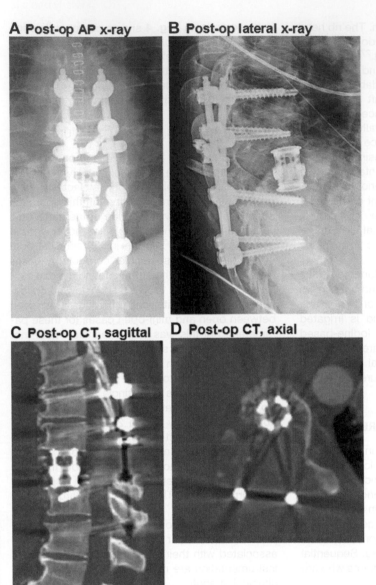

A Post-op AP x-ray

B Post-op lateral x-ray

C Post-op CT, sagittal

D Post-op CT, axial

Fig. 4. Postoperative imaging. (A) Anteroposterior radiograph and (B) lateral radiograph demonstrate good hardware placement with expandable cage placement toward the ventral extent of the corpectomy, as intended. (C) Sagittal and (D) axial CT, bone window, show complete vertebral body resection before cage placement.

in **Fig. 5**).[33] Transthoracic approaches traditionally included open thoracotomy but have evolved to minimally invasive video-assisted thoracoscopy (VAT). Advantages include direct access for complete removal of the vertebral body and graft placement, but disadvantages include lack of spinal cord visibility because of the ventral to dorsal approach, anatomic challenges at the thoracolumbar junction because of the diaphragm, need for a second incision if posterior segmental instrumentation is required, and high complication rates ranging from 14% to 29%.[30] Molina and colleagues[2] reviewed data from 6 studies on minimal access surgeries[34–39] and 5 on VAT surgeries,[40–44] and found these modalities were comparable in

estimated blood loss, operating time, length of stay, pain alleviation, neurologic improvement, and complication rate (**Table 1**).[2]

The remaining approaches each have their own unique strengths and weaknesses. Retropleural approaches target the thoracic spine via a window between the endothoracic fascia and the parietal pleura. Retropleural approaches share the advantages of VAT in allowing complete decompression of the canal and diaphragmatic challenges at the thoracolumbar junction.[45] Additionally, the working angle is challenging and risks the segmental arteries, and the necessary extensive dissection makes it easy to violate the pleura.[30,45] Posterolateral or lateral extracavitary approaches avoid

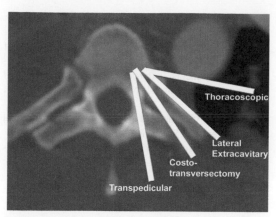

Fig. 5. Minimally invasive approaches to the thoracic spine. (*Modified from* Lall RR, Smith ZA, Wong AP, et al. Minimally invasive thoracic corpectomy: surgical strategies for malignancy, trauma, and complex spinal pathologies. Minim Invasive Surg 2012;2012:213791.)

disruption of the posterior tension band and pleura and allow visualization of the spinal cord by approaching the spine from an oblique angle, but do not allow complete removal of the vertebral body.[30,32]

Table 1
Comparison of minimal access surgery and video assisted thoracoscopy

	Minimal-Access Surgery	Video-Assisted Thoracoscopy
Estimated blood loss, median (range)	905 mL (227–1200 mL)	1113 mL (350–1677 mL)
Operating time, median (range)	3.7 h (2.2–7.0 h)	4.6 h (2.6–6.5 h)
Length of stay, median (range)	5.0 d (4.0–6.25 d)	7.0 d (6.5–7.5 d)
Pain alleviation, median (range)	100% (62.5%–100%)	100% (94%–100%)
Neurologic improvement, median (range)	95% (62.5%–100%)	100% (92%–100%)
Complication rate, median (range)	9% (0%–24%)	0% (0%–54%)

Data from Molina CA, Gokaslan ZL, Sciubba DM. A systematic review of the current role of minimally invasive spine surgery in the management of metastatic spine disease. Int J Surg Oncol 2011;2011:598148.

An important aspect of a minimally invasive or mini-open approach is the lack of arthrodesis at each pedicle screw level. The most destabilized level contains the expandable cage and graft for fusion of the anterior column. Posteriorly, at the pedicle sites, it is possible to dissect down to the facet, decorticate, and place graft material at each segmental level, but this is tedious and adds operative time when performed minimally invasively.[21] Two prospective randomized trials on short-segment pedicle screw instrumentation for thoracolumbar burst fractures found no radiographic or clinical failure at 5- and 7-year follow-up, respectively, in patients who underwent instrumentation without fusion above and below the fractures.[46,47] Decompression and reconstruction cases for spinal metastasis are palliative procedures in patients with limited life expectancy. Therefore, achieving bony fusion is not as paramount a goal as in nontumor clinical settings. Before the advent of expandable titanium cages, anterior column reconstruction was commonly completed with methylmethacrylate and did not even involve arthrodesis at the corpectomy site.[17,48]

The posterior mini-open transpedicular corpectomy offers circumferential decompression and complete metastatic tumor removal from a single midline incision.[21,30] Although prospective and large case series are lacking, initial data suggest rates of neurologic improvement comparable to those of open cases, with low complication rates. Further study is needed to determine if one minimally invasive approach is superior to others. The authors anticipate the continued need for multiple corridors of entry toward the spine, depending on the exact nature and anatomy of the metastatic lesion.

SUMMARY

Metastatic epidural spinal cord compression is an important clinical problem with up to 25,000 cases per year. For patients with greater than 3 months' life expectancy and neurologic deficits, circumferential surgical decompression plus adjuvant radiotherapy is the standard of care. When tumor invades the vertebral body, transpedicular corpectomy allows for this circumferential decompression and anterior column reconstruction from a single posterior approach. Through avoiding invasion of the chest cavity, transpedicular corpectomy represents a less-invasive approach that can be performed without an approach surgeon. Mini-open techniques involve minimally invasive pedicle screw placement, and further minimize disruption of soft tissues. Although class I and II data are lacking, initial data show adequate decompression and neurologic improvement with low estimated blood loss and complication rates.[2,21]

SUPPLEMENTARY DATA

Supplementary data related to this article can be found at http://dx.doi.org/10.1016/j.nec.2013.12.008.

REFERENCES

1. Lu DC, Lau D, Lee JG, et al. The transpedicular approach compared with the anterior approach: an analysis of 80 thoracolumbar corpectomies. J Neurosurg Spine 2010;12:583–91.

2. Molina CA, Gokaslan ZL, Sciubba DM. A systematic review of the current role of minimally invasive spine surgery in the management of metastatic spine disease. Int J Surg Oncol 2011;2011:598148.

3. Patchell RA, Tibbs PA, Regine WF, et al. Direct decompressive surgical resection in the treatment of spinal cord compression caused by metastatic cancer: a randomised trial. Lancet 2005;366:643–8.

4. Mak KS, Lee LK, Mak RH, et al. Incidence and treatment patterns in hospitalizations for malignant spinal cord compression in the United States, 1998-2006. Int J Radiat Oncol Biol Phys 2011;80: 824–31.

5. Schiff D. Spinal cord compression. Neurol Clin 2003; 21:67–86, viii.

6. Witham TF, Khavkin YA, Gallia GL, et al. Surgery insight: current management of epidural spinal cord compression from metastatic spine disease. Nat Clin Pract Neurol 2006;2:87–94 [quiz: 116].

7. Sciubba DM, Petteys RJ, Dekutoski MB, et al. Diagnosis and management of metastatic spine disease. A review. J Neurosurg Spine 2010;13:94–108.

8. Brihaye J, Ectors P, Lemort M, et al. The management of spinal epidural metastases. Adv Tech Stand Neurosurg 1988;16:121–76.

9. Constans JP, de Divitiis E, Donzelli R, et al. Spinal metastases with neurological manifestations. Review of 600 cases. J Neurosurg 1983;59:111–8.

10. Helweg-Larsen S, Sorensen PS. Symptoms and signs in metastatic spinal cord compression: a study of progression from first symptom until diagnosis in 153 patients. Eur J Cancer 1994;30A:396–8.

11. Bilsky MH, Lis E, Raizer J, et al. The diagnosis and treatment of metastatic spinal tumor. Oncologist 1999;4:459–69.

12. Black P. Spinal metastasis: current status and recommended guidelines for management. Neurosurgery 1979;5:726–46.

13. Young RF, Post EM, King GA. Treatment of spinal epidural metastases. Randomized prospective comparison of laminectomy and radiotherapy. J Neurosurg 1980;53:741–8.

14. Lau D, Leach MR, La Marca F, et al. Independent predictors of survival and the impact of repeat surgery in patients undergoing surgical treatment of spinal metastasis. J Neurosurg Spine 2012;17: 565–76.

15. Byrne TN. Spinal cord compression from epidural metastases. N Engl J Med 1992;327:614–9.

16. Harel R, Angelov L. Spine metastases: current treatments and future directions. Eur J Cancer 2010;46: 2696–707.

17. Gokaslan ZL, York JE, Walsh GL, et al. Transthoracic vertebrectomy for metastatic spinal tumors. J Neurosurg 1998;89:599–609.

18. Dhall SS, Wang MY, Mummaneni PV. Clinical and radiographic comparison of mini-open transforaminal lumbar interbody fusion with open transforaminal lumbar interbody fusion in 42 patients with long-term follow-up. J Neurosurg Spine 2008;9:560–5.

19. Kim DY, Lee SH, Chung SK, et al. Comparison of multifidus muscle atrophy and trunk extension muscle strength: percutaneous versus open pedicle screw fixation. Spine (Phila Pa 1976) 2005;30:123–9.

20. Hansen-Algenstaedt N, Knight R, Beyerlein J, et al. Minimal-invasive stabilization and circumferential spinal cord decompression in metastatic epidural spinal cord compression (MESCC). Eur Spine J 2013;22(9):2142–4.

21. Chou D, Lu DC. Mini-open transpedicular corpectomies with expandable cage reconstruction. Technical note. J Neurosurg Spine 2011;14:71–7.

22. Laufer I, Iorgulescu JB, Chapman T, et al. Local disease control for spinal metastases following "separation surgery" and adjuvant hypofractionated or high-dose single-fraction stereotactic radiosurgery: outcome analysis in 186 patients. J Neurosurg Spine 2013;18:207–14.

23. Charles YP, Barbe B, Beaujeux R, et al. Relevance of the anatomical location of the Adamkiewicz artery in spine surgery. Surg Radiol Anat 2011;33:3–9.

24. Resnick DK, Benzel EC. Lateral extracavitary approach for thoracic and thoracolumbar spine trauma: operative complications. Neurosurgery 1998;43:796–802 [discussion: 802–3].

25. Ryken TC, Hurlbert RJ, Hadley MN, et al. The acute cardiopulmonary management of patients with cervical spinal cord injuries. Neurosurgery 2013; 2(Suppl 72):84–92.

26. Upadhyaya CD, Wu JC, Chin CT, et al. Avoidance of wrong-level thoracic spine surgery: intraoperative localization with preoperative percutaneous fiducial screw placement. J Neurosurg Spine 2012;16:280–4.

27. Chou D, Wang VY. Trap-door rib-head osteotomies for posterior placement of expandable cages after transpedicular corpectomy: an alternative to lateral

extracavitary and costotransversectomy approaches. J Neurosurg Spine 2009;10:40–5.

28. Wang MY, Mummaneni PV. Minimally invasive surgery for thoracolumbar spinal deformity: initial clinical experience with clinical and radiographic outcomes. Neurosurg Focus 2010;28:E9.

29. Fessler RG, Sturgill M. Review: complications of surgery for thoracic disc disease. Surg Neurol 1998;49: 609–18.

30. Lall RR, Smith ZA, Wong AP, et al. Minimally invasive thoracic corpectomy: surgical strategies for malignancy, trauma, and complex spinal pathologies. Minim Invasive Surg 2012;2012:213791.

31. Faciszewski T, Winter RB, Lonstein JE, et al. The surgical and medical perioperative complications of anterior spinal fusion surgery in the thoracic and lumbar spine in adults. A review of 1223 procedures. Spine (Phila Pa 1976) 1995;20:1592–9.

32. Kim DH, O'Toole JE, Ogden AT, et al. Minimally invasive posterolateral thoracic corpectomy: cadaveric feasibility study and report of four clinical cases. Neurosurgery 2009;64:746–52 [discussion: 752–3].

33. Mummaneni PV, Rodts GE, Subach BR, et al. Management of thoracic disc disease. Contemp Neurosurg 2001;23:1–8.

34. Deutsch H, Boco T, Lobel J. Minimally invasive transpedicular vertebrectomy for metastatic disease to the thoracic spine. J Spinal Disord Tech 2008;21:101–5.

35. Huang TJ, Hsu RW, Li YY, et al. Minimal access spinal surgery (MASS) in treating thoracic spine metastasis. Spine (Phila Pa 1976) 2006;31:1860–3.

36. Kan P, Schmidt MH. Minimally invasive thoracoscopic approach for anterior decompression and stabilization of metastatic spine disease. Neurosurg Focus 2008;25:E8.

37. Muhlbauer M, Pfisterer W, Eyb R, et al. Minimally invasive retroperitoneal approach for lumbar corpectomy and anterior reconstruction. Technical note. J Neurosurg 2000;93:161–7.

38. Payer M, Sottas C. Mini-open anterior approach for corpectomy in the thoracolumbar spine. Surg Neurol 2008;69:25–31 [discussion: 31–2].

39. Taghva A, Li KW, Liu JC, et al. Minimally invasive circumferential spinal decompression and stabilization for symptomatic metastatic spine tumor: technical case report. Neurosurgery 2010;66: E620–2.

40. Huang TJ, Hsu RW, Sum CW, et al. Complications in thoracoscopic spinal surgery: a study of 90 consecutive patients. Surg Endosc 1999;13:346–50.

41. Le Huec JC, Lesprit E, Guibaud JP, et al. Minimally invasive endoscopic approach to the cervicothoracic junction for vertebral metastases: report of two cases. Eur Spine J 2001;10:421–6.

42. McLain RF. Spinal cord decompression: an endoscopically assisted approach for metastatic tumors. Spinal Cord 2001;39:482–7.

43. Mobbs RJ, Nakaji P, Szkandera BJ, et al. Endoscopic assisted posterior decompression for spinal neoplasms. J Clin Neurosci 2002;9:437–9.

44. Rosenthal D, Marquardt G, Lorenz R, et al. Anterior decompression and stabilization using a microsurgical endoscopic technique for metastatic tumors of the thoracic spine. J Neurosurg 1996;84:565–72.

45. Uribe JS, Dakwar E, Cardona RF, et al. Minimally invasive lateral retropleural thoracolumbar approach: cadaveric feasibility study and report of 4 clinical cases. Neurosurgery 2011;68:32–9 [discussion: 39].

46. Dai LY, Jiang LS, Jiang SD. Posterior short-segment fixation with or without fusion for thoracolumbar burst fractures. A five to seven-year prospective randomized study. J Bone Joint Surg Am 2009;91: 1033–41.

47. Wang ST, Ma HL, Liu CL, et al. Is fusion necessary for surgically treated burst fractures of the thoracolumbar and lumbar spine?: a prospective, randomized study. Spine (Phila Pa 1976) 2006;31:2646–52 [discussion: 2653].

48. Fourney DR, Abi-Said D, Rhines LD, et al. Simultaneous anterior-posterior approach to the thoracic and lumbar spine for the radical resection of tumors followed by reconstruction and stabilization. J Neurosurg 2001;94:232–44.

Minimally Invasive Anterolateral Corpectomy for Spinal Tumors

Michael S. Park, MD*, Armen R. Deukmedjian, MD, Juan S. Uribe, MD

KEYWORDS

- Minimally invasive • Tumor • Retropleural • Transthoracic • Lateral • Corpectomy

KEY POINTS

- Thoracic tumors can be treated by a variety of different surgical approaches, both anterior and posterior, each of which is associated with morbidity and limitations that can lead to increased recovery time and rate of complications.
- Endoscopic (thoracoscopic) approaches that reduce approach-related morbidity but have a steep learning curve have been described.
- The mini-open anterolateral approach provides direct visualization of the ventral spine and neural elements without the morbidity associated with more traditional approaches.

INTRODUCTION

Surgical approaches for disorders of the thoracolumbar spine have traditionally included an anterior or posterior approach, or some combination of the two. The technique used generally depends on surgeon preference, lesion location, pathologic process, and affected level. Spine tumors are classified as extradural, intradural-extramedullary, or intramedullary. Most of these include benign intradural-extramedullary tumors that may grow to compress neural elements to cause symptoms. In the era of modern medicine, treatment options for primary or metastatic spine tumors include radiation, radiation plus chemotherapy, stereotactic radiosurgery, hormonal therapy, or surgical decompression followed by radiation.[1] However, vertebral tumors often require surgical treatment to obtain tissue for diagnosis, decompress neural elements, control pain, improve quality of life, alleviate symptoms, and address spinal instability pursuant to encroachment of the osseous anatomy. Radiation and chemotherapy alone are options for patients either with palliation in mind, or with newly diagnosed disease that shows no evidence of neurologic compromise or spinal instability. When surgery is indicated, the surgeon must consider histologic type of the tumor, prior treatments, tumor location (in the global spinal picture but also within the vertebral body or spinal column), and the patient's life expectancy.

More than 90% of spinal column tumors in the United States are metastatic, most commonly from breast, lung, and prostate, while 30% to 70% of patients with cancer have vertebral involvement.[2–6] The thoracic spine is most commonly involved with neoplasm (70%), followed by lumbar (20%) and cervical (10%), while multiple levels are affected in up to one-third of cases.[2,5] Approximately half of all spinal tumors are extradural, 35% to 40% are intradural-extramedullary, and the remaining 5% to 10% are intramedullary.[7,8]

Disclosure: J.S. Uribe is a consultant for NuVasive, Inc and Orthofix.
Department of Neurosurgery & Brain Repair, Morsani College of Medicine, University of South Florida, 2 Tampa General Circle, 7th Floor, Tampa, FL 33606, USA
* Corresponding author.
E-mail address: mpark1@health.usf.edu

In comparison with metastatic disease, primary osseous neoplasms are uncommon and are classified as benign or malignant. Such tumors can include osteoid osteoma, osteoblastoma, osteochondroma, aneurysmal bone cyst, eosinophilic granuloma, and cavernous hemangioma among the benign lesions; malignant pathology can include giant cell tumor, plasma cell tumor, lymphoma, osteosarcoma, chondrosarcoma, chordoma, and Ewing sarcoma.[9] Patients most commonly present to their physician with complaints of progressive back or neck pain, although weakness may be a presenting symptom in cases where neural elements are compressed. Treatment options vary based on complete or incomplete deficits. One of the greatest stimuli for the advent of minimally invasive surgical (MIS) approaches is the reduction of morbidity through traditional surgery. This aspect is especially evident in the thoracic spine, where traditional anterior and posterior approaches are associated with significant morbidity. This article describes MIS anterolateral corpectomy in the treatment of spinal tumors, and reviews the current literature.

ANTERIOR-BASED APPROACHES

Traditional surgical approaches for the treatment of spinal tumors include anterior-based and posterior-based approaches, or a combination of both.[10–14] Anterior transthoracic approaches have long been established in the management of many pathologic conditions of the anterior thoracic spine. The anterior approach offers easier access to the ventral aspect of the spine and allows decompression without the associated risks of spinal cord or nerve root manipulation,[13–15] but often requires a thoracotomy. There is significant morbidity associated with a thoracotomy, including pain from a large incision and increased muscle dissection, prolonged chest drainage, pulmonary complications such as contusions, atelectasis, effusions, hemothorax and chylothorax, and an extended hospital stay.[16] Major complications with use of the thoracotomy approach have been shown in as many as 79% of patients.[17,18] A lateral retropleural approach aims to be less destructive to the surrounding tissues by not compromising the pleura and using serial dilation as a course to the abnormality. In a more anterior approach the abnormality is encountered first, and the neural elements cannot be visualized until ventral decompression is completed. However, in the lateral retropleural approach the surgeon is able to visualize the thecal sac during the approach to the lesion, affording access to both the thecal sac and the abnormality at the same time. Occasionally the

anterior longitudinal ligament may need to be resected, potentially leading to destabilization.

To mitigate some of the morbidity of the anterior approaches, MIS thoracoscopic techniques were developed and have proved to be effective, but challenging, in terms of learning curve and application. These approaches have been adopted as a means of gaining anterior access to the thoracic spine without requiring large incisions or rib resection.[19–24] Complications, including transient intercostal neuralgia, postoperative atelectasis, pneumothorax and hemothorax, and pleural effusion, are considered to occur with a lower incidence than for open thoracotomies, with a reported range of 14.1% to 29.4%.[23] The lateral retropleural MIS approach to the thoracolumbar spine is considered a variant of the thoracotomy, but combines many of the positive attributes of both anterolateral transthoracic approaches and the lateral extracavitary approach. It affords the surgeon the ability to remain outside the pleura while achieving a ventral decompression of the dural sac, which is especially important with centrally located abnormalities.

POSTERIOR-BASED APPROACHES

Indications for posterior approaches in spine oncologic surgery, which were first introduced by Capener[25] and later modified by Larson and colleagues,[10] include tumors involving the posterior elements or extending into the anterior column. Resection of the posterior elements, epidural tumor, and involved vertebral bodies can be performed through the transpedicular, costotransversectomy, or lateral extracavitary approach, depending on the location of the tumor and how far lateral and anterior the surgeon wishes to be. In general, posterior approaches to perform a corpectomy for tumor resection require the surgeon to visualize and occasionally manipulate the neural elements before encountering the abnormality.[26] These approaches have the advantage of being familiar to most neurosurgeons, allowing for vertebral reconstruction and simultaneous posterior spinal instrumentation and fixation, and are especially suitable for upper thoracic lesions and multilevel disease, or in the setting of multiple medical comorbidities.[27] However, visualization of the dural elements is limited to an oblique view. Extensive muscle dissection is required, and may be associated with copious blood loss. Sectioning of nerve roots may be required for placement of an interbody device, and its size or footprint is limited secondary to constraints imposed by a posterior approach, potentially leading to an increased rate of subsidence or pseudarthrosis.

Surgical decompression of ventrally located cord-compressive lesions and the durability of kyphosis correction in patients with significant ventral column destruction from a solely posterior approach have been unsatisfactory.[11,28]

The lateral retropleural extracavitary approach[10,11,29] is a posterior-based option that provides access to the ventral vertebral column, but is associated with dissection of the lateral paravertebral musculature. It permits a direct view of the dura, neural elements, and any anterior abnormality simultaneously, and allows exposure of the lateral canal without potentially sacrificing the intercostal nerve or intraforaminal radiculomedullary artery.[22,24] The dissection remains extrapleural, in contrast to the transthoracic approach, with a decreased risk of injury to the aorta, vena cava, and sympathetic plexus, as well as development of a duropleural cerebrospinal fluid (CSF) fistula.[11,30,31] This approach is less destabilizing, with preservation of the anterior and posterior longitudinal ligaments and the posterior ligamentous structures. Just as for the other open techniques, a relatively large incision and extensive rib resection are again required.

In either case, proceeding through a traditional open approach leads to longer incisions than those required through a MIS approach. Larger wounds may prove more difficult to heal, particularly in this patient population who are often subjected to immunosuppressive chemotherapy and radiation for treatment of their underlying neoplasms.[32,33] Patient pain and discomfort are also minimized through a less invasive approach from decreased surgical trauma. The advancement of several technologies, including tubular and expandable retractors, specialized instruments, and fiber-optic light sources, have allowed for the development of MIS techniques. In the following sections, the authors present their technique for MIS anterolateral approaches for the treatment of spinal tumors.

LATERAL-BASED APPROACHES

In an effort to avoid the morbidity related to a thoracotomy/thoracoscopic approach and the limited access/extensive tissue dissection associated with posterior approaches, McCormick[11] developed the lateral retropleural thoracotomy. This technique permits a direct view of the neural elements without the need to dissect or potentially sacrifice the intercostal nerve or intraforaminal radiculomedullary artery.[1,22,24] Because of the extrapleural nature of the approach, there is less risk of injury to the aorta, vena cava, and sympathetic plexus, and a reduced risk of developing a

duropleural CSF fistula.[11,30] The anterior and posterior longitudinal ligaments are preserved, in addition to the posterior ligamentous structures, which provides for a less destabilizing surgery. However, this approach requires a significant incision and extensive rib resection (**Fig. 1**).

The MIS lateral approach uses the already outlined fundamental principles that provide a benefit from using the lateral retropleural approach. However, because of technological advances in retraction and instrumentation as well as fiber-optic light sources, the MIS version allows for a much smaller incision and a smaller amount of rib resection (**Fig. 2**). Blood loss, postoperative pain, time to mobilization, and hospital stay are all reduced with MIS approaches.[34–37] However, they demand a significant amount of experience and entail a steep learning curve. The next section outlines the steps used in this procedure.

Surgical Technique and Anatomic Considerations

Preoperative planning

Initial evaluation begins with the history and physical examination. Pain, usually progressive in nature and either localized to the back or in a radicular distribution, is the most common presenting symptom. Neurologic deficit manifesting as motor weakness and/or sensory derangement can occur from compression or involvement of the spinal cord or nerve root, particularly for intradural tumors. Progressive spinal deformity may also occur.[1,9]

Radiographic evaluation nearly always includes magnetic resonance imaging (MRI) with and without contrast or, if MRI is precluded, a computed tomography (CT) myelogram, to delineate the lesion and assess the degree of neural compression. CT is recommended to determine the extent of vertebral involvement and for surgical planning. Standing scoliosis radiographs can be

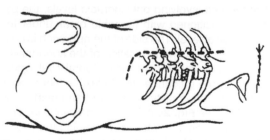

Fig. 1. Lateral extrapleural thoracotomy approach. (*From* Schmidt MH, Larson SJ, Maiman DJ. The lateral extracavitary approach to the thoracic and lumbar spine. Neurosurg Clin N Am 2004;15:438; with permission.)

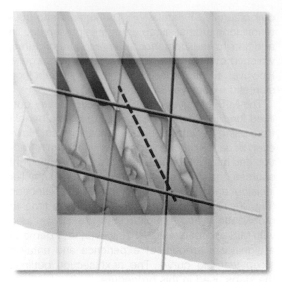

Fig. 2. Minimally invasive surgical approach with smaller incision and rib resection.

obtained to assess for any deformity, and flexion-extension films are appropriate if there are questions regarding instability. Radioisotope bone scans are sensitive for spinal column tumors demonstrating osteolytic or osteoblastic activity, and are frequently used for small lesions such as osteoid osteoma or for detecting metastases in the setting of known malignancy.[38] Angiography is useful for hypervascular tumors, such as aneurysmal bone cyst, hemangioma, renal cell carcinoma, melanoma, or chordoma, to determine their blood supply and for preoperative embolization to reduce intraoperative blood loss.[39–41]

Preparation and patient positioning

The surgical techniques for the MIS lateral approach for access to the thoracic spine have been described previously.[1,42,43] The patient is positioned under fluoroscopic guidance and is secured in a true and direct lateral decubitus position on a flexible radiolucent surgical table. For procedures involving only thoracic levels, the patient is positioned with the table break under the midsurgical level. The side of the approach is chosen depending on the location of the abnormality, surrounding viscera, and the vertebral level. Under fluoroscopic guidance, the index vertebral body level and abnormality are located and marked on the skin (see **Fig. 2**). A 3- to 6-cm oblique incision is marked parallel to the rib traversing the pathologic vertebral body at the midaxillary line.

Surgical approach

The incision is made obliquely over the rib across the region delineated by the skin markings made previously. Dissection is carried down through the subcutaneous tissue to the ribs or intercostal space. Five centimeters of the immediately underlying rib, directly over the lesion, is dissected in a subperiosteal fashion. Using a rib dissector or Cobb elevator, the rib is removed from the underlying pleura and neurovascular bundle, removed, and saved for autograft. The intercostal muscles and parietal pleura are incised to enter the thoracic cavity for a transthoracic approach, while the parietal pleura is swept anteriorly with blunt finger dissection for a retropleural approach. Further rib resection may be required if a larger exposure is needed. The rib resected for access to the thoracolumbar junction usually corresponds to 2 levels above the desired vertebral level (ie, 10th rib for access to T12, 11th rib for L1, and 12th rib for L2).[43]

An index finger is used to enter the pleural space (for a transpleural approach) or the plane between the endothoracic fascia and pleura (for a retropleural approach). The appropriate plane is developed, and diaphragm and/or lung are mobilized anteriorly using a finger and/or sponge stick until the lateral face of the vertebral body, pedicle, and adjacent intervertebral discs are exposed. For access to the thoracolumbar junction, it should be noted that removal of the diaphragmatic-costal attachment may be required. Because of the lateral (costal) diaphragmatic insertion, and for access to L1, the lumbar or posterior attachments of the diaphragm must be sharply transected off the transverse process of L1. The intervening attachment between the medial and lateral arcuate ligaments must also be cut to fully expose the lateral vertebral body. If more anterior exposure of the vertebral body is needed, the ipsilateral crus, which extends along the anterolateral spine to L2 on the left and L3 on the right, may also be transected.[43] Complications arising from this technique have yet to be reported, but further analysis may be mandated. For a left-sided approach, the aorta and hemiazygos vein are also retracted anteriorly. Segmental vessels are ligated as proximally as possible. Sequential tubular dilators are then inserted, and an expandable retractor system (MaXcess; NuVasive, Inc, San Diego, CA) is inserted over the largest dilator and secured with a flexible table-mounted arm assembly (**Fig. 3**).

Surgical procedure

With the retractor placed and adequate exposure obtained, the operation is continued using standard surgical techniques. Resection of tumor, decompression of neural elements, and, when necessary, stabilization of the spine can be performed using this approach. For a guide to the

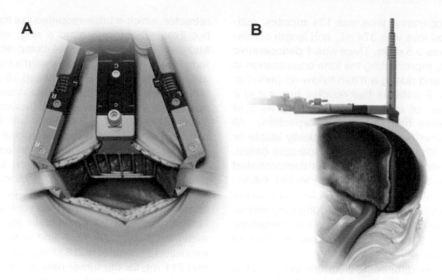

Fig. 3. (*A*) Operative view of expandable retractor. (*B*) Cross-sectional depiction of lateral approach with table-mounted retractor system.

location and proximity of the spinal canal, dural exposure is performed before the corpectomy by removing the pedicle with rongeurs and a high-speed drill. The intervertebral discs above and below the vertebral body of interest are then removed, and osteotomes are used to delineate the area of the corpectomy. At this point, bony removal can be achieved using a combination of rongeurs, curettes, high-speed drills, and osteotomes. A thin layer of bone on the ventral and contralateral sides of the body and the anterior longitudinal ligament are preserved to protect mediastinal and thoracic structures.

For corpectomies, ventral reconstruction is performed using expandable titanium cages, biological allograft, and the rib autograft harvested during the approach. Spinal instrumentation is completed using ventrolateral plate/screw fixation through the expandable retractor and/or percutaneous posterior pedicle screw/rod fixation. Dural repair, when necessary after resection of intradural tumor, is performed with a running 5-0 suture. The dural repair is reinforced with fibrin glue, and CSF is drained through a lumbar catheter.

Following a transthoracic approach or in the event of a pleural violation air must be removed from the pleural cavity, which is traditionally accomplished by placement of a chest tube. Alternatively, a red rubber catheter can be situated in the pleural space through the wound, and placed under a water trap (ie, with the distal end submerged under water). The surgical wound is closed in standard fashion, including the muscular and fascial layers. The red rubber catheter is secured with a purse-string stitch, and a Valsalva

maneuver with end-inspiratory hold is performed until no more air bubbles are observed to emanate from the submerged distal end of the catheter, representing evacuation of all air from the thoracic cavity. The red rubber catheter is removed as the purse string is tied. This technique obviates the use of a chest tube.

Postoperative care

A chest radiograph is obtained in the recovery room and on the morning of postoperative day 1, to verify the absence of pneumothorax if the aforementioned red rubber technique was used, or to verify placement and position of a chest tube if one was placed intraoperatively. In this case, it is initially placed on suction and weaned to water seal; serial chest radiographs are obtained to confirm reexpansion of the lung before removal of the chest tube. Declining oxygen saturation or recurrence of a pneumothorax warrants further evaluation and, if necessary, surgical reexploration. It is the authors' practice to mobilize patients postoperatively with thoracolumbosacral orthoses, and obtain upright radiographs to verify hardware placement and stability.

Outcomes Using a Minimally Invasive Anterolateral Approach

Uribe and colleagues[1] presented a series of 21 consecutive patients treated for thoracic spine tumors via an MIS lateral approach, 13 of who required corpectomy. Overall, the mean operating time was 117 minutes, estimated blood loss was 291 mL, and length of hospital stay was 2.9 days; for the group undergoing corpectomy, the mean operating time was 124 minutes, estimated blood loss was 374 mL, and length of hospital stay was 3.5 days. There was 1 perioperative pneumonia, representing the lone complication in the series, and during a mean follow-up period of 21 months, 2 patients had residual tumor and 2 patients died of extraspinal metastasis. All 5 of these patients had undergone corpectomy. All patients either remained neurologically stable or improved with regard to their preoperative deficit, and pain and outcome measures demonstrated improvement from preoperatively to last follow-up. All patients required rib resection. No patient required single-lung ventilation during the procedure. However, subtotal resection of metastatic tumors (5 of 21) was not considered a failure of the technique.

Comparable data in the literature are scarce. A MEDLINE search performed on July 21, 2013 including the terms "corpectomy," "spinal fractures," "spinal fusion," "thoracic vertebrae," "postoperative complications," "lumbar vertebrae," "spinal cord compression," "minimally invasive," "MIS," and "tumor" revealed 367 articles, more than 95% of which pertained to intracranial, cervical, or peritoneal visceral disease, were not available in English, or were limited to percutaneous vertebroplasty or kyphoplasty. There are several series of MIS approaches for spinal tumor, but in each case the approach was posterior or posterolateral for epidural or intradural-extramedullary tumors.[44–46] There was one series of 8 transpedicular partial vertebrectomies without vertebral reconstruction,[47] and one case report of a transpedicular vertebrectomy with expandable titanium cage placement and percutaneous posterior instrumentation and fusion from T1 to T8.[48] The latter case reported a blood loss of 1400 mL with a total operative time of 7 hours; the patient had a good neurologic outcome and was discharged on postoperative day 5.

Outcomes with the MIS anterolateral approach compare favorably with those of thoracoscopic techniques; Ragel and colleagues[49] reported on a series of 21 anterior vertebral body reconstructions, 6 for tumor. Operative time, estimated blood loss, and length of hospital stay in this subset of patients were 4.9 hours, 758 mL, and 8.2 days, respectively. There was no difference with regard to these variables in a comparison with another group of 10 patients from the same institution who also underwent anterior vertebral body reconstruction via a traditional, open approach.[49]

Perhaps the best comparison can be found in a series of 39 patients undergoing corpectomy, 11 for tumor, by mini-open approaches using the SynFrame (Stratec Medical, Oberdorf, Switzerland)

retractor, which is table-mounted like the MaXcess but fixes retractors around a ring, whereas the MaXcess is an expandable tubular retractor system. Five of the patients underwent a transthoracic approach for abnormality between T5 and T11; 3 patients underwent a transthoracic transdiaphragmatic approach for abnormality between T12 and L2; and the remaining 3 patients with lumbar abnormality underwent a retroperitoneal approach. Aside from use of a double-lumen endotracheal tube for ipsilateral lung deflation on entering the pleural cavity, slightly longer incisions and rib resections (6–10 cm in this series vs 6 cm), and chest-tube placement, the technique was largely similar. Including all patients in the series the mean total operative time and estimated blood loss was 181 minutes and 632 mL, and 188 minutes and 711 mL for the tumor patients. For the transthoracic patients, inclusive of both tumor and trauma patients, the mean total operative time and estimated blood loss were 178 minutes and 535 mL; for those undergoing the transthoracic transdiaphragmatic approach, 178 minutes and 644 mL. Complications included a durotomy repaired with fibrin glue and muscle patch, a superficial wound infection, a postoperative ileus, and 2 cases of ilioinguinal hypesthesia.[50]

An earlier study also using the SynFrame reviewed the outcomes of 65 consecutive cases of anterior vertebral reconstruction via mini-open transthoracic approach (for thoracic or thoracolumbar abnormality) or retroperitoneal approach (for lumbar abnormality), 6 of which were for metastatic disease. The overall mean operating time was 170 minutes and blood loss was 912 mL; in the tumor cases the mean operative time was 112 minutes, which extended to 153 minutes in cases when removal of intracanal tumor or debris was necessary. In 4 of the metastatic cases, the reconstruction was performed using expandable Synex cages (Stratec Medical, Switzerland); the other 2 reconstructions were performed with steel plates filled with acrylic cement. In none of the 65 cases was single-lung ventilation necessary, nor were there any cases of intercostal neuralgia or post-thoracotomy complications.[51]

Mühlbauer and colleagues[52] presented a small series of 5 lumbar anterior reconstructions, 1 for metastatic prostate tumor. The mean operative time in their series was 6 hours (5.1 hours for the anterior decompression and 7.25 hours for the 360° fusion) and the mean estimated blood loss was 1120 mL. To facilitate exposure, the MIASPAS self-retaining retractor system was used. This system does not require table mounting, but is instead secured in place with 2 anchoring screws at the adjacent vertebral levels, analogous to a Caspar pin retraction system for anterior cervical discectomy. The surgical approach used was similar to the description given herein of the lateral access to the lumbar spine,[53] except that the investigators transected the medial insertions of the psoas and retracted the muscle dorsally. The tumor patient was fully ambulatory at 1 year.[52]

Advantages of the Minimally Invasive Lateral Approach

The MIS lateral approach offers the advantages of using smaller incisions, leading to fewer wound-related complications and somatic pain, earlier mobilization, and shorter recovery times, which have been shown for other spine indications to increase pulmonary and metabolic function and decrease the risk of medical complications related to inactivity.[54] Decreased blood loss, reduced incidence of unintended CSF leak, greater preservation of biomechanically important spinal anatomy, and decreased incidence of postoperative spinal instability and deformity are additional advantages of MIS approaches to spinal tumors.[9] In comparison with more traditional approaches, adequate exposure to achieve the goals of surgery can be obtained with direct visualization of the abnormality while avoiding the extensive muscle dissection associated with posterior approaches or single-lung ventilation, large incision, and extensive rib resection required by anterior approaches. Furthermore, for a retropleural approach, tumor cell dissemination into the chest cavity is limited or prevented in comparison with open thoracotomy.[1]

Limitations of the Minimally Invasive Lateral Approach

One major drawback of the MIS lateral approach is that the working distance is long in a relatively narrow working space. Familiarity with MIS techniques and experience working through these retractor systems is recommended. Dissection through the retropleural space may be rendered difficult if adhesions from previous ipsilateral thoracotomy are present. Similarly, spinal osteomyelitis and/or metastases can manifest with adhesive thickening of the parietal pleura and/or infiltration of the pleura by tumor or inflammatory fibrous tissue. In addition, if posterior instrumentation is required, a second incision must be made.

It must be kept in mind that the MIS lateral approach is not a silver bullet intended to uniformly treat all neoplastic spinal abnormalities; depending on the location of the abnormality, more traditional approaches may be favorable. The posterior approach would be chosen for primarily posterior element involvement or tumor with or without bilateral pedicle invasion, as well as for lesions of the upper thoracic levels (T1–T4), given the anatomic constraints imposed by the mediastinum anteriorly and the axilla laterally at these levels.

SUMMARY

The MIS anterolateral approach offers direct visualization of the ventral and lateral spine, with surgical access to vertebral body and neural elements without the morbidity concomitant with either anterior or posterior approaches. Its safety and efficacy have been demonstrated in the treatment of spinal tumors, including corpectomy and vertebral reconstruction, with results comparable with or superior to more traditional approaches. It is an excellent option as choice of surgical approach and should be in the armamentarium of all spine surgeons.

REFERENCES

1. Uribe JS, Dakwar E, Le TV, et al. Minimally invasive surgery treatment for thoracic spine tumor removal: a mini-open, lateral approach. Spine (Phila Pa 1976) 2010;35(Suppl 26):S347–54.
2. Klimo P Jr, Schmidt MH. Surgical management of spinal metastases. Oncologist 2004;9(2):18–96.
3. Medin PM, Solberg TD, De Salles AA, et al. Investigations of a minimally invasive method for treatment of spinal malignancies with LINAC stereotactic radiation therapy: accuracy and animal studies. Int J Radiat Oncol Biol Phys 2002; 52(4):1111–22.
4. Yao KC, Boriani S, Gokaslan ZL, et al. En bloc spondylectomy for spinal metastases: a review of techniques. Neurosurg Focus 2003;15(5):E6.
5. Byrne TN. Spinal cord compression for epidural metastases. N Engl J Med 1992;327(9):614–9.
6. Wolcott WP, Malik JM, Shaffrey CI, et al. Differential diagnosis of surgical disorders of the spine. In: Benzel EC, editor. Spine surgery: techniques, complication avoidance, and management, vol. 1, 2nd edition. Philadelphia: Elsevier; 2005. p. 33–60.
7. Parsa AT, Lee J, Parney IF, et al. Spinal cord and intradural-extraparenchymal spinal tumors: current best care practices and strategies. J Neurooncol 2004;69(1–3):291–318.
8. Tredway TL, Santiago P, Hrubes MR, et al. Minimally invasive resection of intradural-extramedullary spinal neoplasms. Neurosurgery 2006;58(Suppl 1): ONS52–8.
9. O'Toole JE, Eichholz KM, Fessler RG. Minimally invasive approaches to vertebral column and spinal cord tumors. Neurosurg Clin N Am 2006;17: 491–506.

10. Larson SJ, Holst RA, Henny DC, et al. Lateral extracavitary approach to traumatic lesions of the thoracic and lumbar spine. J Neurosurg 1976;45: 628–37.

11. McCormick PC. Retropleural approach to the thoracic and thoracolumbar spine. Neurosurgery 1995;37(5):908–14.

12. Scheufler KM. Technique and clinical results of minimally invasive reconstruction and stabilization of the thoracic and thoracolumbar spine with expandable cages and ventrolateral plate fixation. Neurosurgery 2007;61:798–808.

13. Rosenthal D, Marquardt G, Lorenz R, et al. Anterior decompression and stabilization using a microsurgical endoscopic technique for metastatic tumors of the thoracic spine. J Neurosurg 1996;84:565–72.

14. Sundaresan N, Shah J, Foley KM, et al. An anterior surgical approach to the upper thoracic vertebrae. J Neurosurg 1984;61:686–90.

15. Chen LH, Chen WJ, Niu CC, et al. Anterior reconstructive spinal surgery with Zielke instrumentation for metastatic malignancies of the spine. Arch Orthop Trauma Surg 2000;120:27–31.

16. Gokaslan ZL, York JE, Walsh GL, et al. Transthoracic vertebrectomy for metastatic spinal tumors. J Neurosurg 1998;89:599–609.

17. Dimar JR 2nd, Wilde PH, Glassman SD, et al. Thoracolumbar burst fractures treated with combined anterior and posterior surgery. Am J Orthop (Belle Mead NJ) 1996;25(2):159–65.

18. Lu DC, Lau D, Lee JG, et al. The transpedicular approach compared with the anterior approach: an analysis of 80 thoracolumbar corpectomies. J Neurosurg Spine 2010;12(6):583–91.

19. Huang TJ, Hsu RW, Liu HP, et al. Video-assisted thoracoscopic surgery to the upper thoracic spine. Surg Endosc 1999;13(2):123–6.

20. Huang TJ, Hsu RW, Li YY, et al. Minimal access spinal surgery (MASS) in treating thoracic spine metastasis. Spine 2006;31(16):1860–3.

21. Kan P, Schmidt MH. Minimally invasive thoracoscopic approach for anterior decompression and stabilization of metastatic spine disease. Neurosurg Focus 2008;25(2):E8.

22. Mack MJ, Regan JJ, Bobechko WP, et al. Application of thoracoscopy for diseases of the spine. Ann Thorac Surg 1993;56(3):736–8.

23. Dickman CA, Rosenthal D, Karahalios DG, et al. Thoracic vertebrectomy and reconstruction using a microsurgical thoracoscopic approach. Neurosurgery 1996;38:279–93.

24. Regan JJ, Mack MJ, Picetti GD 3rd. A technical report on video-assisted thoracoscopy in thoracic spinal surgery. Preliminary description. Spine (Phila Pa 1976) 1995;20(7):831–7.

25. Capener N. The evolution of lateral rhachotomy. J Bone Joint Surg Br 1954;36:173–9.

26. Bilsky MH, Boland P, Lis E, et al. Single-stage posterolateral transpedicle approach for spondylectomy, epidural compression, and circumferential fusion of spinal metastases. Spine 2000;25: 2240–9.

27. Wiggins CC, Mirza S, Bellabarba C, et al. Perioperative complications with costotransversectomy and anterior approaches to thoracic and thoracolumbar tumors. Neurosurg Focus 2001;11:e4.

28. Fessler RG, Sturgill M. Review: complications of surgery for thoracic disc disease. Surg Neurol 1998;49:609–18.

29. Schmidt MH, Larson SJ, Maiman DJ. The lateral extracavitary approach to the thoracic and lumbar spine. Neurosurg Clin N Am 2004;15:437–41.

30. Bohlman HH, Zdeblick TA. Anterior excision of herniated thoracic discs. J Bone Joint Surg Am 1988; 70(7):1038–47.

31. Thiel W. Photographic atlas of practical anatomy. 2nd edition. New York: Springer; 2003.

32. Street J, Fisher C, Sparkes J, et al. Single-stage posterolateral vertebrectomy for the management of metastatic disease of the thoracic and lumbar spine: a prospective study of an evolving surgical technique. J Spinal Disord Tech 2007; 20:509–20.

33. Ghogawala Z, Mansfield FL, Borges LF. Spinal radiation before surgical decompression adversely affects outcomes of surgery for symptomatic metastatic spinal cord compression. Spine 2001;26: 818–24.

34. Oppenheimer JH, DeCastro I, McDonnell DE. Minimally invasive spine technology and minimally invasive spine surgery: a historical review. Neurosurg Focus 2009;27(3):E9.

35. Khoo LT, Palmer S, Laich DT, et al. Minimally invasive percutaneous posterior lumbar interbody fusion. Neurosurgery 2002;51(Suppl 5):S166–81.

36. Amin BY, Tu TH, Mummaneni PV. Mini-open transforaminal lumbar interbody fusion. Neurosurg Focus 2013;35(Suppl 2):Video2.

37. Mummaneni PV, Rodts GE Jr. The mini-open transforaminal lumbar interbody fusion. Neurosurgery 2005;57(Suppl 4):256–61 [discussion: 256–61].

38. Gates GF. SPECT bone scanning of the spine. Semin Nucl Med 1998;28(1):78–94.

39. Broaddus WC, Grady MS, Delashaw JB, et al. Preoperative superselective arteriolar embolization: a new approach to enhance resectability of spinal tumors. Neurosurgery 1990;27(5):755–9.

40. Harrison MJ, Eisenberg MB, Ullman JS, et al. Symptomatic cavernous malformations affecting the spine and spinal cord. Neurosurgery 1995; 37(2):195–204.

41. Manke C, Bretschneider T, Lenhart M, et al. Spinal metastases from renal cell carcinoma: effect of preoperative particle embolization on intraoperative

blood loss. AJNR Am J Neuroradiol 2001;22(5): 997–1003.

42. Uribe JS, Dakwar E, Cardona RF, et al. Minimally invasive lateral retropleural thoracolumbar approach: cadaveric feasibility study and report of 4 clinical cases. Neurosurgery 2011;68(ONS Suppl 1):32–9.

43. Dakwar E, Ahmadian A, Uribe JS. The anatomical relationship of the diaphragm to the thoracolumbar junction during the minimally invasive lateral extracoelomic (retropleural/retroperitoneal) approach. J Neurosurg Spine 2012;16:359–64.

44. Lu DC, Dhall SS, Mummaneni PV. Mini-open removal of extradural foraminal tumors of the lumbar spine. J Neurosurg Spine 2009;10:46–50.

45. Lu DC, Chou D, Mummaneni PV. A comparison of mini-open and open approaches for resection of thoracolumbar intradural spinal tumors. J Neurosurg Spine 2011;14:758–64.

46. Haji FA, Cenic A, Crevier L, et al. Minimally invasive approach for the resection of spinal neoplasm. Spine 2011;36(15):E1018–26.

47. Deutsch H, Boco T, Lobel J. Minimally invasive transpedicular vertebrectomy for metastatic disease to the thoracic spine. J Spinal Disord Tech 2008;21:101–5.

48. Taghva A, Li KW, Liu JC, et al. Minimally invasive circumferential spinal decompression and stabilization for symptomatic spine tumor: technical case report. Neurosurgery 2010;66:E620–2.

49. Ragel BT, Kan P, Schmidt MH. Blood transfusions after thoracoscopic anterior thoracolumbar vertebrectomy. Acta Neurochir 2010;152:597–603.

50. Payer M, Sottas C. Mini-open anterior approach for corpectomy in the thoracolumbar spine. Surg Neurol 2008;69:25–32.

51. Kossman T, Jacobi D, Trentz O. The use of a retractor system (SynFrame) for open, minimal invasive reconstruction of the anterior column of the thoracic and lumbar spine. Eur Spine J 2001;10:396–402.

52. Mühlbauer M, Pfisterer W, Eyb R, et al. Minimally invasive retroperitoneal approach for lumbar corpectomy and anterior reconstruction. J Neurosurg 2000;93(Spine 1):161–7.

53. Ozgur BM, Aryan HE, Pimenta L, et al. Extreme Lateral Interbody Fusion (XLIF): a novel surgical technique for anterior lumbar-interbody fusion. Spine 2006;6:435–43.

54. Rampersaud YR, Annand N, Dekutoski MB. Use of minimally invasive surgical techniques in the management of thoracolumbar trauma: current concepts. Spine 2006;31:S96–102.

Minimally Invasive Approaches for the Treatment of Intramedullary Spinal Tumors

Trent L. Tredway, MD

KEYWORDS

- Minimally invasive spine surgery • Intramedullary tumors • Ependymoma • Astrocytoma
- Juvenile pilocytic astrocytoma • Hemangioblastoma

KEY POINTS

- Identify and differentiate between the various types of intramedullary tumors including astrocytomas, ependymomas, juvenile pilocytic astrocytomas (JPAs), and hemangioblastomas.
- Determine surgical treatment options for the different types of intramedullary tumors including ependymomas, astrocytomas, JPAs, and hemangioblastomas.
- Describe the surgical procedure for minimally invasive resection of an intramedullary spinal cord tumor as well as the potential advantages.

INTRODUCTION

Primary tumors of the spinal cord are 10 to 15 times less common than primary intracranial tumors, and overall represent 2% to 4% of all primary tumors of the central nervous system (CNS). There are an estimated 850 to 1700 new adult cases of primary spinal cord tumors diagnosed each year in the United States.[1] The histology of spinal cord tumors is similar to that of their intracranial counterparts; however, unlike primary intracranial tumors, spinal cord tumors show no association between increasing grade of malignancy and age at diagnosis. Most primary spinal cord tumors are classified as low grade (grades 1 and 2) according to the World Health Organization (WHO) pathologic classification.

Primary spinal cord tumors are divided into 3 categories based on anatomic location: intramedullary, intradural extramedullary, and extradural.[2] Intramedullary spinal cord tumors (IMSCT) constitute 8% to 10% of all primary spinal cord tumors, with the majority comprising gliomas (80%–90%), of which 60% to 70% are ependymomas and 30% to 40% are astrocytomas.[3] The third most common IMSCT is hemangioblastoma, representing approximately 3% to 8% of all IMSCTs, of which 15% to 25% are associated with von Hippel–Lindau (VHL) syndrome.[4–6]

The clinical presentation of primary spinal cord tumors is determined in part by the location of the tumor, and in nearly all clinical instances pain is the predominant presenting symptom. In a recent series of IMSCT, pain was the most common presenting symptom (72%), manifesting as back pain (27%), radicular pain (25%), or central pain (20%). Motor disturbance was the next most common presenting symptom (55%), followed by sensory loss (39%).[7] Diagnosis of a primary spinal cord tumor requires a high index of suspicion based on clinical signs and symptoms, in addition to spine-directed magnetic resonance imaging (MRI).

INTRAMEDULLARY SPINAL CORD TUMORS

Astrocytomas and ependymomas represent the most common intramedullary neoplasms. It is estimated that the intracranial to spinal ratio for astrocytomas and ependymomas are 10:1 and 3:1 to

NeoSpine, 901 Boren Avenue, Suite 600, Seattle, WA 98104, USA
E-mail addresses: ttredway@NeoSpine.net; ttredway@hotmail.com

Neurosurg Clin N Am 25 (2014) 327–336
http://dx.doi.org/10.1016/j.nec.2013.12.010

20:1, respectively (depending on the histologic variant).[8] The clinical presentation of an intramedullary tumor is variable, but pain and a mixed sensorimotor tract disturbance (segmental sensory level, upper motor neuron signs) are usually present.

MRI of the spine is the diagnostic modality of choice; however, patients unable to undergo MRI (ie, patients with a cardiac pacemaker) may require computed tomography (CT) myelography. An intramedullary tumor is radiographically recognized by focal, and sometimes holocord, spinal cord expansion with associated T2-weighted (T2W) and fluid-attenuated inversion recovery (FLAIR) image hyperintensity, T1-weighted (T1W) hypointensity or isointensity, variable contrast enhancement, and occasional tumor-associated syrinx.[9]

Ependymoma

Ependymomas are the most frequently encountered intramedullary spinal cord tumor in adults.[1,10] Histologically there are 2 distinct pathologic types: cellular (WHO grades 2 and 3) and myxopapillary (WHO grade 1). Cellular (classic) ependymoma arises from the intraspinal canal of the cervical and thoracic cord. Myxopapillary ependymomas arise from the filum terminale and occur almost exclusively at the conus medullaris. The treatment and prognosis for spinal cord ependymomas is often excellent, as these tumors may be resected completely and in such instances manifest a low risk of recurrence.[7,11,12]

On MRI ependymomas appear as a focal enlargement of the cord and hyperintense on T2W and FLAIR images, and hypointense or isointense to normal spinal cord on T1W images with heterogeneous contrast enhancement.[9] These tumors may also be associated with cystic changes, hemosiderin suggestive of previous hemorrhage, and syrinx (**Fig. 1**).

Ependymomas most often are of low grade with a benign indolent course, although malignant histologic subtypes (anaplastic ependymoma; WHO grade 3) rarely occur. Surgery is the most effective treatment, with complete surgical resection yielding reported local control rates of 90% to 100%, although gross total resection is not achieved in most patients.[12–14] Intraoperative monitoring of motor and somatosensory evoked potentials are often used to assist in achieving a more safe and complete resection.[15–17] Involved-field external beam radiotherapy at a dose of 45 to 54 Gy is indicated for partially resected or biopsied WHO grade 2 ependymomas or malignant WHO grade 3 tumors.[14,18,19] Overall, spinal cord ependymomas are associated with prolonged progression-free and overall survival, with a median of 82 months and 180 months, respectively.[20]

Astrocytoma

Approximately 40% of IMSCTs are astrocytomas.[10,21] The majority (75%) are low-grade (WHO grade 2) fibrillary astrocytomas with 5-year survivorship exceeding 70%.[7,10,22] Histology is the most important prognostic variable.[23–25] Juvenile pilocytic astrocytoma (JPA) is a low-grade (WHO grade 1) variant that more commonly presents in younger patients. High-grade spinal cord gliomas (WHO grades 3 and 4, 25%) are less common and associated with a poor survival. Regardless of WHO grade, spinal cord astrocytomas are

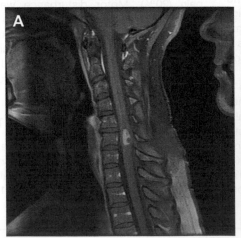
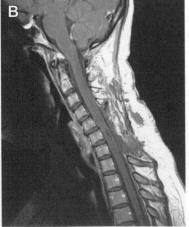

Fig. 1. (*A*) Preoperative sagittal T1-weighted magnetic resonance (MR) image with gadolinium, showing characteristics of an intramedullary ependymoma. (*B*) Postoperative sagittal T1-weighted MR image with gadolinium, showing complete resection of ependymoma with associated postoperative changes.

infiltrative and associated with poorly characterized boundaries, and consequently are typically biopsied only. However, a recent case report of cordectomy yielded survival of longer than 15 months in one patient.[26]

Astrocytomas appear on MRI as fusiform expansion of the cord with an indistinct and, occasionally, cystic component.[9] Associated edema or syrinx (seen in 40%) may be present. The tumor is hypointense to isointense on T1W images and hyperintense on T2W and FLAIR images, with variable contrast enhancement. In general, the distinction between astrocytomas and ependymomas by MRI is not always possible (**Fig. 2**).

Initial treatment consists of maximal safe surgical resection or biopsy followed by observation or external beam radiotherapy. Because spinal cord gliomas are infiltrative, gross total resection is rarely accomplished (in approximately 12% of WHO grade 2 and 0% of grade 3 or 4 astrocytomas).[7] The optimal extent of surgical resection and need for postoperative radiotherapy is controversial. Tumor histology, extent of resection, and functional status at time of presentation seem to be the primary determinants of outcome.[10,13] Nonetheless, radiotherapy is indicated for patients with high-grade histology, tumors in which a substantial resection cannot be performed, biopsied-only tumors, and those with progressive disease. Though rare in adults, most spinal cord JPAs can occasionally be completely resected (up to 80%).[7]

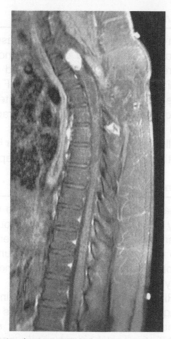

Fig. 2. Sagittal T1-weighted MR image with gadolinium, showing characteristics of recurrent intramedullary juvenile pilocytic astrocytoma.

Hemangioblastoma

Hemangioblastomas, the third most common IMSCT, are rare vascular tumors that occur as a solitary tumor or as part of VHL syndrome.[4–7] Approximately 10% to 30% of patients with hemangioblastoma of the spinal cord have VHL syndrome, an autosomal dominant disorder caused by a deletion on chromosome 3p. Other tumors associated with VHL include retinal hemangiomas, renal and pancreatic cysts, pheochromocytomas, and renal cell carcinomas. Regardless of whether hemangioblastoma occurs as part of the VHL syndrome or solitarily, the clinical and histopathologic characteristics are identical. There is a male predominance, and presentation is usually in the fourth decade.[5,27]

Most hemangioblastomas arise from the dorsal or dorsolateral portion of the spinal cord.[3,5,27] As such, presenting symptoms are usually sensory, especially slowly progressive proprioception deficits. There may also be other long tract signs and radicular symptoms. Rarely, patients present with subarachnoid or intramedullary hemorrhage.[28–32]

On MRI, the hemangioblastomas appear as a homogeneously enhancing hypervascular nodule with associated cyst or syrinx and peritumoral edema.[5] Spinal angiography demonstrates enlarged feeding arteries, intense nodular stains, and early draining veins.[9] Hemangioblastoma can be differentiated from ependymoma by the vascular abnormalities on MRI, and the presence of tumor hypervascularity with feeding arteries and draining veins on a spinal angiogram if performed. Hemangioblastoma is differentiated from a spinal cord vascular malformation by associated syrinx and tumor enhancement on MRI (**Fig. 3**).

Surgical resection is the primary treatment. There are often well-defined margins allowing for a complete resection. Excessive intraoperative bleeding that obscures the operative field is the limiting factor for subtotal resection.[5] In contrast to posterior fossa hemangioblastomas, preoperative embolization is usually not performed, as complications have been reported.[33–36] Serial MRI should be obtained because de novo lesions can appear in patients with VHL. There is a limited role for radiotherapy, and experience with chemotherapy is almost nonexistent. Stereotactic radiosurgery is an option for patients with recurrent or unresectable tumors.[37]

Ganglioglioma

Ganglioglioma is a glial-neuronal tumor that usually occurs in the brain, but may arise from the intramedullary spinal cord. The tumor is typically

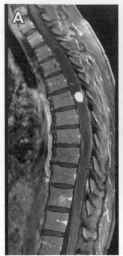
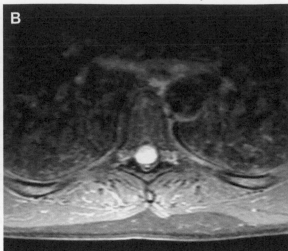
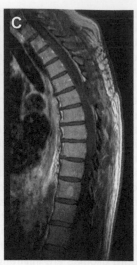

Fig. 3. (*A*) Preoperative sagittal T1-weighted MR image with gadolinium, showing characteristics of intramedullary hemangioblastoma. (*B*) Preoperative axial T1-weighted MR image with gadolinium, showing characteristics of intramedullary hemangioblastoma. (*C*) Postoperative sagittal T1-weighted MR image with gadolinium, showing complete resection of hemangioblastoma.

slow growing, but rarely may have an aggressive course. Adult cases of spinal cord ganglioglioma are rare, and paraparesis and radicular pain are the most common presenting symptoms.[11]

On T1W MRI the tumor is hypointense or has mixed signal characteristics, and has homogeneous or heterogeneous hyperintensity on T2W/FLAIR images, with variable contrast enhancement. Tumor cysts, scoliosis, and bone erosion/scalloping may be present.[38]

Maximal surgical resection is the optimal treatment for spinal cord gangliogliomas. Complete or near complete resection is associated with excellent long-term survival and minimal morbidity.[11,38] Postoperative radiotherapy is not recommended, even in patients who undergo a subtotal resection. Despite the apparent benign nature, the progression-free survival rate in the largest case series (56 pediatric patients) was only 67%.[11] Rarely, there is transformation to a higher-grade tumor (ie, anaplastic ganglioglioma).[39,40]

Lymphoma

Primary CNS lymphoma rarely (<1% of all CNS lymphomas) presents as an isolated spinal cord intramedullary tumor.[41–45] On MRI, lymphoma appears as single or multifocal, ill-defined T2W/FLAIR hyperintense lesions with homogeneous contrast enhancement on T1W images. Because of high cell tumor density, diffusion-weighted MRI often demonstrates restriction and a correspondingly high signal, that is, hyperintensity. Following histologic diagnosis, a careful search for other sites of CNS disease (including slit-lamp eye examination, brain MRI, total spine MRI, and cerebrospinal fluid [CSF] flow cytometry/cytology) should be performed. Because CNS lymphoma is a diffuse disease most often affecting the entire neuraxis, treatment should include high-dose methotrexate-based chemotherapy similar to regimens used to treat CNS lymphoma involving the brain.[46]

Germinoma

Several investigators have described cases of primary intramedullary spinal cord germinoma.[47–52] Age at presentation is between 10 and 40 years old. Craniospinal axis imaging and CSF cytology should be obtained to look for other sites of disease. Because germinoma is usually radiosensitive and chemosensitive, treatment includes biopsy followed by radiotherapy alone or in combination with platinum-based chemotherapy.[52]

Melanoma

Melanoma can arise and be isolated to the intramedullary spinal cord region; numerous cases have been reported.[53–60] Clinical presentation is similar to that of other intramedullary tumors, but often evolves more rapidly than ependymomas or astrocytomas.

On MRI, melanoma is usually hyperintense on T1W images, isointense or hypointense on T2W/FLAIR images, and with mild contrast enhancement.[55] Intratumoral hemorrhage is common at presentation, and may lead to the erroneous diagnosis of cavernous angioma or other vascular malformation.[54,57,60] The MRI features are variable depending on intratumoral bleeding and melanin content. Because there is no straightforward MRI method to differentiate primary spinal cord melanoma from metastatic tumor, a careful examination of skin, squamous mucosa, and eyes should be performed as well as contrast-enhanced CT imaging of the chest, abdomen, and pelvis.

Surgery establishes the diagnosis and may provide long-term palliation if the tumor is resected completely.[56] As complete image-verified resection is rarely achieved, most patients receive postoperative radiotherapy.

Others

Other rare primary IMSCTs include primitive neuroectodermal tumor (PNET), paraganglioglioma, teratoma, dermoid cyst, epidermoid cyst, lipoma, and hamartoma. Treatment following maximal safe resection is similar to that of intracranial counterparts, and in most instances surgery suffices as primary therapy (PNET being the exception).

SURGICAL TREATMENT OF INTRAMEDULLARY TUMORS

The treatment of intramedullary spinal cord tumors has been largely based on open surgical biopsy or resection if possible. Successful surgical resections with good clinical outcomes have been reported in the literature with traditional open surgery.[61–65] However, surgical morbidity should also be considered when resecting these lesions.

Open surgical intervention requires adequate exposure with removal of the posterior spinal elements. These structures are also important in maintaining alignment of the spinal column. Extensive removal of the posterior elements can be associated with increased pain and increased blood loss, and can lead to worsening kyphotic deformities of the spine.[66] This anomaly is more pronounced in the cervical spine, but can also occur in the thoracic spine. It has been reported in the literature that there was an increased risk of kyphosis in the pediatric population after patients underwent surgeries that required greater than 3 levels of laminectomy for the intradural tumor resection.[66] Therefore, some neurosurgeons perform laminoplasties in the pediatric population to decrease the risk of postsurgical kyphotic deformity as the patient ages.

MINIMALLY INVASIVE RATIONALE AND TECHNIQUE

The term minimally invasive surgery has been credited to a British urologist, J.E.A. Wickham,

who in his 1987 article describing the new surgery prophetically proclaimed, "this means that surgeons will need to be trained as microendoscopists and bioengineers rather than as butchers and carpenters."[67] Over the past few decades, neurosurgeons have been exploiting advances in surgical instrumentation, surgical optics, and endoscopy, as well as adjunct hemostatic agents, dural substitutes, sutures, and surgical clips, to perform spinal surgery with less morbidity, faster and less painful recovery, and excellent patient outcomes. The technological advancements combined with the pioneering ingenuity of surgeons have allowed treatment of a wide variety of spinal disorders using minimally invasive concepts and techniques. Disc herniations, lumbar stenosis, spondylolisthesis, extradural and intradural extramedullary tumors, and surgeries for the treatment of traumatic fractures, spinal column metastases, tethered cords, and syringomyelia can all be treated with minimally invasive techniques.[68–78] These advancements have also allowed clinicians to treat selected patients harboring intramedullary abnormality, including tumors, as was first reported by Ogden and Fessler.[79]

SURGICAL TECHNIQUE
Preoperative Planning

Patients presenting with signs/symptoms consistent with an intramedullary process should be evaluated with MRI with and without contrast to determine the imaging characteristics of the lesion, including the size and location as well as associated factors including edema, presence/absence of a cyst, and presence of a well-delineated lesion versus a diffuse lesion without well-defined borders. This evaluation will enable the surgeon to determine the feasibility of resection of the lesion rather than obtaining a biopsy for histologic confirmation (**Fig. 4**A, B). It is also important to obtain anteroposterior, lateral, and flexion/extension radiographs to determine whether there is any preoperative instability or kyphosis that may worsen with the surgical removal of the posterior elements. This step may help determine whether surgical stabilization is required at the time of the tumor resection. After obtaining the information, the surgeon can then weigh the feasibility of removing the tumor through a minimally invasive approach. Typically, lesions spanning over 2 spinal levels may be too difficult to treat using minimally invasive approaches.

Preparation and Patient Positioning

Consent should be requested from all patients undergoing minimally invasive resection of an

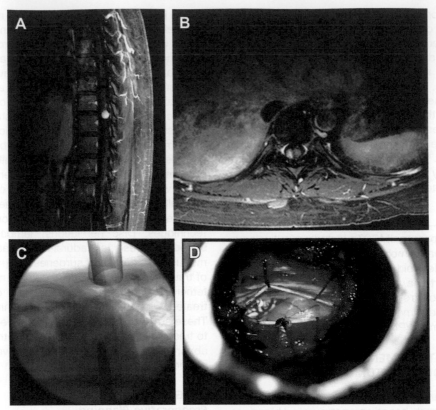

Fig. 4. (*A*) Preoperative sagittal T1-weighted MR image with gadolinium, demonstrating neurofibromatosis type 2, with an intradural, extramedullary lesion (schwannoma) as well as an intramedullary lesion (ependymoma). (*B*) Axial preoperative T1-weighted MR image with gadolinium, showing both lesions (schwannoma and ependymoma). (*C*) Intraoperative fluoroscopy showing tubular retractor access to the intradural lesions. (*D*) Intraoperative view of dural opening with extramedullary schwannoma.

intramedullary tumor, for both surgical resection and intraoperative monitoring including the use of motor evoked potentials (MEPs) and somatosensory evoked potentials (SSEPs). Such monitoring will enable the surgeon to have some real-time feedback when resecting the lesion in the operative suite. The author prefers to initiate a methylprednisolone protocol consisting of an initial load of 30 mg/kg over 15 minutes, followed by a maintenance dose of 5.4 mg/kg/h during the surgical procedure, which is continued for 24 hours in the postoperative period. Patients are also started on a proton-pump inhibitor, pantoprazole (Protonix; Pfizer, New York City, NY) to reduce the risks of gastric ulceration from the steroid therapy. All patients are also given preoperative antibiotics, and a discussion with anesthesia colleagues is initiated with the goal of keeping the mean arterial pressure (MAP) higher than 60 to 70 mm Hg. This action will help ensure adequate perfusion of the spinal cord during surgical resection and inadvertent spinal cord manipulation.

Patients harboring tumors in the cervical spinal cord or upper thoracic (T1–T3) are placed in a prone position using cranial-fixation tongs with the neck placed in a neutral position, thus enabling access to the spinal canal easier than if the patient is placed in a lordotic position. Patients who have thoracic intramedullary lesions below T4 are placed on a chest frame, with the arms in a "Superman" position so that anesthesiologists have access to the intravenous sites and arterial lines. This position also allows for easier fluoroscopic confirmation of the correct levels undergoing surgical intervention. All bony prominences are well protected with gel or foam barriers, and an effort to keep the patient's eyes from pressure-related incidents is paramount during the prone operative procedures. Finally, intraoperative monitoring needles are placed and baseline MEP and SSEP responses are recorded.

Surgical Approach

After verification of the correct surgical level with lateral fluoroscopy, a paramedian incision is made in the skin, subcutaneous tissue, and fascia to allow for entry of the tubular retractor system (see **Fig. 4C**). Once the incision is completed, serial dilators are used to dock overlying lamina where the intramedullary tumor is located. The soft tissue is removed with monopolar electrocautery, and a hemilaminectomy with undercutting of the spinous process is performed to allow for a midline durotomy. The dura is incised with a dural knife and the edges are tacked back using a 4-0 braided nylon suture to expose the spinal cord. As with open surgical resection of intramedullary lesions, care is taken to identify the midline and enter the cord between the dorsal columns so as to reduce the risk of postoperative dorsal column dysfunction. If the lesion is present on the surface, the tumor can be accessed through the shortest, most direct route, thus limiting damage to the spinal cord. Laterally based lesions can be accessed through the dorsal root entry zone with minimal damage to the cord. The lesion is identified, and a surgical plane is developed between the lesion and the spinal cord proper. The author prefers to not use pial sutures, as this may lead to some decreased perfusion of the spinal cord. Once the lesion is gently dissected from the spinal cord proper, it can be removed using an en bloc technique, if possible, or it can be resected in a piecemeal fashion using an ultrasonic aspirator. Ultrasonography can be helpful in identifying the lesion before removal and for documenting the complete resection after surgery. Intraoperative MRI can also be helpful if the operative suite has the capability (**Fig. 5**). Once the tumor is resected, the dura is closed with either a running 4-0 braided nylon suture or dural clips, as has been reported in the literature.[80] The use of bayoneted instruments, which can be used through the tubular retractor system, is of utmost importance to obtain a watertight closure of the dural. The suture knot is thrown outside of the tube and the knot is advanced with the use of a knot pusher, commonly used in laparoscopic surgery. A small, rounded needle can also prove useful when reapproximating the dural edges. The suture line is reinforced with a small piece of dural substitute (Duragen; Integra, Plainsboro, NJ) and fibrin sealant (Tisseel; Baxter, Deerfield, IL) to decrease the risk of a postoperative pseudomeningocele. The tubular retractor and endoscope/microscope is removed, the fascia and muscle are reapproximated with a 2-0 resorbable suture, and the subdermal region is reapproximated with a 3-0 resorbable suture. The skin is closed with a 4-0 resorbable suture using a subcuticular closure, and the skin is covered with 2-octyl cyanoacrylate (Dermabond; Ethicon, Somerville, NJ).

Immediate Postoperative Care

Patients undergoing a minimally invasive resection of an intramedullary tumor are observed in the intensive care unit (ICU) for the first 24 hours with close attention to their neurologic examination,

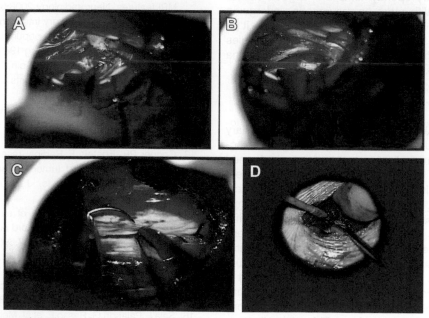

Fig. 5. Intraoperative views of surgery. (*A*) Minimally invasive resection of intramedullary ependymoma. (*B*) Completely resected intramedullary ependymoma. (*C*) Minimally invasive dural closure. (*D*) Incision after removal of tubular retractor.

blood pressure with goals of a MAP higher than 60 mm Hg, as well as their blood glucose response to the high-dose steroid therapy. MRI with and without contrast is performed to determine the extent of resection and to obtain a baseline imaging study for possible future adjunct therapy, if necessary.

Rehabilitation and Recovery

After transfer from the ICU to the ward, the patient is evaluated by physical therapists and occupational therapists to determine the need for inpatient versus outpatient rehabilitation. Important factors in determining patients' clinical disposition include ambulatory status, hand function, bowel/bladder function, ability to perform transfers if needed, and the amount of assistance required for their activities of daily living.

CLINICAL RESULTS IN THE LITERATURE

Although there have been reports of minimally invasive treatment of intradural extramedullary tumors with good clinical outcomes, there are few reports in the literature regarding the minimally invasive treatment of intramedullary tumors.[75,81,82] Minimally invasive resection of intramedullary tumors is relatively new to the neurosurgeon's armamentarium, and thus clinical outcome measures are sparse in the literature to date. Ogden and Fessler[79] reported on the resection of an intramedullary ependymoma with a good clinical outcome. With more neurosurgeons undergoing training in minimally invasive techniques, it is hoped that more reports and outcomes studies regarding this exciting new neurosurgical arena will be forthcoming.

SUMMARY

The mainstay of the treatment of intramedullary tumors is surgical resection. Open surgical resection of intramedullary tumors has been performed with good clinical outcomes. However, recent advances in surgical instrumentation, optics, endoscopy, and minimally invasive approaches have allowed neurosurgeons to resect intramedullary tumors safely and efficaciously using these less invasive techniques. With reduction of damage to the surrounding soft tissue and bony structures, these techniques may reduce the amount of hospitalization and postoperative pain, and may eliminate the need for larger surgical interventions and stabilization procedures. The minimally invasive approaches offer a feasible alternative to traditional open procedures.

REFERENCES

1. Campello C, Parker F, et al. Neuroepithelial intramedullary spinal cord tumors in adults: study of 70 cases, in American Academy of Neurology Annual Meeting. Seattle, 2009.
2. Elsberg CA. Some aspects of the diagnosis and surgical treatment of tumors of the spinal cord: with a study of the end results in a series of 119 operations. Ann Surg 1925;81(6):1057–73.
3. Miller DJ, McCutcheon IE. Hemangioblastomas and other uncommon intramedullary tumors. J Neurooncol 2000;47(3):253–70.
4. Browne TR, Adams RD, Roberson GH. Hemangioblastoma of the spinal cord. Review and report of five cases. Arch Neurol 1976;33(6):435–41.
5. Lee DK, Choe WJ, Chung CK, et al. Spinal cord hemangioblastoma: surgical strategy and clinical outcome. J Neurooncol 2003;61(1):27–34.
6. Lonser RR, Weil RJ, Wanebo JE, et al. Surgical management of spinal cord hemangioblastomas in patients with von Hippel-Lindau disease. J Neurosurg 2003;98(1):106–16.
7. Raco A, Esposito V, Lenzi J, et al. Long-term follow-up of intramedullary spinal cord tumors: a series of 202 cases. Neurosurgery 2005;56(5):972–81 [discussion: 972–81].
8. Parsa AT, Miller JI, Eggers AE, et al. Autologous adjuvant linked fibroblasts induce anti-glioma immunity: implications for development of a glioma vaccine. J Neurooncol 2003;64(1–2):77–87.
9. Abul-Kasim K, Thurnher MM, McKeever P, et al. Intradural spinal tumors: current classification and MRI features. Neuroradiology 2008;50(4):301–14.
10. Helseth A, Mork SJ. Primary intraspinal neoplasms in Norway, 1955 to 1986. A population-based survey of 467 patients. J Neurosurg 1989;71(6):842–5.
11. Jallo GI, Freed D, Epstein FJ. Spinal cord ganglio-gliomas: a review of 56 patients. J Neurooncol 2004;68(1):71–7.
12. McCormick PC, Torres R, Post KD, et al. Intramedullary ependymoma of the spinal cord. J Neurosurg 1990;72(4):523–32.
13. Cooper PR, Epstein F. Radical resection of intramedullary spinal cord tumors in adults. Recent experience in 29 patients. J Neurosurg 1985;63(4):492–9.
14. Volpp PB, Han K, Kagan AR, et al. Outcomes in treatment for intradural spinal cord ependymomas. Int J Radiat Oncol Biol Phys 2007;69(4):1199–204.
15. Yanni DS, Ulkatan S, Deletis V, et al. Utility of neurophysiological monitoring using dorsal column mapping in intramedullary spinal cord surgery. J Neurosurg Spine 2010;12(6):623–8.
16. Sala F, Palandri G, Basso E, et al. Motor evoked potential monitoring improves outcome after surgery for intramedullary spinal cord tumors: a historical

control study. Neurosurgery 2006;58(6):1129–43 [discussion: 1129–43].

17. Quinones-Hinojosa A, Gulati M, Lyon R, et al. Spinal cord mapping as an adjunct for resection of intramedullary tumors: surgical technique with case illustrations. Neurosurgery 2002;51(5):1199–206 [discussion: 1206–7].

18. Isaacson SR. Radiation therapy and the management of intramedullary spinal cord tumors. J Neurooncol 2000;47(3):231–8.

19. Linstadt DE, Wara WM, Leibel SA, et al. Postoperative radiotherapy of primary spinal cord tumors. Int J Radiat Oncol Biol Phys 1989;16(6):1397–403.

20. Gomez DR, Missett BT, Wara WM, et al. High failure rate in spinal ependymomas with long-term follow-up. Neuro Oncol 2005;7(3):254–9.

21. Guidetti B. Intramedullary tumours of the spinal cord. Acta Neurochir (Wien) 1967;17(1):7–23.

22. Rodrigues GB, Waldron JN, Wang CS, et al. A retrospective analysis of 52 cases of spinal cord glioma managed with radiation therapy. Int J Radiat Oncol Biol Phys 2000;48(3):837–42.

23. Minehan KJ, Brown PD, Scheithauer BW, et al. Prognosis and treatment of spinal cord astrocytoma. Int J Radiat Oncol Biol Phys 2009;73(3):727–33.

24. Kim MS, Chang CK, Choe G, et al. Intramedullary spinal cord astrocytoma in adults: postoperative outcome. J Neurooncol 2001;52(1):85–94.

25. Innocenzi G, Salvati M, Cervoni L, et al. Prognostic factors in intramedullary astrocytomas. Clin Neurol Neurosurg 1997;99(1):1–5.

26. Ewelt C, Stummer W, Klink B, et al. Cordectomy as final treatment option for diffuse intramedullary malignant glioma using 5-ALA fluorescence-guided resection. Clin Neurol Neurosurg 2010;112(4): 357–61.

27. Murota T, Symon L. Surgical management of hemangioblastoma of the spinal cord: a report of 18 cases. Neurosurgery 1989;25(5):699–707 [discussion: 708].

28. Cerejo A, Vaz R, Feyo PB, et al. Spinal cord hemangioblastoma with subarachnoid hemorrhage. Neurosurgery 1990;27(6):991–3.

29. Dijindjian M, Dijindjian r, Houdart R, et al. Subarachnoid hemorrhage due to intraspinal tumors. Surg Neurol 1978;9(4):223–9.

30. Kormos RL, Tucker WS, Bilbao JM, et al. Subarachnoid hemorrhage due to a spinal cord hemangioblastoma: case report. Neurosurgery 1980;6(6):657–60.

31. Minami M, Hanakita J, Suma H, et al. Cervical hemangioblastoma with a past history of subarachnoid hemorrhage. Surg Neurol 1998;49(3):278–81.

32. Yu JS, Short MP, Schumacher J, et al. Intramedullary hemorrhage in spinal cord hemangioblastoma. Report of two cases. J Neurosurg 1994;81(6):937–40.

33. Eskridge JM, McAuliffe W, Harris B, et al. Preoperative endovascular embolization of craniospinal hemangioblastomas. AJNR Am J Neuroradiol 1996;17(3):525–31.

34. Standard SC, Ahuja A, Livingston K, et al. Endovascular embolization and surgical excision for the treatment of cerebellar and brain stem hemangioblastomas. Surg Neurol 1994;41(5):405–10.

35. Tampieri D, Leblanc R, TerBrugge K. Preoperative embolization of brain and spinal hemangioblastomas. Neurosurgery 1993;33(3):502–5 [discussion: 505].

36. Vazquez-Anon V, Botella C, Beltan A, et al. Preoperative embolization of solid cervicomedullary junction hemangioblastomas: report of two cases. Neuroradiology 1997;39(2):86–9.

37. Ryu SI, Kim DH, Chang SD. Stereotactic radiosurgery for hemangiomas and ependymomas of the spinal cord. Neurosurg Focus 2003;15(5):E10.

38. Patel U, Pinto RS, Miller DC, et al. MR of spinal cord ganglioglioma. AJNR Am J Neuroradiol 1998;19(5): 879–87.

39. Amini A, Chin SS, Schmidt MH. Malignant transformation of conus medullaris ganglioglioma: case report. J Neurooncol 2007;82(3):313–5.

40. Di Patre PL, Payer M, Bruneq M, et al. Malignant transformation of a spinal cord ganglioglioma—case report and review of the literature. Clin Neuropathol 2004;23(6):298–303.

41. Bekar A, Cordan T, Evrensel T, et al. A case of primary spinal intramedullary lymphoma. Surg Neurol 2001;55(5):261–4.

42. Heran NS, Yong RL, Heran MS, et al. Primary intradural extraarachnoid Hodgkin lymphoma of the cervical spine. Case report. J Neurosurg Spine 2006;5(1):61–4.

43. Itami J, Mori S, Arimizu N, et al. Primary intramedullary spinal cord lymphoma: report of a case. Jpn J Clin Oncol 1986;16(4):407–12.

44. Machiya T, Yoshita M, Iwasa K, et al. Primary spinal intramedullary lymphoma mimicking ependymoma. Neurology 2007;68(11):872.

45. Pels H, Vogt I, Klockgether T, et al. Primary non-Hodgkin's lymphoma of the spinal cord. Spine (Phila Pa 1976) 2000;25(17):2262–4.

46. Abrey LE, Yahalom J, DeAngelis LM. Treatment for primary CNS lymphoma: the next step. J Clin Oncol 2000;18(17):3144–50.

47. Aoyama T, Hida K, Ishii N, et al. Intramedullary spinal cord germinoma—2 case reports. Surg Neurol 2007;67(2):177–83 [discussion: 183].

48. Chute DJ, Burton EC, Klement IA, et al. Primary intramedullary spinal cord germinoma: case report. J Neurooncol 2003;63(1):69–73.

49. Hata M, Ogino I, Sakata K, et al. Intramedullary spinal cord germinoma: case report and review of the literature. Radiology 2002;223(2):379–83.

50. Itoh Y, Ogino I, Sakata K, et al. Intramedullary spinal cord germinoma: case report and review of the literature. Neurosurgery 1996;38(1):187–90 [discussion: 190–1].

51. Matsuyama Y, Nagasaka T, Mimatsu K, et al. Intramedullary spinal cord germinoma. Spine (Phila Pa 1976) 1995;20(21):2338–40.

52. Yang KY, Li SH, Lin JW, et al. Concurrent chemoradiotherapy for primary cervical spinal cord germinoma. J Clin Neurosci 2009;16(1):115–8.

53. Connolly ES Jr, Winfree CJ, McCormick PC, et al. Intramedullary spinal cord metastasis: report of three cases and review of the literature. Surg Neurol 1996;46(4):329–37 [discussion: 337–8].

54. Denaro L, Pallini R, DiMuro L, et al. Primary hemorrhagic intramedullary melanoma. Case report with emphasis on the difficult preoperative diagnosis. J Neurosurg Sci 2007;51(4):181–3.

55. Farrokh D, Fransen P, Faverly D. MR findings of a primary intramedullary malignant melanoma: case report and literature review. AJNR Am J Neuroradiol 2001;22(10):1864–6.

56. Francois P, Lioret E, Jan M. Primary spinal melanoma: case report. Br J Neurosurg 1998;12(2):179–82.

57. Larson TC 3rd, et al. Primary spinal melanoma. J Neurosurg 1987;66(1):47–9.

58. Salpietro FM, Alafaci C, Gervasio O, et al. Primary cervical melanoma with brain metastases. Case report and review of the literature. J Neurosurg 1998;89(4):659–66.

59. Vaquero J, de Prado F, Pedrosa M. Primary intraparenchymatous spinal cord melanoma. Spinal Cord 1998;36(5):363–5.

60. Yamasaki T, Kikuchi H, Yamashita J, et al. Primary spinal intramedullary malignant melanoma: case report. Neurosurgery 1989;25(1):117–21.

61. Epstein F, Epstein N. Surgical treatment of spinal cord astrocytomas of childhood. A series of 19 patients. J Neurosurg 1982;57(5):685–9.

62. Epstein FJ, Farmer JP. Pediatric spinal cord tumor surgery. Neurosurg Clin N Am 1990;1(3):569–90.

63. Epstein FJ, Farmer JP, Freed D. Adult intramedullary spinal cord ependymomas: the result of surgery in 38 patients. J Neurosurg 1993;79(2):204–9.

64. Constantini S, Miller DC, Allen JC, et al. Radical excision of intramedullary spinal cord tumors: surgical morbidity and long-term follow-up evaluation in 164 children and young adults. J Neurosurg 2000;93(Suppl 2):183–93.

65. Jallo GI, Kothbauer KF, Epstein FJ. Intrinsic spinal cord tumor resection. Neurosurgery 2001;49(5):1124–8.

66. Sciubba DM, Chaichana KL, Woodworth GF, et al. Factors associated with cervical instability requiring fusion after cervical laminectomy for intradural tumor resection. J Neurosurg Spine 2008;8(5):413–9.

67. Wickham JE. The new surgery. Br Med J (Clin Res Ed) 1987;295(6613):1581–2.

68. Foley KT, Smith MM, Rampersaud YR. Microendoscopic approach to far-lateral lumbar disc herniation. Neurosurg Focus 1999;7(5):e5.

69. Perez-Cruet MJ, Foley KT, Isaacs RE, et al. Microendoscopic lumbar discectomy: technical note. Neurosurgery 2002;51(Suppl 5):S129–36.

70. Khoo LT, Fessler RG. Microendoscopic decompressive laminotomy for the treatment of lumbar stenosis. Neurosurgery 2002;51(Suppl 5):S146–54.

71. Khoo LT, Fessler RG. Minimally invasive percutaneous posterior lumbar interbody fusion. Neurosurgery 2002;51(Suppl 5). S166–1.

72. Khoo LT, Beisse R, Potulski M. Thoracoscopic-assisted treatment of thoracic and lumbar fractures: a series of 371 consecutive cases. Neurosurgery 2002;51(Suppl 5):S104–17.

73. Isaacs RE, Podichetty V, Fessler RG. Microendoscopic discectomy for recurrent disc herniations. Neurosurg Focus 2003;15(3):E11.

74. Isaacs RE, Podichetty VK, Santiago P, et al. Minimally invasive microendoscopy-assisted transforaminal lumbar interbody fusion with instrumentation. J Neurosurg Spine 2005;3(2):98–105.

75. Tredway TL, Santiago P, Hrubes MR, et al. Minimally invasive resection of intradural-extramedullary spinal neoplasms. Neurosurgery 2006;58(Suppl 1):ONS52–8 [discussion: ONS52–8].

76. Tredway TL, Musleh W, Christie SD, et al. A novel minimally invasive technique for spinal cord untethering. Neurosurgery 2007;60(2 Suppl 1):ONS70–4 [discussion: ONS74].

77. O'Toole JE, Eichholz KM, Fessler RG. Minimally invasive insertion of syringosubarachnoid shunt for posttraumatic syringomyelia: technical case report. Neurosurgery 2007;61(5 Suppl 2):E331–2 [discussion: E332].

78. Deutsch H, Boco T, Lobel J. Minimally invasive transpedicular vertebrectomy for metastatic disease to the thoracic spine. J Spinal Disord Tech 2008;21(2):101–5.

79. Ogden AT, Fessler RG. Minimally invasive resection of intramedullary ependymoma: case report. Neurosurgery 2009;65(6):E1203–4 [discussion: E1204].

80. Park P, Leveque JC, LaMarca F, et al. Dural closure using the U-clip in minimally invasive spinal tumor resection. J Spinal Disord Tech 2010;23(7):486–9.

81. Pompili A, Caroli F, Telera S, et al. Minimally invasive resection of intradural-extramedullary spinal neoplasms. Neurosurgery 2006;59(5):E1152.

82. Haji FA, Cenic A, Crevier L, et al. Minimally invasive approach for the resection of spinal neoplasm. Spine (Phila Pa 1976) 2011;36(15):E1018–26.

Percutaneous Pedicle Screw Fixation for Thoracolumbar Fractures

Nader S. Dahdaleh, MD[a],*, Zachary A. Smith, MD[a],
Patrick W. Hitchon, MD[b]

KEYWORDS

- Thoracolumbar fractures • Thoracic fractures • Lumbar fractures • Minimally invasive spine surgery
- Percutaneous pedicle screws

KEY POINTS

- A thorough knowledge of the current classification system is key to successful management of various thoracolumbar fractures.
- Percutaneous pedicle screw fixation is an option for a wide variety of thoracolumbar fractures in patients who are neurologically normal and do not require decompression of neural elements.

INTRODUCTION

Percutaneous spinal techniques have gained wide popularity in the degenerative spinal arena over the past 2 decades. Supported by an immense and still growing amount of evidence, the main principle of avoiding unnecessary muscle dissection and tissue disruption[1] translates into faster recovery, decreased blood loss, decreased complications, shorter hospitalization, and improved cost-effectiveness when compared with traditional open surgical techniques,[2–7] obviously without compromising efficacy and long-term outcome.

In parallel, percutaneous pedicle screw fixation has been gaining popularity in the management of a variety of thoracic, thoracolumbar junction, and lumbar fractures.[8–12] With goals beyond sparing muscle and tissue disruption, percutaneous surgery for spinal fractures offers the option of internal fixation, stabilization, and fracture healing while sparing fusion and maintaining motion at the segments above and below the fracture. To date, clinical studies have shown that instrumentation without fusion in the treatment of thoracolumbar burst fractures is viable.[13] Thoracolumbar burst fractures with fusion in 37 fractures and without fusion in 36 fractures did equally well at 5 years' follow-up. Operative time and blood loss were less in the nonfusion group, and the operative time was shorter. There was no hardware failure in the nonfusion group. Both groups showed improvement in kyphosis and neurologic performance.

In general, the immediate goals of treating any spinal fracture include the achievement of spinal stability with anatomic or near anatomic alignment, and the ability to expedite patient mobilization. Long-term goals include healing of the fracture with maintenance of alignment, avoidance of posttraumatic kyphosis, and, if possible, sparing motion at the segments above and below the fracture.[14]

Sources of Support: None.
[a] Department of Neurological Surgery, Northwestern University Feinberg School of Medicine, 676 North St Clair Street, Suite 2210, Chicago, IL 60611, USA; [b] Department of Neurosurgery, Carver School of Medicine, 200 Hawkins Drive, University of Iowa, Iowa City, IA 52242, USA
* Corresponding author.
E-mail address: ndahdale@nmff.org

Neurosurg Clin N Am 25 (2014) 337–346
http://dx.doi.org/10.1016/j.nec.2013.12.011
1042-3680/14/$ – see front matter © 2014 Elsevier Inc. All rights reserved.

CLASSIFICATION OF THORACOLUMBAR SPINE FRACTURES

An in-depth knowledge of the current and popular systems that classify spinal fractures is of utmost importance. The first step in the management of thoracolumbar fractures requires the ability to differentiate between stable fractures that can be treated safely with or without bracing, and unstable fractures that require operative intervention. The second step in the decision making requires the selection of the appropriate surgical technique and approach (or approaches) in fractures that require operative intervention.

One classification that has stood the test of time because of its ease of use and applicability is the one devised by Denis[15] that divides the spine into 3 columns: anterior, middle, and posterior. Based on this and other classification systems that take into account the integrity of the posterior ligaments, neurologic state, and persistent pain, the Iowa algorithm has been successfully used at the authors' institution (**Fig. 1**).[16] This classification simply identifies 4 types of fractures based on the Denis columns involved. Compression fractures, also known as flexion compression fractures, involve the fracture of the anterior column. These injuries are usually treated conservatively with or without bracing. Two-column injuries, also known as burst fractures, occur because of axial loading and involve fractures of the anterior and middle Denis columns. Identification of instability in this category is more challenging and is based on the neurologic state, degree of kyphosis, and disruption of the posterior ligamentous complex. When operative treatment is required it might require anterior column reconstruction, as explained later. Three-column injuries include fracture dislocations and flexion (or extension) distraction injuries. These fractures are inherently clinically and biomechanically unstable, and always require operative internal fixation.

FRACTURES TREATABLE BY PERCUTANEOUS PEDICLE SCREW FIXATION

Percutaneous pedicle screw fixation provides an appropriate option to internally fix a spinal fracture until the healing of the fracture takes place. Fractures most suited for minimally invasive surgery (MIS) instrumentation are intact with or without pain. Obviously a fracture that lends itself as treatable by MIS is one that does not require reduction or decompression (Magerl type A1, A2, and some A3 fractures, and Thoracolumbar Injury Classification and Severity [TLICS] score <5). Fractures with disruption of the posterior ligamentous complex without subluxation or dislocation (some Magerl type B fractures) are also suited for percutaneous screw fixation (**Fig. 2**). Fracture dislocations that are irreducible percutaneously because of locked facets require open reduction. Fractures such as bursts with bone in the canal and neurologic deficit (TLICS score >5) also require open decompression.

After fracture healing or union takes place, the surgeon has the option to remove the screws without compromising alignment, and hence maintain the mobility of segments cranial and caudal to the fracture. Most investigators agree that the appropriate time for hardware removal is after 9 months to 1 year following the injury and operative fixation.

TECHNIQUE FOR PERCUTANEOUS PEDICLE SCREW PLACEMENT

The fractured level is identified using C-arm fluoroscopy. The anteroposterior (AP) view is then used. A good AP image would show the spinous

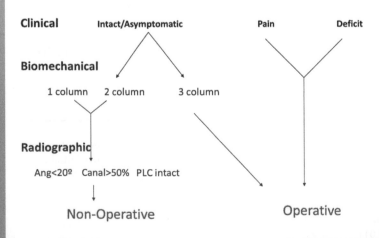

Fig. 1. Iowa algorithm for the management of thoracolumbar fractures. PLC, posterior ligament complex.

A

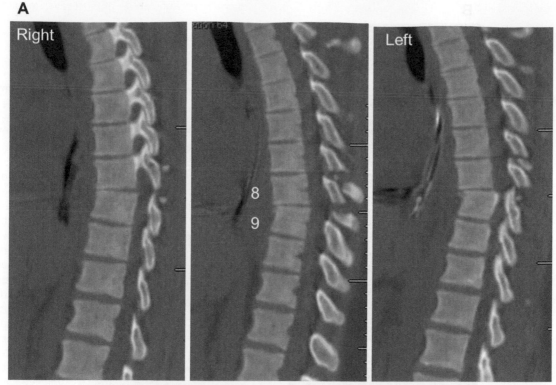

Fig. 2. A 23-year-old man, the restrained driver involved in a roll-over accident at highway speed. He was intact neurologically, but complained of spinal and chest pain. (*A*) Sagittal computed tomography (CT) shows fractured facets and laminae with minimal anterior subluxation and kyphosis. (*B*) Sagittal T2-weighted and short-tau inversion recovery (STIR) magnetic resonance (MR) images show disruption of the posterior ligamentous complex. He was managed with percutaneous pedicle screw fixation. (*C*) One and a half years later, anteroposterior and lateral radiographs show good alignment and no hardware complications. The patient had been released to return to work.

process in midline and a well-demarcated superior end plate above the pedicles of interest (**Fig. 3**A). A 1- to 2-cm incision is proposed and marked just lateral to the lateral border of the pedicle. The incision is then made down to the fascia. The dorsolumbar fascia is then incised with scissors or monopolar cautery.

While viewing the AP fluoroscopic view, the following is performed. First, the Jamshidi needle is introduced until bone is encountered. The entry point is usually selected to be at or just lateral to the lateral border of the pedicle in the AP view. The Jamshidi needle is introduced parallel to the disc space, and is triangulated relative to the sagittal plane. At the thoracolumbar junction, triangulation can be around 10°, with triangulation increasing to as much as 30° toward the top of the thoracic spine and the bottom of the lumbar spine. The tip of the needle should not violate the medial border of the pedicle following 20-mm introduction. Once the needle is within the body and past the pedicle, the lateral fluoroscopic view is chosen.

A K-wire is then introduced through the Jamshidi needle. This wire acts as a guide for all subsequent instruments, including the pedicle screw. Thus it is necessary to keep the guide wire in place without inadvertently withdrawing or advancing it. The Jamshidi needle is withdrawn and the K-wire is kept in place. A dilator is then advanced along the guide wire, followed by a cannulated awl to penetrate the cortical bone at the point of entry. The awl is withdrawn, and an appropriately sized cannulated tap is introduced through the K-wire and used to create the path for the screw in a direction parallel to the end plate. The pedicle is tapped, with only the tip of the tap reaching into the body. Undertapping the pedicle is advised for a snugger fit of the screw. Maintaining the trajectory of the guide wire is necessary such that it is not transected or bent by the tap or screw. The tap is withdrawn and a cannulated screw, the diameter and length of which are based on the computed tomography images, introduced through the K-wire (**Fig. 3**B).

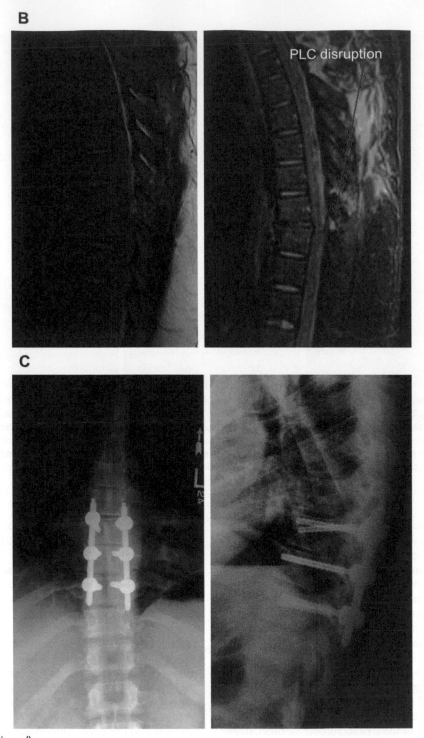

Fig. 2. (continued)

Rod measurement is accomplished by using a compass or through trial and error in estimating length and curvature. The rod is contoured, lordotic for lumbar, straight for thoracolumbar, and kyphotic for thoracic, and attached to the introducer (**Fig. 3**C). The rod is introduced subfascially, rostrally, or caudally, and advanced through the slots of the pedicle screws. The screws are

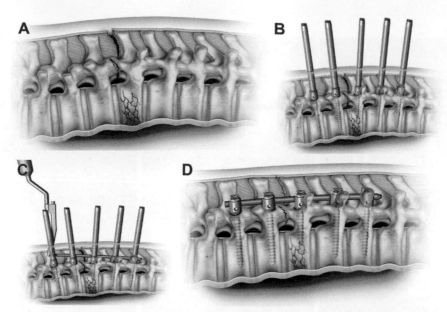

Fig. 3. Sequence of steps in percutaneous screw fixation. (*A*) The patient is prone on the operating-room table and ready for posteroanterior and lateral fluoroscopy. (*B*) Pedicle screws with extended tabs are inserted. (*C*) Contoured rod is inserted subfascially. (*D*) Set screws are tightened on the rod.

then inserted, and under compression are tightened while the rod is held in the inserter to prevent the rod from flipping from a lordotic to a kyphotic position. Final tightening is performed with the antitorque in place to prevent rod rotation in the coronal plane (**Fig. 3**D). The authors usually obtain an intraoperative multiplanar image to verify appropriate screw placement in 3 dimensions without medial or lateral violation of the pedicle. Afterward, the screw holders are removed or the extended tabs broken off.

APPLICATIONS AND PRELIMINARY RESULTS

A cage can be supplemented with posterior percutaneous pedicle screw fixation. A variety of fractures can be treated successfully with percutaneous pedicle screw fixation, including flexion or extension-distraction injuries, compression fractures, and burst fractures. To date, minimally invasive percutaneous screw fixation has been undertaken in 30 patients at the authors' institution, only 1 of whom has required revision of hardware the following day for misplaced hardware, without sequelae.

Flexion-Distraction Injuries

These fractures are best treated with percutaneous pedicle screws with the goal of restoring the disrupted posterior tension band formed by the posterior ligamentous complex, allowing for

the fractured pedicle and middle columns to heal. In 2 reports, Beringer and colleagues[10] and Schizas and Kosmopoulos[9] treated a total of 4 Chance fractures successfully with hardware removal after 6 to 9 months. An example is presented in **Fig. 4**, which illustrates a flexion-distraction fracture of L1. A recent article by Grossbach and colleagues[17] demonstrated similar efficacy, less blood loss, and a trend toward less hospitalization for flexion-distraction injuries treated percutaneously in comparison with open techniques.

Burst Fractures

Burst fractures with low load-sharing scores can be treated with purely percutaneous pedicle screw fixation. Fractures requiring anterior column reconstructions can be supplemented with posterior percutaneous pedicle screw fixation. Growing evidence is emerging showing the feasibility of percutaneous pedicle screw fixation for these fractures. Ni and colleagues[11] treated 36 Magerl type A3 (burst) fractures and a load-sharing score of 6 or less with percutaneous short-segment fixation. After a mean follow-up of 48.5 months, 31 (86.1%) patients had a satisfactory result (19 excellent and 12 good), and the remaining 5 fair. A few reports also demonstrated the option of percutaneous pedicle screw fixation as an adjunct to kyphoplasty,[18,19] an example of which is presented in **Fig. 5**.

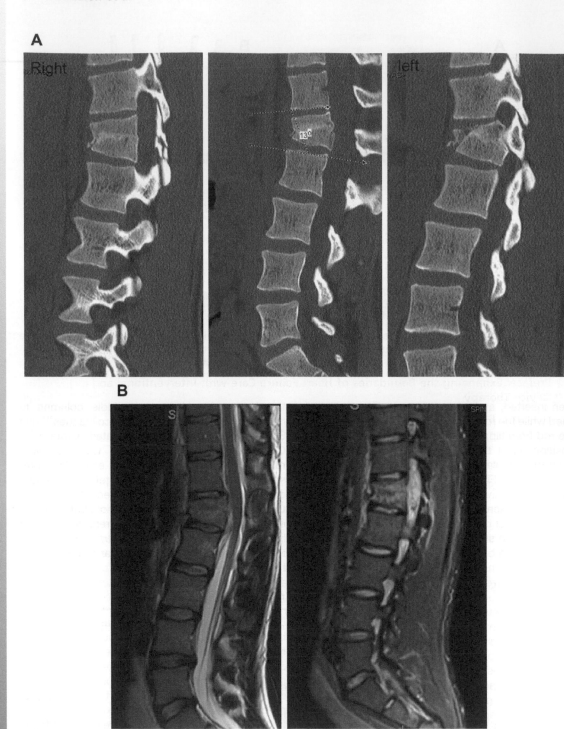

Fig. 4. A 26-year-old man who jumped and landed on his feet from a 6-m high parking structure. The patient suffered severe back pain, but continued to ambulate after his injury without deficit. (*A*) Sagittal CT scans show the flexion-distraction fracture of L1, with facet fracture on the right, compression fracture of the body, and kyphosis. (*B*) T2-weighted and STIR MR sequences show the kyphosis and compression fracture. The true extent of the ligamentous disruption is uncertain. The patient was managed with percutaneous pedicle screw fixation. Two months later the patient returned to the clinic with minimal discomfort and returned to light duty. (*C*) The entry wounds are well healed. (*D*) Radiographs show satisfactory alignment with hardware intact.

C

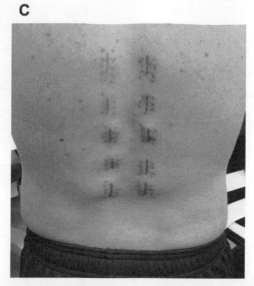

D

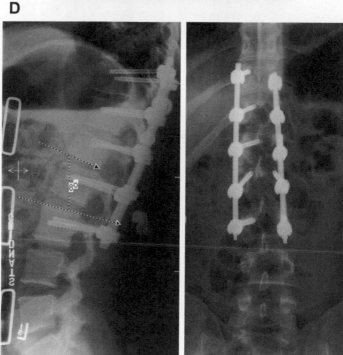

Fig. 4. (*continued*)

Controversy still abounds over the management of burst fractures in patients who are neurologically normal, as these patients can be braced or treated operatively. To date the literature lacks any studies comparing percutaneous pedicle screw fixation with external bracing.

Compression Fractures

Most of these fractures are stable, requiring an external brace and sometimes no bracing at all.

In patients whose pain prevents them from being mobilized, percutaneous short-segment fixation improves pain and enhances earlier mobilization. Palmisani and colleagues[8] retrospectively reviewed 51 patients who suffered 64 thoracolumbar fractures and were treated with percutaneous pedicle screw fixation. The mean follow-up period was 14.2 months. T12 and L2 constituted 66% of fracture levels involved. Thirty (46.9%) were Magerl/AO type A1 and A2 fractures, whereas the rest were a combination of

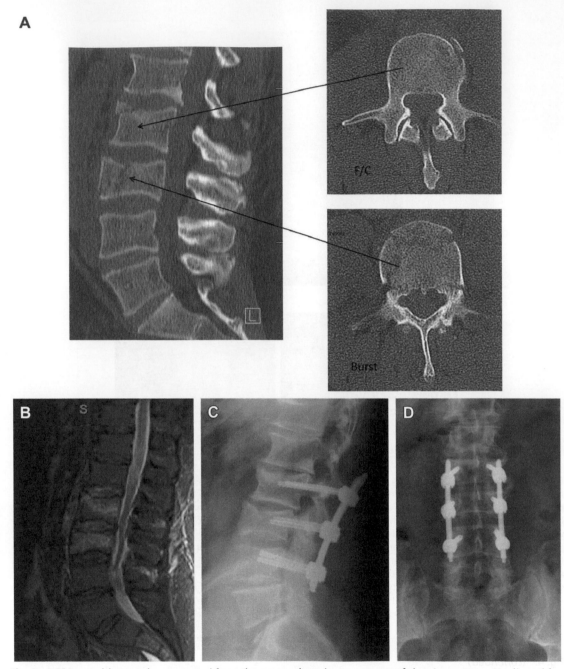

Fig. 5. A 59-year-old man who presented from the scene where he was on a roof cleaning gutters. He slipped forward off edge of the roof and fell 14 feet (4.27 m), and hit the ground feet first, knees bent up to the chest. He complained of back pain, but was intact. (*A*) CT image shows the compression fracture of L2 and the burst fracture of L3. There is minimal retropulsion of bone into the canal. (*B*) STIR MR image shows no disruption of the posterior ligament complex. The patient underwent percutaneous screw fixation, and 2 years later he is symptom-free. (*C, D*) Lateral and anteroposterior plain films show the alignment preserved and the hardware intact.

A3, B1, B2, C1, and C2 fractures. There was improvement and maintenance of improvement in postoperative kyphosis, except for constructs that used polyaxial screws. Of 64 fractures, 63 fused with resolution of back pain at follow-up.

Two constructs showed mechanical failure and one fracture did not heal, requiring the patient to undergo anterior arthrodesis. Ten of the 51 patients had their instrumentation removed. An example is presented in **Fig. 5**.

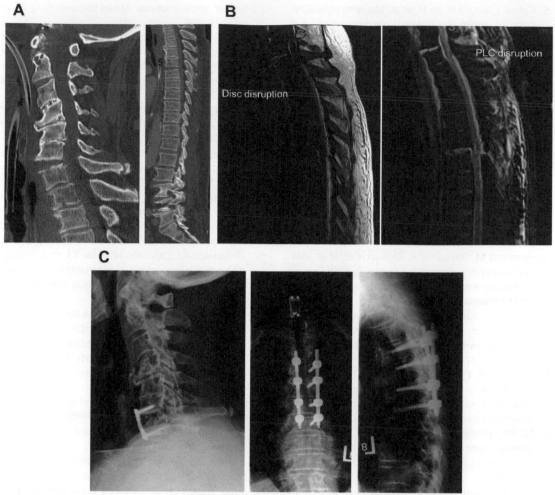

Fig. 6. An 85-year-old man was logging on his farm when a tree fell, pinning him to the ground. He was pinned there for about 5 minutes before onlookers were able to remove the tree. He was unresponsive and intubated. Emergency needle decompression of the left chest was done. The patient was spontaneously moving all 4 extremities. (*A*) CT image demonstrates extension injuries to the spine at C6-7 and T5-6. (*B*) T2-weighted and STIR MR images show disc disruption at both levels, with some displacement and posterior ligamentous disruption at T5-6. (*C*) Postoperative plain films 5 months later show stable alignment and intact hardware.

Extension-Distraction Injuries

These 3-column injuries occur in the setting of ankylosing spondylitis or diffuse idiopathic skeletal hyperostosis.[20] Unlike for other types of fractures, the authors recommend long-segment fixation because most or all of the segments above and below the fractures are autofused, forming a large lever arm. For optimal biomechanical stability, it is prudent to have multiple points of fixation. An example is shown in **Fig. 6**.

REFERENCES

1. Kim DY, Lee SH, Chung SK, et al. Comparison of multifidus muscle atrophy and trunk extension muscle strength: percutaneous versus open pedicle screw fixation. Spine 2005;30(1):123–9.
2. Parker SL, Lerner J, McGirt MJ. Effect of minimally invasive technique on return to work and narcotic use following transforaminal lumbar inter-body fusion: a review. Prof Case Manag 2012;17(5):229–35.
3. Wang J, Zhou Y, Feng Zhang Z, et al. Comparison of clinical outcome in overweight or obese patients after minimally invasive versus open transforaminal lumbar interbody fusion. J Spinal Disord Tech 2012. [Epub ahead of print].
4. Lee KH, Yue WM, Yeo W, et al. Clinical and radiological outcomes of open versus minimally invasive transforaminal lumbar interbody fusion. Eur Spine J 2012;21(11):2265–70.

5. Kotani Y, Abumi K, Ito M, et al. Mid-term clinical results of minimally invasive decompression and posterolateral fusion with percutaneous pedicle screws versus conventional approach for degenerative spondylolisthesis with spinal stenosis. Eur Spine J 2012;21(6):1171–7.

6. Parker SL, Adogwa O, Bydon A, et al. Cost-effectiveness of minimally invasive versus open transforaminal lumbar interbody fusion for degenerative spondylolisthesis associated low-back and leg pain over two years. World Neurosurg 2012;78(1–2):178–84.

7. Wang MY, Cummock MD, Yu Y, et al. An analysis of the differences in the acute hospitalization charges following minimally invasive versus open posterior lumbar interbody fusion. J Neurosurg Spine 2010; 12(6):694–9.

8. Palmisani M, Gasbarrini A, Brodano GB, et al. Minimally invasive percutaneous fixation in the treatment of thoracic and lumbar spine fractures. Eur Spine J 2009;18(Suppl 1):71–4.

9. Schizas C, Kosmopoulos V. Percutaneous surgical treatment of chance fractures using cannulated pedicle screws. Report of two cases. J Neurosurg Spine 2007;7(1):71–4.

10. Beringer W, Potts E, Khairi S, et al. Percutaneous pedicle screw instrumentation for temporary internal bracing of nondisplaced bony Chance fractures. J Spinal Disord Tech 2007;20(3):242–7.

11. Ni WF, Huang YX, Chi YL, et al. Percutaneous pedicle screw fixation for neurologic intact thoracolumbar burst fractures. J Spinal Disord Tech 2010; 23(8):530–7.

12. De Iure F, Cappuccio M, Paderni S, et al. Minimal invasive percutaneous fixation of thoracic and lumbar spine fractures. Minim Invasive Surg 2012; 2012:141032.

13. Dai LY, Jiang LS, Jiang SD. Posterior short-segment fixation with or without fusion for thoracolumbar burst fractures. A five to seven-year prospective randomized study. J Bone Joint Surg Am 2009;91(5): 1033–41.

14. Kim YM, Kim DS, Choi ES, et al. Nonfusion method in thoracolumbar and lumbar spinal fractures. Spine 2011;36(2):170–6.

15. Denis F. The three column spine and its significance in the classification of acute thoracolumbar spinal injuries. Spine 1983;8(8):817–31.

16. Dahdaleh NS, Hitchon PW. Classification of thoracolumbar spine fractures. In: Benzel EC, editor. Spine surgery: techniques, complication avoidance, and management. Philadelphia: Elsevier; 2012. p. 593–9.

17. Grossbach AJ, Dahdaleh NS, Abel TJ, et al. Flexion-distraction injuries of the thoracolumbar spine: open fusion versus percutaneous pedicle screw fixation. Neurosurg Focus 2013;35(2):E2.

18. Bironneau A, Bouquet C, Millet-Barbe B, et al. Percutaneous internal fixation combined with kyphoplasty for neurologically intact thoracolumbar fractures: a prospective cohort study of 24 patients with one year of follow-up. Orthop Traumatol Surg Res 2011;97(4):389–95.

19. Fuentes S, Blondel B, Metellus P, et al. Percutaneous kyphoplasty and pedicle screw fixation for the management of thoraco-lumbar burst fractures. Eur Spine J 2010;19(8):1281–7.

20. Burkus JK, Denis F. Hyperextension injuries of the thoracic spine in diffuse idiopathic skeletal hyperostosis. Report of four cases. J Bone Joint Surg Am 1994;76(2):237–43.

Miniopen Pedicle Subtraction Osteotomy
Surgical Technique and Initial Results

Michael Y. Wang, MD[a,b,*]

KEYWORDS

- Minimally invasive • Spinal deformity • Osteotomy • Scoliosis • Kyphosis • Pedicle screw
- Percutaneous • Sagittal balance

KEY POINTS

- Adult spinal deformity surgery is becoming increasingly common, in part as a result of the aging of the population in the developed world as well as the increasing recognition that deformities can severely affect the quality of life of afflicted patients.
- The traditional open surgical procedures for adult spinal deformity are highly effective. However, they are associated with high morbidity and complication rates.
- Correction and maintenance of proper sagittal balance is a key determinant of success with spinal fusion surgeries.
- A new miniopen approach for using pedicle subtraction osteotomy to achieve sagittal realignment is a promising option for adult patients with deformity.

INTRODUCTION: NATURE OF THE PROBLEM

Throughout the developed world, the past century has seen phenomenal advances in medicine, safety, and sanitation. The result has been a substantially lengthened average life span, and it is now not uncommon for spinal surgery patients to be in their late 80s or 90s. In concert with this development has been the increasing expectation from patients that they will have not only a prolonged life span but also an associated full functional ability during most of that time. In the United States, the fastest growing population is between the ages of 80 and 100 years.[1] These forces are shaping the future for spinal surgeons and creating ever more challenges.

Adult spinal deformities (ASD), particularly those associated with kyphosis in the thoracolumbar spine, are commonly associated with advancing age. ASD is a common reason for presentation to the neurosurgeon or orthopedic surgeon, and the National Health and Nutrition Examination Survey database has identified that up to 8.3% of the adult population harbors a scoliosis of 10° or more.[2] Symptoms at presentation can include leg pain from radiculopathy, neurogenic claudication from spinal stenosis, back pain from degenerative arthritis, or postural complaints. Numerous modern spinal surgical techniques have been developed to treat symptomatic ASD, and most of these rely on some form of anterior column height restoration or osteotomy to improve lordosis and correct scoliosis.[3–9] However, these methods often require severe disruption of the soft tissue envelope through a subperiosteal to expose the spinal anatomy. This situation leads to substantial blood loss, prolonged

Disclosure statement: M.Y. Wang serves as a consultant and receives royalty payments from Depuy Spine.
[a] Department of Neurological Surgery, University of Miami Miller School of Medicine, Miami, FL, USA;
[b] Department of Rehabilitation Medicine, University of Miami Miller School of Medicine, Miami, FL, USA
* Department of Neurological Surgery, Lois Pope Life Center, 1095 NW 14th Terrace, D4-6, Lois Pope LIFE Center, Miami, FL 33136.
E-mail address: MWang2@med.miami.edu

hospitalizations, and higher risk for the patient. In many instances, the risks involved require a staged operation.

When coupled with the fact that patients with ASD are often aged with multiple medical comorbidities, such surgeries pose a challenge for surgeons managing their care. The major complication rate from these interventions is reported to vary between 25% and 60% in large reported series.[10–12] One of the future challenges for spinal deformity surgeons is to develop newer methods for minimizing the risks of the surgical intervention to improve the safety profile of these interventions.

Over the past decade, new minimally invasive surgical (MIS) techniques have been developed to improve the clinical outcomes of spinal surgery. It is becoming apparent that reduced blood loss and infection rates are benefits of minimizing soft tissue injury.[13–15] MIS techniques for treating ASD thus offer the potential for reducing complication rates and morbidity associated with these surgeries. Over the past 5 years, spinal surgeons have been using a combined approach with lateral MIS interbody fusion followed by percutaneous pedicle screws to correct ASD.[16–19] However, this approach has been proved to be limited for correcting regional or global lumbar lordosis or sagittal balance.[20] Traditionally, a 3-column osteotomy such as a pedicle subtraction osteotomy (PSO) has been necessary for correction of kyphosis or flat back syndrome. This approach has been previously described in a cadaveric model by Voyadis and colleagues.[21] More recently, the clinical feasibility of this approach in patients has been reported using a miniopen PSO and percutaneous spinal fixation.[22]

SURGICAL TECHNIQUE

The miniopen PSO that we have been using at the University of Miami incorporates 3 distinct elements. The osteotomy site is approached with a bilateral open subperiosteal dissection. Thus, it is achieved in a manner similar to an open PSO. This strategy overcomes the problem of control of bleeding and the management of neural structures intrinsic to 3-column osteotomies. However, the total soft tissue envelope disruption is similar to a 1-level posterolateral fusion or a 2-level open laminectomy. The surgery caudal to the PSO is performed with MIS transforaminal interbody fusions (TLIFs) with interbody cages, and potentially with percutaneous iliac screws.[23] Above the PSO site, the construct is achieved with percutaneous screws supplemented with facet or interlaminar fusions.

The difficulty with previous MIS sagittal deformity correction was the result of an inability to pass a lordotic rod through a kyphotic or flat spine. This procedure had been a geometric impossibility without further soft tissue elevation or placement of a rod above the fascia. With the mini-PSO, a technique was borrowed from the open surgical methods. Use of a 4-rod cantilever construct allowed for 2 rods to be passed from above and 2 from below (**Figs. 1** and **2**). The rod tips protruded through the central incision (at the mini-PSO site) and were connected after the osteotomy site was fractured to surgically introduce lumbar lordosis. The 4-rod technique provided 4 unique advantages. First, as mentioned earlier, the appropriate amount of lordosis can be introduced into the rod construct. Second, the spine can be mechanically controlled after the destabilizing osteotomy. In open surgery, this control is accomplished with a temporary rod. In the mini-PSO, the rod-screw articulations are used to break the wedge osteotomy and the final destabilizing maneuver (lateral or posterior cortical bone removal) is performed only after the rods have been affixed to the screws in a semirigid manner. Third, the use of 4 rods allows the spine to be managed as 2 distinct segments: cranial and caudal. The screws and rods above work as a single unit, and the screws and rods below work as another unit. This factor reduces the risk of screw pullout, which is more likely in segmental correction maneuvers. This situation is clearly beneficial when treating osteoporotic patients. The amount of rod bending before placement can be reduced on any part of its length. This goal is achieved by distributing half the total bend on the caudal rod and half on the cranial rod. The amount of lordosis is the same, but there is a reduction in the amount or metal fretting and etching as a result (**Fig. 3**). The result is simultaneous correction of the sagittal and coronal deformities, with the correction occurring through the PSO site (see **Fig. 3**).

Surgical procedure steps:
1. Minimally invasive interbody fusion at levels caudal to the planned mini-PSO
2. Exposure of the mini-PSO site (typically L2 or L3), with exposure to the transverse process at that level
3. Full laminectomy and bilateral full facetectomies at the mini-PSO level
4. Skeletonization of the roots above and below the mini-PSO pedicles
5. Disconnection of the transverse processes and removal of the pedicles bilaterally
6. Cancellous decandellation at the mini-PSO level

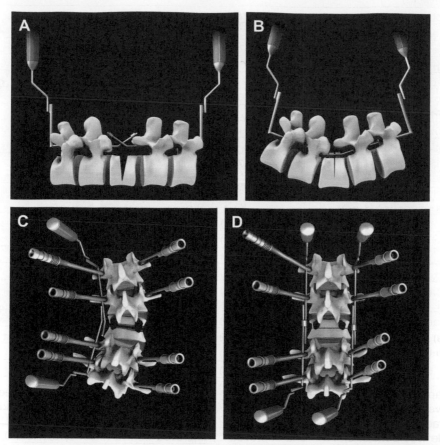

Fig. 1. Artist's depiction of a miniopen PSO correction before (*A, B*) and after (*C, D*) osteotomy closure.

7. Removal of the posterior vertebral cortex and posterior longitudinal ligament
8. Optional removal of the caudal disk for an extended PSO
9. Percutaneous spinal fixation at all levels necessary
10. Placement of 4 subfascial rods and set screw application
11. Removal of final PSO bone (lateral vertebral cortical walls)
12. Fracture across the PSO site
13. Connection of cranial rods to caudal rods
14. Facet and interlaminar fusion at proximal levels
15. Closure

CLINICAL AND RADIOGRAPHIC OUTCOMES

The first 7 patients treated at the University of Miami with a minimum of 12-month follow-up were evaluated. The mean age was 65.9 years (range 58–84 years) and the male/female ratio was 3:4. The total number of levels instrumented and fused was a mean of 8.1 (range 8–9), and the total mean number of interbody fusion levels was 2.6 (range 1–4). Surgical parameters included a mean operative time of 364 ± 57 minutes (range 300–450 minutes), and a mean intraoperative blood loss of 793 ± 303 mL (range 400–1200 mL). Three patients had elective allogeneic blood transfusions, with a mean of 0.86 ± 1.1 units of packed red blood cells (range 0–2 units). There were no intraoperative complications, but 1 patient had a return to the operative room for cage repositioning on postoperative day 3. Mean length of stay in the hospital was 5.4 days.

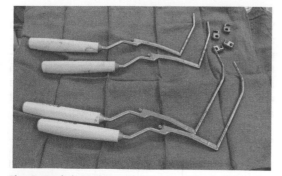

Fig. 2. Rods bent into the appropriate configuration for mini-PSO with rod connectors on a Mayo stand.

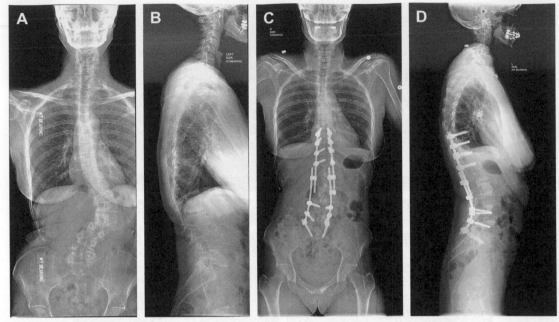

Fig. 3. (*A*, *B*) Preoperative and (*C*, *D*) postoperative 91-cm (36-in) standing radiographs of a patient who underwent a mini-PSO with facet fusion and MIS TLIF.

Radiographic outcomes were determined on preoperative and postoperative 91-cm (36-in) standing radiographs. The preoperative coronal Cobb angle was a mean of 44.4° and improved to 15.9° at last follow-up (**Table 1**). The preoperative coronal alignment was a mean of 5.5 cm and improved to 1.8 cm at last follow-up. The preoperative lumbar lordosis angle (L1-S1) was a mean of 16.1° and improved to 45.3° at last follow-up. This situation resulted in an average increase of 29.2° of lumbar lordosis (range 17–44°). The preoperative sagittal vertical axis was a mean of 9.5 cm and improved to 3.2 cm at last follow-up. Pelvic tilt was a mean of 35.6° and improved to 26.0° at last follow-up.

Clinical outcomes were determined using the Visual Analog Scale (VAS) for leg and back pain and the Oswestry Disability Index (ODI). Leg VAS improved from a mean of 5.4 to 1.0; axial back pain VAS improved from a mean of 9.3 to 4.2. The mean ODI improved from 39.3 to 13.7.

COMPLICATIONS AND CONCERNS

This new technique for MIS spinal deformity correction is still in its early stages. The technique relies on the use of osteobiological agents, particularly to promote facet and interlaminar fusions in the proximal construct. The presence of previous posterior spinal instrumentation can also impede surgery using this technique. In addition, longer-term follow-up is needed to show the maintenance of deformity correction over time and satisfactory bony fusion rates. Delayed nonunions and hardware fracture occur with a high prevalence even at 5 or more years after ASD surgery. It can be expected that a proportion of the MIS treated patients will also have these untoward events. In addition, larger case series at multiple institutions are needed not only to validate this technique but also to determine its ease of adoption.

SUMMARY

This new mini-PSO technique is a hybrid method that respects the tremendous clinical experience of open deformity surgeons. Those deformity

Table 1
Radiographic parameters

	Preoperative (Mean ± SD)	Postoperative (Mean ± SD)
Coronal Cobb angle	44.4° ± 14.2	15.8° ± 6.2
Coronal alignment	5.5 ± 3.9 cm	1.8 ± 1.1 cm
Lumbar lordosis angle (L1-S1)	16.1° ± 13	45.3° ± 11.8
Sagittal vertical axis	9.5 ± 10.4 cm	3.2 ± 5.2
Pelvic tilt	35.6° ± 11.1	26.0° ± 7.0

principles for ASD include the need to maintain or establish global sagittal balance, serious attempts to achieve a bony arthrodesis, and rigid fixation over a long segment construct. By reducing blood loss and disruption of the soft tissue envelope, this method has great promise. However, techniques and technology are in constant evolution and future developments will create more effective and safer interventions. Methods for destabilizing the stiff ASD spine, achieving adequate fixation in osteoporotic bone, correcting the deformity with less tissue trauma, and promoting bony arthrodesis are needed in the future with an ever aging and challenged population of patients with ASD.

REFERENCES

1. Krach C. Centenarians in the United States, in: US Department of Health & Human Services, US Department of Commerce, US Census Bureau, 1990, Vol P23-199RV. p. 1–24.
2. Carter O, Haynes S. Prevalence rates for scoliosis in US adults: results from the First National Health and Nutrition Examination Survey. Int J Epidemiol 1987;16:537–44.
3. Bridwell KH, Lewis SJ, Lenke LG, et al. Pedicle subtraction osteotomy for the treatment of fixed sagittal imbalance. J Bone Joint Surg Am 2003;85-A:454–63.
4. Heary RF, Bono CM. Pedicle subtraction osteotomy in the treatment of chronic, posttraumatic kyphotic deformity. J Neurosurg Spine 2006;5:1–8.
5. Kim Y, Bridwell K, Lenke L, et al. Results of lumbar pedicle subtraction osteotomies for fixed sagittal imbalance: a minimum 5-year follow-up study. Spine 2007;32:2189–97.
6. Mummaneni P, Dhall S, Ondra S, et al. Pedicle subtraction osteotomy. Neurosurgery 2008;63:S171–6.
7. Ondra SL, Marzouk S, Koski T, et al. Mathematical calculation of pedicle subtraction osteotomy size to allow precision correction of fixed sagittal deformity. Spine 2006;31:E973–9.
8. van Loon PJ, van Stralen G, van Loon CJ, et al. A pedicle subtraction osteotomy as an adjunctive tool in the surgical treatment of a rigid thoracolumbar hyperkyphosis; a preliminary report. Spine J 2006;6:195–200.
9. Wang MY, Berven SH. Lumbar pedicle subtraction osteotomy. Neurosurgery 2007;60:ONS140–6 [discussion: ONS146].
10. Charosky S, Guigui P, Blamoutier A, et al. Complications and risk factors of primary adult scoliosis surgery: a multicenter study of 306 patients. Spine 2012;37:693–700.
11. Smith J, Shaffrey C, Glassman S, et al. Risk-benefit assessment of surgery for adult scoliosis. Spine 2011;36:817–24.
12. Weistroffer J, Perra J, Lonstein J, et al. Complications in long fusions to the sacrum for adult scoliosis: minimum five-year analysis of fifty patients. Spine 2008;33:1478–83.
13. Fessler R. Minimally invasive percutaneous posterior lumbar interbody fusion. Neurosurgery 2003;52:1512.
14. Holly L, Foley K. Percutaneous placement of posterior cervical screws using three-dimensional fluoroscopy. Spine 2006;31:536–41.
15. Khoo L, Palmer S, Laich D, et al. Minimally invasive percutaneous posterior lumbar interbody fusion. Neurosurgery 2003;S2:166–81.
16. Anand N, Rosemann R, Khalsa B, et al. Mid-term to long-term clinical and functional outcomes of minimally invasive correction and fusion for adults with scoliosis. Neurosurg Focus 2010;28:E6.
17. Dakwar E, Cardona R, Smith D, et al. Early outcomes and safety of the minimally invasive, lateral retroperitoneal transpsoas approach for adult degenerative scoliosis. Neurosurg Focus 2010;28:E8.
18. Hsieh P, Koski T, Sciubba D, et al. Maximizing the potential of minimally invasive spine surgery in complex spinal disorders. Neurosurg Focus 2008;25:E19.
19. Wang MY, Mummaneni PV. Minimally invasive surgery for thoracolumbar spinal deformity: initial clinical experience with clinical and radiographic outcomes. Neurosurg Focus 2010;28:E9.
20. Acosta F, Liu J, Slimack N, et al. Changes in coronal and sagittal plane alignment following minimally invasive direct lateral interbody fusion for the treatment of degenerative lumbar disease in adults: a radiographic study. J Neurosurg 2011;15:92–6.
21. Voyadis J, Gala V, O'Toole J, et al. Minimally invasive posterior osteotomies. Neurosurgery 2008;63:A204–10.
22. Wang M, Madhavan K. Mini-open pedicle subtraction osteotomy: surgical technique. World Neurosurg 2012. [Epub ahead of print].
23. Wang MY. Improvement of sagittal balance and lumbar lordosis following less invasive adult spinal deformity surgery with expandable cages and percutaneous instrumentation. J Neurosurg Spine 2013;18:4–12.

Lateral Transpsoas Lumbar Interbody Fusion
Outcomes and Deformity Correction

Nader S. Dahdaleh, MD[a],*, Zachary A. Smith, MD[a],
Laura A. Snyder, MD[b], Randall B. Graham, MD[a],
Richard G. Fessler, MD, PhD[b], Tyler R. Koski, MD[a]

KEYWORDS

- Minimally invasive • Lateral transpsoas lumbar interbody fusion • Deformity
- Direct lateral interbody fusion • Extreme lateral interbody fusion • DLIF • XLIF

KEY POINTS

- The lateral transpsoas approach for interbody fusion is a minimally invasive technique that has been successfully used in the treatment of a variety of spinal degenerative disorders.
- There is growing evidence that this technique can be used in the management of adult deformity with good results and acceptable risks.
- It is more powerful in correcting coronal deformity than sagittal deformity if used as the sole approach or technique.

INTRODUCTION

The lateral transpsoas approach for interbody fusion was first described by McAffee and colleagues[1] and later on further advanced by Ozgur and colleagues.[2] Through a small incision, a lateral window through the psoas muscle is created; through a table-mounted working channel, lumbar interbody fusion can be completed using large cages with footprints that span the vertebral body from side to side.

This minimally invasive technique, which lacks an open counterpart, has been increasingly used to accomplish interbody fusions for a wide variety of spinal degenerative disorders that include spondylolisthesis and degenerative disk disease with reportedly excellent outcomes and an acceptable risk profile (**Fig. 1**). Following the interbody fusion, most surgeons supplement the construct with percutaneous pedicle screws placed though a posterior or dorsal approach because this has been proven to be biomechanically superior to stand-alone lateral interbody fusions.[3,4] Moreover, pedicle screw supplementation improves correction and decreases the risk of graft subsidence.[5]

The degree of segmental correction in the coronal plane ranges from 3.0° to 5.9°. The average segmental correction in the sagittal plane varied between 2.2° and 3.3°.[6–10] Following the increasing successful use of this interbody fusion technique in the degenerative arena, reports of its application to adult deformity and mainly adult degenerative scoliosis started to emerge as an alternative way to open traditional corrections, where blood loss and muscle dissection are not insignificant.[11] This article presents a review of the literature analyzing clinical and radiographic studies using the lateral lumbar transpsoas

Sources of support: none.
[a] Department of Neurological Surgery, Northwestern University, Feinberg School of Medicine, 676 North St Clair Street, Chicago, IL 60611, USA; [b] Department of Neurological Surgery, Rush University Medical Center, 1725 W. Harrison Street, Suite 855, Chicago, IL 60612, USA
* Corresponding author. Department of Neurological Surgery, Northwestern University Feinberg School of Medicine, 676 North St. Clair Street, Suite 2210, Chicago, IL 60611, USA.
E-mail address: nsdahdaleh@gmail.com

neurosurgery.theclinics.com

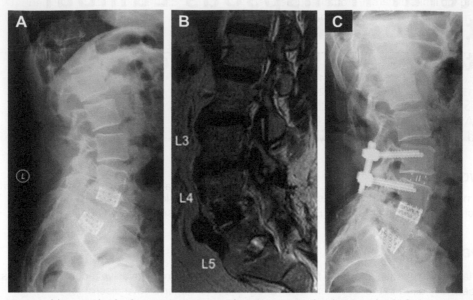

Fig. 1. A 65-year-old man who had a previous L4-5 and L5-S1 anterior lumbar interbody fusion with L4 and L5 laminectomies presented with progressive low back and bilateral lower extremity pain. Plain radiographs and magnetic resonance imaging demonstrated adjacent segment disease at L3-4 with loss of disk height and foraminal stenosis (*A, B*). Following L3-4 direct lateral interbody fusion and posterior percutaneous instrumentation (*C*), disk height and foraminal height were restored with relief of the patient's symptoms.

approach in the correction of adult degenerative scoliosis.

MATERIALS AND METHODS

A computerized literature search of the National Library of Medicine's database, Cochrane database, and Google Scholar was performed for published material between January 1966 and August 2013 using keywords and medical subject headings. The keywords included the following: lateral lumbar interbody fusion, direct lateral interbody fusion, extreme lateral interbody fusion, lateral transpsoas interbody fusion, DLIF (direct lateral interbody fusion), and XLIF (extreme lateral interbody fusion). The search yielded 546 citations. The authors then selected for English citations and reviewed all abstracts generated in the search.

Among the citations reviewed, the authors identified 10 articles that primarily focused on radiographic and clinical outcomes following lateral transpsoas interbody fusion for the correction of spinal deformity. All 10 citations were retrospective studies (**Table 1**). The articles are summarized in the results section.

RESULTS

Table 1 summarizes all 10 studies focusing on radiographic and clinical outcomes following

lateral transpsoas interbody fusion for the correction of spinal deformity.

Anand and colleagues[12] reported a series of 12 patients who underwent lateral interbody fusion and posterior percutaneous instrumentation for the treatment of adult scoliosis. They reported improvement of an average preoperative coronal Cobb angle of 18.9° to 6.1° postoperatively along with clinical improvement of Visual Analogue Score (VAS) and treatment intensity scores.

Tormenti and colleagues[13] compared 8 patients who underwent combined lateral interbody fusion and posterior fusion with 4 patients who underwent posterior-only approaches. In the combined group, the median Cobb angle was 38.5° and improved to 10.0° with 70.2% correction. The apical vertebral translation (AVT) improved from 3.6 to 1.8 cm. The mean preoperative lordosis was 47.3°, and the mean postoperative lordosis was 40.4°. Pertaining to the posterior-only group, the mean preoperative coronal Cobb angle was 19° and improved to 11° postoperatively with 44.7% degree of correction. The mean operative AVT in the posterior-only group was 2.2 cm and changed to 1.1 cm postoperatively. The mean preoperative lumbar lordosis was 30.0° and improved to 37.7°.

Wang and Mummaneni[14] reported 23 patients treated with lateral transpsoas interbody fusion and percutaneous pedicle screw fixation for adult degenerative scoliosis. The mean preoperative coronal Cobb angle improved from 31.4° to

Table 1
Summary of studies on lateral lumbar interbody fusion for deformity correction

Author, Year	Number of Patients	Follow-up (mo)	Average Lateral Interbody Fusion Segments	Coronal Cobb Angle Preoperative	Coronal Cobb Angle Postoperative	Sagittal Cobb Angle Preoperative	Sagittal Cobb Angle Postoperative	Outcomes Improved	Blood Loss (mL)	Hospital Stay (d)
Anand et al,[12] 2008	12	2.5	3.6	18.9	6.1	N/A	N/A	VAS, TIS	257	8.6
Tormenti et al,[13] 2010	8	10.5	2.8	38.5	10.0	47.3	40.4	VAS	N/A	N/A
Wang & Mummaneni,[14] 2010	23	13.4	3.7	31.4	11.5	37.4	45.5	VAS	447	6.2
Dakwar et al,[15] 2010	25	11.0	3.0	21.1	6.4	N/A	N/A	VAS, ODI	53/level	6.2
Karikari et al,[16] 2011	11	16.4	N/A	22.0	14.0	39.0	44.0	VAS, ODI	228	4.8
Sharma et al,[10] 2011	25	12.0	N/A	24.0	13.6	47.8	48.3	VAS,ODI, SF-12 P	N/A	N/A
Acosta et al,[9] 2011	8	21.0	N/A	21.4	9.7	42.1	46.2	VAS, ODI	N/A	N/A
Kotwal et al,[17] 2012	31	24.0 minimum	N/A	24.8	13.6	N/A	N/A	VAS, ODI, SF-12 P	537	7.7
Johnson et al,[6] 2013	15	6.0 minimum	N/A	13.0	7.1	42.8	44.4	VAS, ODI, SF-36	N/A	N/A
Anand et al,[18] 2013	66	39.0	4.0	24.7	9.5	N/A	N/A	VAS, TIS, ODI, SF-36	314 for lateral interbody fusion	7.6

Abbreviations: N/A, not available; ODI, Oswestry Disability Index; P, Physical; SF-12, Short Form-12; SF-36, 36-Item Short Form Health Survey; TIS, treatment intensity score; VAS, Visual analogue score.

11.5°. They also reported improvement of their mean postoperative VAS scores.

Dakwar and colleagues[15] reported on 25 patients who underwent lateral interbody fusion for adult degenerative scoliosis. Sixteen patients had only lateral plate supplementation, and 8 patients had posterior fixation. In their cohort, the average preoperative coronal Cobb angle was 21.1°, and their average postoperative coronal Cobb angle was 6.4°.

Karikari and colleagues[16] reported 22 patients, 11 of whom underwent lateral interbody fusions for degenerative scoliosis. In these patients, the preoperative Cobb angle improved from 22° to 14° postoperatively. Sagittally, the mean preoperative Cobb angle was 39° and improved to 44°. Outcomes including Oswetry Disability Index (ODI) and VAS pain also improved.

Sharma and colleagues[10] retrospectively reviewed 43 patients who underwent lateral interbody fusion. Twenty-five of these patients underwent this operation for adult scoliosis correction. In that group, the mean preoperative coronal Cobb angle was 24.0° and improved to 13.6° during the last follow-up. VAS for back pain, ODI, and Short Form-12 (SF-12) physical component significantly improved postoperatively.

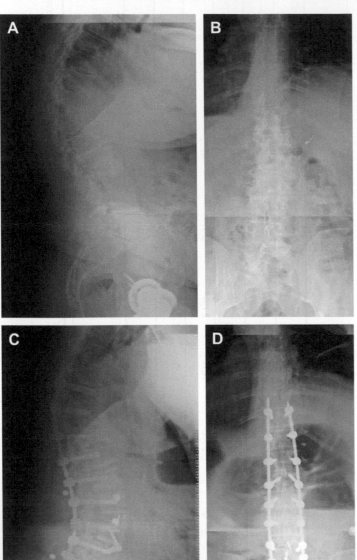

Fig. 2. A 70-year-old man presented with back pain, lower extremity pain, and neurogenic claudications. Lateral (A) and anteroposterior (B) radiographs demonstrated degenerative lumbar dextroscoliosis measuring 11°. After a period of conservative therapy, the patient underwent staged L1/2, L2/3, L3/4 minimally invasive lateral interbody fusion, L4/5 and L5/S1 anterior lumbar interbody fusions, and percutaneous posterior T10 to sacrum fixation (C, D).

Acosta and colleagues[9] reviewed 36 patients who underwent lateral transpsoas lumbar interbody fusion. The study included 8 patients with adult degenerative scoliosis. In these patients, the preoperative coronal Cobb angle was 21.4° and improved to 9.7° postoperatively. The mean global coronal alignment was 19.1 mm preoperatively and improved to 12.5 mm postoperatively. In the sagittal plane, the mean preoperative lumbar lordosis was 42.1° and 46.2° postoperatively.

Kotwal and colleagues[17] recently reviewed their series of patients who underwent lateral interbody fusions and had a minimum 2-year follow-up. Their retrospective series included 118 patients, 31 of whom had degenerative scoliosis. In this subgroup of patients, the coronal Cobb angle improved from 24.8° preoperatively to 13.6° postoperatively. The ODI, SF-12 physical component, and VAS pain showed improvement postoperatively.

Johnson and colleagues[6] recently reviewed their cohort of 30 patients who underwent lateral lumbar interbody fusion. Fifteen patients had degenerative lumbar scoliosis. In this subset of patients, the coronal Cobb angle improved from 13.0° to 7.1° postoperatively. Although segmental lumbar lordosis improved following surgery, there was no change in global lumbar lordosis. Moreover, other pelvic parameters, including sacral slope and pelvic tilt, remained unchanged postoperatively. There were significant improvements in ODI, VAS pain, and the 36-Item Short Form Health Survey at 2 and 6 months postoperatively.

Finally, Anand and colleagues[18] recently reported their cohort of 71 patients who underwent minimally invasive correction for scoliosis. 54 patients had degenerative scoliosis. 66 patients underwent lateral interbody fusion as part of their correction strategy and 67 underwent posterior percutaneous pedicle screw fixation. The minimum follow-up was 2 years, and some patients were followed up for up to 5 years. The mean preoperative Cobb angle was 24.7° and improved to 9.5° postoperatively. The mean preoperative coronal balance was 25.5 mm and improved to 12 mm postoperatively. The mean preoperative sagittal balance was 31.7 mm and improved to 10.7 mm postoperatively. Pertaining to complications, 4 patients had pseudoarthrosis, 4 had persistent stenosis, one suffered from osteomyelitis, one from adjacent segment discitis, one had a late wound infection, one suffered from proximal junctional kyphosis, one had screw prominence, one had idiopathic cerebellar hemorrhage, and 2 suffered from a wound dehiscence.

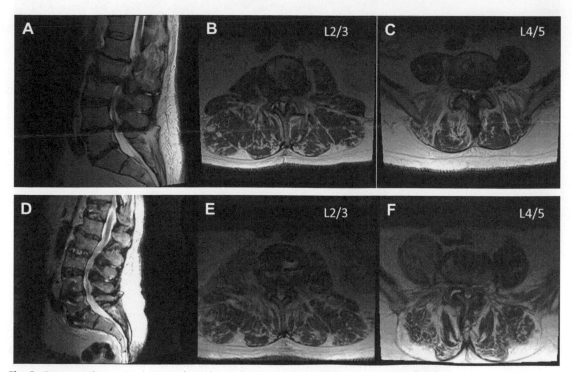

Fig. 3. Preoperative sagittal T2- and axial-weighted magnetic resonance imaging (MRI) scan demonstrating preoperative scoliosis and multilevel stenosis most severe at L2/3 and L4/5. (*A–C*) Postoperative T2-weighted MRI demonstrating improvement in the central canal diameter in the sagittal plane (*D*) and axial plane at L2/3 (*E*) and L4/5 (*F*).

DISCUSSION

Minimally invasive spinal techniques have been gaining popularity as treatment options for a wide variety of degenerative, traumatic, and neoplastic spinal disorders.[19–21] The hallmark of minimizing unnecessary muscle dissection, soft tissue damage, and trauma has unequivocally translated into lesser wound infections, blood loss, cerebrospinal fluid leaks, hospital stay, and even cost-effectiveness, while maintaining similar long-term outcomes.[22–25] With the recent development of the lateral transpsoas approaches as extreme lateral interbody fusion (XLIF) and direct lateral interbody fusion (DLIF), enthusiasm of applying these techniques to scoliosis correction has increased, especially knowing that traditional open surgeries involve significant tissue dissection, blood loss, and longer hospitalization (**Fig. 2**).

Patients with adult degenerative scoliosis often present with axial and lower extremity pain and/or claudication that are caused by a variety of reasons, such as concavity foraminal stenosis, central canal stenosis, and segmental lateral or sagittal spondylolisthesis. Lateral interbody fusion offers an attractive solution addressing these concurrent issues through one approach. Successful indirect decompression of the foramina and central canal even independent of graft position has been demonstrated.[26] Moreover, for the restoration of lumbar lordosis, Lateral Lumbar Interbody Fusion

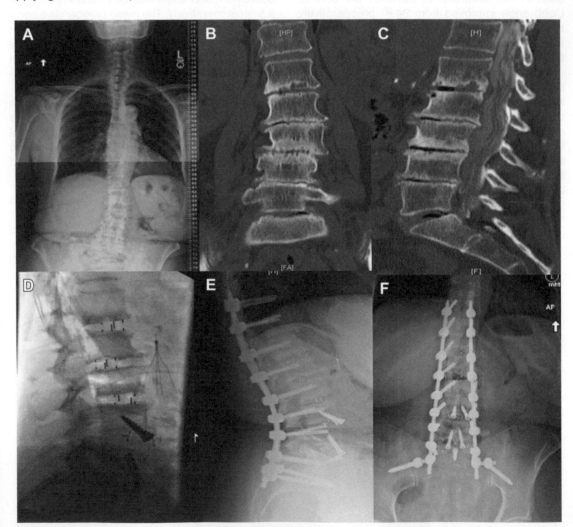

Fig. 4. A 70 year old woman presented with chronic back pain and bilateral lower extremity radiculopathy of a few years in duration. She failed conservative measures. Standing scoliosis xrays demonstrated mild lumbar scoliosis (A), CT of the lumbar spine showed degenerative disk disease involving all segments of the lumbar spine as well as multilevel bilateral foraminal stenosis (B, C). The patient underwent Anterior lumbar interbody fusion at L4/5 and L5/S1 as well as lateral lumbar interbody fusion at L1/2, L2/3, L3/4 (D), followed by percutaneous pedicle screw fixation from T11 to Sacrum/Ilium (E, F).

(LLIF) has been found to be superior to transforaminal lumbar interbody fusion (**Figs. 3** and **4**).[8]

The results of the studies reviewed are encouraging. All studies agree that successful correction for coronal deformity can be achieved using lateral interbody fusions (see **Table 1**). Moreover, most of the studies demonstrate improved short- and long-term clinical outcomes. The impact of improving lumbar lordosis and sagittal balance is less. Recently, efforts have been made to improve sagittal correction through the release of the anterior longitudinal ligament.[27]

The authors' approach to patients with adult degenerative kyphoscoliosis or scoliosis starts with the calculation of pelvic parameters, including sagittal and coronal balance, pelvic incidence, lumbar lordosis, and pelvic tilt.[28] The aim of any corrective surgery is the restoration of appropriate sagittal balance of less than 5 cm and a coronal balance of close to zero. Lumbar lordosis should match the pelvic incidence, and increased pelvic tilt is taken into consideration when calculating the exact amount of correction patients need to restore balance in both planes.

In patients who are sagittally balanced and their symptoms are mainly caused by scoliosis, pure lateral transpsoas lumbar interbody fusion LLIF and posterior percutaneous fixation is a powerful approach for the restoration of coronal balance. In patients whose sagittal balance is compromised, dorsal releases and osteotomy are used along with hybrid techniques that use LLIF as part of the surgical strategy.

COMPLICATIONS

The complications of the lateral transpsoas approach are well documented. Most of the complications are related to lumbar plexus injuries. These complications most commonly manifest as anterolateral thigh or groin pain and or numbness and also weakness with the ipsilateral iliopsoas or quadriceps. The frequency of thigh numbness postoperatively ranges from 17.8% to more than 40.0% immediately postoperatively.[29–31] Weakness ranges from 25.0% to 54.9%.[30,32] Most reports agree that symptoms usually resolve by 6 months to a year.[29,32]

SUMMARY

Lateral transpsoas lumbar interbody fusion is a minimally invasive option for the correction of degenerative scoliosis. Evidence suggests that adequate radiographic correction and improved clinical outcomes can be achieved using this approach.

REFERENCES

1. McAfee PC, Regan JJ, Geis WP, et al. Minimally invasive anterior retroperitoneal approach to the lumbar spine. Emphasis on the lateral BAK. Spine 1998;23(13):1476–84.
2. Ozgur BM, Aryan HE, Pimenta L, et al. Extreme lateral interbody fusion (XLIF): a novel surgical technique for anterior lumbar interbody fusion. Spine J 2006;6(4):435–43.
3. Cappuccino A, Cornwall GB, Turner AW, et al. Biomechanical analysis and review of lateral lumbar fusion constructs. Spine 2010;35(Suppl 26):S361–7.
4. Nayak AN, Gutierrez S, Billys JB, et al. Biomechanics of lateral plate and pedicle screw constructs in lumbar spines instrumented at two levels with laterally placed interbody cages. Spine J 2013;13(10):1331–8.
5. Karikari IO, Grossi PM, Nimjee SM, et al. Minimally invasive lumbar interbody fusion in patients older than 70 years of age: analysis of peri- and postoperative complications. Neurosurgery 2011;68(4):897–902 [discussion].
6. Johnson RD, Valore A, Villaminar A, et al. Pelvic parameters of sagittal balance in extreme lateral interbody fusion for degenerative lumbar disc disease. J Clin Neurosci 2013;20(4):576–81.
7. Le TV, Vivas AC, Dakwar E, et al. The effect of the retroperitoneal transpsoas minimally invasive lateral interbody fusion on segmental and regional lumbar lordosis. ScientificWorldJournal 2012;2012:516706.
8. Watkins RG 4th, Hanna R, Chang D, et al. Sagittal alignment after lumbar interbody fusion: comparing anterior, lateral, and transforaminal approaches. J Spinal Disord Tech 2013. [Epub ahead of print].
9. Acosta FL, Liu J, Slimack N, et al. Changes in coronal and sagittal plane alignment following minimally invasive direct lateral interbody fusion for the treatment of degenerative lumbar disease in adults: a radiographic study. J Neurosurg Spine 2011;15(1):92–6.
10. Sharma AK, Kepler CK, Girardi FP, et al. Lateral lumbar interbody fusion: clinical and radiographic outcomes at 1 year: a preliminary report. J Spinal Disord Tech 2011;24(4):242–50.
11. Caputo AM, Michael KW, Chapman TM Jr, et al. Clinical outcomes of extreme lateral interbody fusion in the treatment of adult degenerative scoliosis. ScientificWorldJournal 2012;2012:680643.
12. Anand N, Baron EM, Thaiyananthan G, et al. Minimally invasive multilevel percutaneous correction and fusion for adult lumbar degenerative scoliosis: a technique and feasibility study. J Spinal Disord Tech 2008;21(7):459–67.
13. Tormenti MJ, Maserati MB, Bonfield CM, et al. Complications and radiographic correction in adult scoliosis following combined transpsoas extreme lateral

interbody fusion and posterior pedicle screw instrumentation. Neurosurg Focus 2010;28(3):E7.

14. Wang MY, Mummaneni PV. Minimally invasive surgery for thoracolumbar spinal deformity: initial clinical experience with clinical and radiographic outcomes. Neurosurg Focus 2010;28(3):E9.

15. Dakwar E, Cardona RF, Smith DA, et al. Early outcomes and safety of the minimally invasive, lateral retroperitoneal transpsoas approach for adult degenerative scoliosis. Neurosurg Focus 2010;28(3):E8.

16. Karikari IO, Nimjee SM, Hardin CA, et al. Extreme lateral interbody fusion approach for isolated thoracic and thoracolumbar spine diseases: initial clinical experience and early outcomes. J Spinal Disord Tech 2011;24(6):368–75.

17. Kotwal S, Kawaguchi S, Lebl D, et al. Minimally invasive lateral lumbar interbody fusion: clinical and radiographic outcome at a minimum 2-year follow-up. J Spinal Disord Tech 2012. [Epub ahead of print].

18. Anand N, Baron EM, Khandehroo B, et al. Long-term 2- to 5-year clinical and functional outcomes of minimally invasive surgery for adult scoliosis. Spine 2013;38(18):1566–75.

19. Grossbach AJ, Dahdaleh NS, Abel TJ, et al. Flexion-distraction injuries of the thoracolumbar spine: open fusion versus percutaneous pedicle screw fixation. Neurosurg Focus 2013;35(2):E2.

20. Dahdaleh NS, Nixon AT, Lawton CD, et al. Outcome following unilateral versus bilateral instrumentation in patients undergoing minimally invasive transforaminal lumbar interbody fusion: a single-center randomized prospective study. Neurosurg Focus 2013;35(2):E13.

21. Zairi F, Arikat A, Allaoui M, et al. Minimally invasive decompression and stabilization for the management of thoracolumbar spine metastasis. J Neurosurg Spine 2012;17(1):19–23.

22. Adogwa O, Parker SL, Bydon A, et al. Comparative effectiveness of minimally invasive versus open transforaminal lumbar interbody fusion: 2-year assessment of narcotic use, return to work, disability, and quality of life. J Spinal Disord Tech 2011;24(8):479–84.

23. McGirt MJ, Parker SL, Lerner J, et al. Comparative analysis of perioperative surgical site infection after minimally invasive versus open posterior/transforaminal lumbar interbody fusion: analysis of hospital billing and discharge data from 5170 patients. J Neurosurg Spine 2011;14(6):771–8.

24. Parker SL, Adogwa O, Bydon A, et al. Cost-effectiveness of minimally invasive versus open transforaminal lumbar interbody fusion for degenerative spondylolisthesis associated low-back and leg pain over two years. World Neurosurg 2012;78(1–2):178–84.

25. Parker SL, Mendenhall SK, Shau DN, et al. Minimally invasive versus open transforaminal lumbar interbody fusion (TLIF) for degenerative spondylolisthesis: comparative effectiveness and cost-utility analysis. World Neurosurg 2013. [Epub ahead of print].

26. Marulanda GA, Nayak A, Murtagh R, et al. A cadaveric radiographic analysis on the effect of extreme lateral interbody fusion cage placement with supplementary internal fixation on indirect spine decompression. J Spinal Disord Tech 2013. [Epub ahead of print].

27. Deukmedjian AR, Dakwar E, Ahmadian A, et al. Early outcomes of minimally invasive anterior longitudinal ligament release for correction of sagittal imbalance in patients with adult spinal deformity. ScientificWorldJournal 2012;2012:789698.

28. Ondra SL, Marzouk S, Koski T, et al. Mathematical calculation of pedicle subtraction osteotomy size to allow precision correction of fixed sagittal deformity. Spine 2006;31(25):E973–9.

29. Pumberger M, Hughes AP, Huang RR, et al. Neurologic deficit following lateral lumbar interbody fusion. Eur Spine J 2012;21(6):1192–9.

30. Le TV, Burkett CJ, Deukmedjian AR, et al. Postoperative lumbar plexus injury after lumbar retroperitoneal transpsoas minimally invasive lateral interbody fusion. Spine 2013;38(1):E13–20.

31. Sofianos DA, Briseno MR, Abrams J, et al. Complications of the lateral transpsoas approach for lumbar interbody arthrodesis: a case series and literature review. Clin Orthop Relat Res 2012;470(6):1621–32.

32. Moller DJ, Slimack NP, Acosta FL Jr, et al. Minimally invasive lateral lumbar interbody fusion and transpsoas approach-related morbidity. Neurosurg Focus 2011;31(4):E4.

Evidence Basis/Outcomes in Minimally Invasive Spinal Scoliosis Surgery

Neel Anand, MD, Mch Orth[a],*, Eli M. Baron, MD[b],
Sheila Kahwaty, PA-C[c]

KEYWORDS

- Adult scoliosis • Minimally invasive spine surgery • Evidence basis • Outcomes

KEY POINTS

- Minimally invasive spinal surgery (MISS) scoliosis correction may allow for adult scoliosis correction with significantly less tissue destruction and less blood loss than open procedures.
- MISS scoliosis correction without osteotomies has limits using present technologies in terms of correcting sagittal plane deformity and has a ceiling effect of about 40° of coronal Cobb correction.
- MISS scoliosis correction has a different complication profile from traditional open scoliosis correction; this may be largely reflective of the use of the lateral transpsoas approach and reduced blood loss.
- Long-term level II and III studies are needed to compare outcomes between MISS and open adult scoliosis correction.

INTRODUCTION: NATURE OF THE PROBLEM

The principal goal of adult scoliosis surgery is obtaining both sagittal and coronal balance of the spine.[1] However, traditional scoliosis correction has been associated with high-volume blood loss and significant medical complications.[2–4] Given this situation, minimally invasive spinal surgery (MISS) for the treatment of adult scoliosis is particularly attractive. MISS techniques have been used for the treatment of lumbar degenerative scoliosis, iatrogenic scoliosis, and adult idiopathic scoliosis. Theoretically, blood loss can be limited, and medical complication rates can possibly be reduced with less invasive procedures. Nevertheless, clinical and radiographic outcomes of MISS scoliosis correction need to be comparable with open surgery before recommending widespread adoption of these techniques for the treatment of adult scoliosis. MISS principles and surgical techniques used in MISS scoliosis correction are reviewed in this article, as well as outcomes, complications, and limitations of this rapidly evolving area of spinal surgery.

THERAPEUTIC OPTIONS OR SURGICAL TECHNIQUE(S)

Indications for adult scoliosis correction include deformity progression, sagittal or coronal imbalance with unremitting back pain, radiculopathy on the side of the concavity of the curve caused by foraminal stenosis, lumbar hyperlordosis, patients with a history of flat-back syndrome and back pain, fixed lateral listhesis within the degenerative curve when motion is present on side-bending

[a] Department of Surgery, Spine Trauma, Spine Center, Cedars Sinai Medical Center, 444 South San Vicente Boulevard, Suite 800, Los Angeles, CA 90048, USA; [b] Department of Neurosurgery, Spine Center, Cedars Sinai Medical Center, 444 South San Vicente Boulevard, Suite 800, Los Angeles, CA 90048, USA; [c] Department of Surgery, Spine Center, Cedars Sinai Medical Center, 444 South San Vicente Boulevard, Suite 800, Los Angeles, CA 90048, USA
* Corresponding author.
E-mail address: neel.anand@cshs.org

Neurosurg Clin N Am 25 (2014) 361–375
http://dx.doi.org/10.1016/j.nec.2013.12.014

films, and when extensive decompression including facetectomy or the violation of the pars is planned.[5] A relative indication is progressively worsening deformity with pain as the rib cage abuts the pelvis.

In our practice, adult patients who undergo MISS scoliosis surgery are typically being treated for symptomatic back and leg pain (**Fig. 1**). These patients include those with adult idiopathic scoliosis, iatrogenic scoliosis, and lumbar degenerative scoliosis. Patients have tried numerous conservative measures, including physical therapy and epidural and facet injections, before being considered for surgery. The main indication for correction of adult scoliosis is mechanical low back pain. This pain is typified by stiffness in the morning, with progressive worsening of pain with activity that increases throughout the day. Often, but not always, this pain may be accompanied by radiculopathy or claudication.[6]

The main principle of adult scoliosis correction is achieving a balanced spinal alignment and addressing symptomatic levels. Radiographic evaluation of the patient with adult deformity, whether being treated with traditional open correction or MISS, involves measurement of the Cobb angle in the coronal plane, the amount of correction on side-bending films, and the amount of deviation of the apical vertebrae to the central sacral vertical line.[7] In the sagittal plane, a plumb line is drawn from the center of the C7 vertebra to the sacrum. Normally, this line should be within 5 cm of the posterior aspect of the sacrum. In addition, regional alignment and pelvic parameters, such as pelvic incidence and pelvic tilt, are calculated. In planning for adult scoliosis, the patient's symptoms, stenosis, and disk degeneration must be considered.

Interbody fusion techniques are used to improve lordosis, help correct lateral listhesis, and, potentially, increase fusion rates. For lumbar degenerative scoliosis, proximal fusions are typically stopped at a stable vertebra.[7] Others have advocated stopping at T10.[8] In terms of where to begin and end a fusion, this topic has been discussed in detail elsewhere and is not the focus of this article.[7,9] If a thoracolumbar fusion is extended to the sacrum, interbody fusion and pelvic fixation should be considered.[9]

Segmental pedicle screw fixation allows for greater pullout strength than previous generation instrumentation systems (ie, hooks, cables). Pedicle screws may allow for shorter fusion length and less operative blood loss than hooks.[7,10,11]

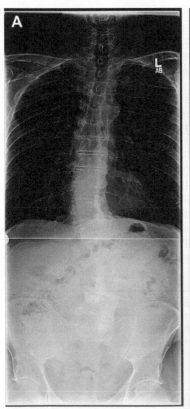
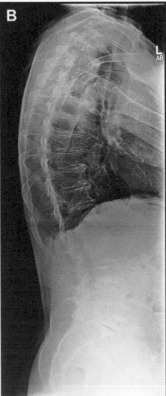

Fig. 1. (*A, B*) Anteroposterior and lateral 91 cm (36-inch) films of a 68-year-old man with a history of back pain and leg pain refractory to conservative measures. He was noted to have lumbar degenerative scoliosis with a curve measuring 37° from L1 to L5, with the apex to the left.

Traditional scoliosis surgery allows for various open corrective maneuvers, such as derotation, vertebral coplanar alignment, and in situ rod bending.[12–14] In addition, open surgery allows for both structural interbody techniques and osteotomies to assist in further deformity correction, with the creation of lumbar lordosis as needed.[1,7]

A systematic review of adult scoliosis surgery showed that adult scoliosis surgery is associated with long-term improvement in patient radiographic and clinical outcomes. At a mean follow-up of 3.6 years, average curve reduction was noted to be 40.7% and mean Oswestry Disability Index (ODI) was reduced by 15.7.[15] In terms of scoliosis deformity correction, sagittal balance improvement seems to be the strongest predictor of improved clinical outcomes, with correction of coronal balance being a lesser factor.[16]

Open adult scoliosis correction has certain limitations. Medical complication rates associated with open adult deformity correction may be as high as 70%.[2] Large volume blood loss is not unusual in these complex procedures. Seo and colleagues[17] reported outcomes in 152 patients older than 20 years undergoing open adult scoliosis correction. These investigators noted a mean blood loss of 2855.8 mL $\pm$ 1822.9 mL. Transfeldt and colleagues[18] noted a mean blood loss of 1538 mL in patients undergoing full fusion and decompression of their degenerative scoliotic curves. The population undergoing adult scoliosis surgery is often elderly, with significant medical comorbidities and high cardiac risk. Given this situation, the decision to proceed operatively with adult surgical deformity correction in the older population must be made carefully.[19] Considering these limitations, MISS options may be attractive if similar results can be obtained with less blood loss and less tissue trauma.

MISS Scoliosis Correction

A portion of the morbidity associated with traditional spinal surgery occurs because of muscle damage associated with exposure and retraction and subsequent muscular devascularization and denervation.[20–23] Tubular approaches for diskectomy, decompression, and minimally invasive surgery posterior fusion were developed to minimize these complications.[24–29] MISS interbody fusion techniques followed. This was an important development, because interbody fusion may have higher fusion rates than posterolateral fusion techniques.[7,30] In addition, diskectomy and graft placement may allow the achievement of anterior deformity release and alignment.[31–34] Current options for MISS interbody fusion techniques include

transforaminal lumbar interbody fusion (TLIF), mini-iopen and MISS anterior lumbar interbody fusion (ALIF), lateral transpsoas interbody fusion and the presacral approach for interbody fusion (Axia-LIF) (**Table 1**). All of these options have subsequently been used in MISS correction of adult scoliosis.[35–41]

The combined use of 3 techniques to facilitate circumferential MISS scoliosis correction was reported in 2008.[42] These techniques included the transpsoas approach for diskectomy and interbody fusion, the presacral approach for L5-S1 fusion, and percutaneous pedicle screw and rod placement. Percutaneous screw and rod placement has proved to be a major determinant of correction of apical vertical translation, even beyond diskectomy and interbody fusion.[6] Subsequently, other series have reported outcomes using a combination of MISS techniques for adult scoliosis.

Most articles reporting MISS scoliosis correction rely heavily on the lateral transpsoas approach. This factor allows the surgeon MISS access to the spine, where diskectomy, deformity release, and interbody fusion can be achieved for multiple levels with minimal tissue disruption. The current technique, as described by Luiz Pimenta and published by Ozgur and colleagues,[43] builds on the experience of other historical approaches in which MISS techniques were used to achieve ALIF.[44–46] The techniques of Thalgott and colleagues[47] and that of McAfee and colleagues[48] served as precursors to the current technique. The current technique does not rely on endoscopy or laparoscopy. It requires less specialized equipment and theoretically has less of a learning curve. The transpsoas approach has subsequently been widely adopted as a technique to achieve release of scoliotic curves and perform interbody fusion (**Fig. 2**).[6,40,41,49,50] However, the lateral approach does place the lumbar plexus and genitofemoral nerve at risk for injury and is not without its own complication profile, reflected in **Table 3**.

The development of multilevel percutaneously placed screws, with freehand rod passage, allowed for deformity correction and fixation with minimal tissue disruption.[42] Percutaneous rod and screw placement results in substantially less disruption of the thoracolumbar fascia than open techniques. This factor is clinically relevant, because the thoracolumbar fascia may be a major stabilizer of the lumbosacral spine and pelvis.[51] Percutaneous screw and rod placement has proved to be crucial in the correction of apical vertical translation, even beyond diskectomy and interbody fusion.[6] In addition, MISS screw techniques have been developed to allow

Table 1
MISS interbody fusion technique

Technique	Advantages	Disadvantages	Sagittal and Coronal Plane Correction with Technique
TLIF	Posterior approach for diskectomy and interbody fusion Reduced risk for neurologic injury/durotomy when compared with posterior lumbar interbody fusion	Potential for neurologic injury and durotomy Time consuming	In 1 large deformity series, change in local lordosis ranging from −1.7° to 4° depending on level treated. May have superior results to ALIF in correction of AP lumbar curve and fractional curves. Mean correction of AP lumbar curve reported at 22.9° and AP fractional lumbosacral curve of 10.3°[78]
ALIF	Large grafting surface, indirect neuroforaminal decompression Avoidance of spinal canal	Potential viscous/vascular injury, often requires approach surgeon, potential sympathetic dysfunction/retrograde ejaculation	Superior sagittal correction when compared with TLIF. In 1 large deformity series, increase in local lordosis ranging from 2.5° to 5.5° was noted with ALIF, depending on level treated. Reduced correction of AP lumbar curve and fractional curve was noted when compared with TLIF; 9.9° for AP lumbar curve and 3.3° AP correction for fractional lumbar curve[78]
Transpsoas interbody fusion	Efficient method of achieving diskectomy, deformity release and interbody fusion; reduced risk of vascular/viscus injury when compared with ALIF, large graft surface, indirect foraminal decompression	Usually cannot be performed at L5-S1, potential for thigh dysesthesias, leg weakness	Mean gain of 2.8° lordosis at each level of transpsoas interbody fusion[63] Controversial as to whether global coronal alignment is improved or not Global sagittal balance seems not improved with this technique[62,63]
AxiaLIF	Minimally invasive corridor to L5-S1	Cannot be performed in cases of prerectal scarring or aberrant vasculature	Data not available

Abbreviation: AP, anteroposterior.

supplemental iliac fixation, allowing rod insertion without connectors or extensive soft tissue dissection.[52,53]

In terms of achieving MISS fusion, series to date have relied heavily on interbody grafting and the off-label use of recombinant human bone morphogenetic protein 2 (rhBMP-2) (Medtronic Sofamor Danek, Memphis, TN) (**Table 2**). Use of rhBMP-2 has facilitated fusion without the need for extensive posterolateral decortication or autogenous bone graft harvesting.

CLINICAL OUTCOMES

In the series mentioned earlier, reporting the combined use of 3 techniques for MISS correction of scoliosis, outcomes for 12 patients were reported (**Fig. 3**).[42] Mean segments operated on were 3.64. Mean blood loss for the transpsoas approach was 164 mL, and for the posterior approach, including pedicle screw placement and AxiaLIF, it was 94 mL. Mean surgical time for anterior procedures was 4 hours. Mean surgical time for posterior

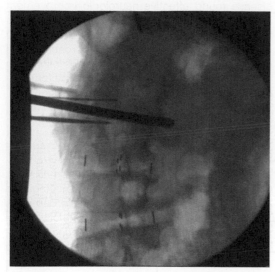

Fig. 2. Anteroposterior fluoroscopic image showing Cobb elevator being used to release contralateral annulus during a direct lateral interbody fusion procedure.

procedures was 3.9 hours. Mean preoperative Cobb was 18.93°. Mean postoperative Cobb was 6.19°. Mean follow-up time was 75.5 days, with clinical improvement documented by a decrease in Visual Analogue Scale (VAS) of 4.8. Although this study was primarily a feasibility study describing the usefulness of MISS techniques in the correction of adult scoliosis, it was also the first study describing multilevel percutaneous screw and freehand rod placement. Subsequently, numerous other series regarding MISS for adult scoliosis have been published (see **Table 2**).

COMPLICATIONS AND CONCERNS

Complication rates and complications commonly seen with MISS deformity correction may be different from those seen with open correction of adult spinal deformity (ASD). Complications noted with MISS scoliosis series are summarized in (**Table 3**).

The complication rates in these series compare favorably with open approach series for lumbar degenerative deformity, in which complication rates of 20% to 80% have been reported.[54–57] Cho and colleagues[58] reported an overall complication rate of 68% in patients undergoing posterior fusion and instrumentation (in addition, 7 patients underwent posterior lumbar interbody fusion) for degenerative scoliosis. These investigators noted an early complication rate of 30%, a mean blood loss of 2.1 L, and a mean hospital stay of 20.7 days. Similarly, Wu and colleagues[59] noted

a mean blood loss of 1.7 L in 29 patients undergoing posterior lumbar interbody fusion for degenerative scoliosis. In a study of 78 articles regarding fusion for lumbar degenerative conditions noted in degenerative scoliosis, Bono and Lee[60] noted a pooled good to excellent outcome rate of 82% with fusion rates of 87%. However, these investigators noted a pooled complication rate of 55%.

Several concerns have been raised regarding MISS correction of adult scoliosis. All the series to date regarding MISS adult scoliosis correction have been classified as level IV data (see **Table 2**). Future level II or III studies may better answer how outcomes compare with open surgery. To date, there has been no direct comparison with open surgery in any trial.

Shaffrey and Smith[61] noted several problems regarding most series and outcomes data for MISS deformity correction. Most series report outcomes of less than 2 years, with limited health-related quality of life data. Even although more of these data have been reported,[37] there are still limited data regarding MISS deformity correction and its relationship to pelvic parameters, lumbar lordosis, and the sagittal vertical axis (SVA). Thus, it is argued that a study needs to be conducted that meets the same standard used in the treatment of open deformity surgery.

Understanding limitations of current techniques in achieving appropriate alignment is mandatory when using MISS technology for deformity correction. Acosta and colleagues[62] reviewed radiographic records of 36 patients undergoing transpsoas diskectomy and interbody fusion for lumbar degenerative disease. Transpsoas diskectomy and interbody fusion was performed on an average of 1.8 levels per patient. Supplemental MISS posterior fixation was used in all but 1 patient. Standing anteroposterior (AP) and lateral 91 cm (36-inch) films were obtained preoperatively and postoperatively for measurement of global coronal and sagittal balance. AP and lateral lumbar standing radiographs were obtained for measurement of segmental and regional sagittal and coronal Cobb angles. The investigators noted transpsoas interbody fusion to significantly improve segmental, regional, and global coronal plane alignment in these patients. However, they noted that regional lumbar lordosis and global sagittal alignment were not improved by these techniques. Similarly, Sharma and colleagues[63] noted a mean gain of 2.8° (P<.001) of lordosis at each level of transpsoas interbody fusion but no significant change in the overall coronal or sagittal plane alignment of the lumbar spine.

Recently, Johnson and colleagues[64] reported on pelvic parameters and sagittal balance after

Table 2
MISS scoliosis series

Author, Year	Number of Patients	Length of Follow-Up	Blood Loss	Radiologic/Clinical Outcomes	Comments	Level of Evidence
Anand et al,[42] 2008	12	75.5 d	164 mL for transpsoas approach; 94 mL for posterior instrumented fusion and AxiaLIF	Decrease in mean Cobb from 18.93° to 6.19° Mean decrease in VAS of 4.8	Retrospective, feasibility study using a combination of the transpsoas lateral approach for diskectomy and interbody fusion, AxiaLIF, and percutaneous pedicle screw and rod placement. Mean segments operated on was 3.64 rhBMP-2 was used for all fusion sites Posterolateral fusion at all fusion sites without interbody fusion and at L5-S1	IV
Anand et al,[38] 2010	28	22 mo	241 mL for transpsoas approach; for posterior procedures (including pedicle screw and rod placement and AxiaLIF) was 231 mL	Decrease in mean Cobb from 22° to 7° ODI improved from 39.13 to 7 VAS improved from 7.05 to 3.03 All patients were noted to maintain correction of their deformity and noted to have arthrodesis on plain radiograph	Retrospective study. MISS correction and fusion over 3 or more levels for adult scoliosis. Combination of the transpsoas lateral approach for diskectomy and interbody fusion, AxiaLIF (if fusing to L5-S1), and percutaneous pedicle screw and rod placement rhBMP-2 was used for all fusion sites. Posterolateral fusion at all fusion sites without interbody fusion	IV

Anand et al,[37] 2013	71	39 mo	Patients with 1-stage same-day surgery had a mean blood loss of 412 mL. Patients with 2-stage surgery had a mean blood loss of 314 mL for transpsoas interbody fusion and 357 mL for posterior instrumentation and axial lumbar interbody fusion	Mean number of levels operated on was 4.4. Mean hospital stay was 7.6 d (mean preoperative Cobb angle was 24.7°, which corrected to 9.5°. Mean preoperative coronal balance was 25.5 mm, which corrected to 11 mm. Mean preoperative sagittal balance was 31.7 mm and corrected to 10.7 mm. Mean preoperative lumbar apical vertical translation was 24 mm and corrected to 12 mm. Fusion rate, as assessed by CT scan was 94%. VAS, ODI, and SF-36 improved significantly: preoperatively, 6.43, 50.3, and 41.8; at last follow-up, 2.35, 41, and 62.7, respectively	Retrospective study. MISS correction and fusion over 2 or more levels for adult scoliosis. Combination of the transpsoas lateral approach for diskectomy and interbody fusion, AxiaLIF (if fusing to L5–S1), and percutaneous pedicle screw and rod placement rhBMP-2 was used for all fusion sites. Posterolateral fusion at all fusion sites without interbody fusion	IV
Caputo et al,[39] 2012	30	1 y	ODI decreasing from 24.8% to 19.0% and VAS leg pain score decreasing from 5.4 to 2.8	Mean Cobb 20.2 preoperatively Postoperatively not reported Mean ODI decreased from 24.8 to 19.0. Mean VAS back decreased; mean VAS leg decreased from 6.8 to 4.6	Patients underwent the transpsoas approach followed by posterior MISS instrumentation for adult degenerative scoliosis. Osteocell used for interbody fusion (Nuvasive, San Diego, CA)	IV
Dakwar et al,[40] 2010	25	80% of patients underwent more than 6 mo of follow-up	53 mL per segment fused	Decrease in mean Cobb from 22.1° to 6.2°. Mean improvement of 5.7 points on the VAS scores and a 23.7% improvement in ODI. All patients with >6 mo follow-up with solid fusion	Patients with adult degenerative deformity. A variety of stabilization techniques were used, including lateral plates, and open and percutaneously placed pedicle screws. At each level, rhBMP-2, tricalcium phosphate, and hydroxy-apatite used as fusion material	IV
Isaacs et al,[79] 2010	107	6 wk	Almost two-thirds (62.5%) of patients had a recorded blood loss of 100 mL, and only 9 patients (8.4%) had a 300 mL blood loss	NA	Multicenter prospective, nonrandomized study of transpsoas lumbar interbody fusion procedures in adult degenerative scoliosis. Perioperative outcome study. Fusion material not specified	IV

(continued on next page)

Table 2
(continued)

Author, Year	Number of Patients	Length of Follow-Up	Blood Loss	Radiologic/Clinical Outcomes	Comments	Level of Evidence
Karikari et al,[80] 2011	22 patients, of whom 11 had degenerative scoliosis	16.4 mo	227.5 mL	In the subset of patients treated for degenerative scoliosis, the mean preoperative and postoperative coronal Cobb angles were 22° and 14°, respectively	Retrospective study. Most patients without supplemental fixation. Lateral screws in 4 patients. Posterior fixation in 1 patient. All patients treated for scoliosis received rhBMP-2 in their cages	IV
Scheufler et al,[81,82] 2010	30 patient with thoracolumbar degenerative kyphoscoliosis	19.6 mo	771.7 mL	Fusion rate was 90% (26 patients available for CT scan at a mean of 6 mo). Average segmental correction of 10°–12° in the coronal and sagittal planes. Mean lumbar sagittal Cobb angle correction was 44.8 ± 10.7°, resulting in a mean postoperative lumbar lordosis of −36 ± 6.9°. Mean preoperative sagittal balance of 31.6 ± 15.2 mm (range, 5–96 mm) was reduced by 63.5 ± 30% to a postoperative mean of 8 ± 8.4 mm (range, −4–25 mm). A mean coronal Cobb angle correction of 31.7 ± 13.7° was sufficient to achieve a final mean postoperative coronal Cobb angle of 10.3 ± 7.8° at 12-mo follow-up. Mean preoperative apical vertebral translation was reduced from 22.3 ± 32 mm (range, 17–78 mm) to 9.9 ± 15.6 mm (range, 8–30 mm). Mean VAS reduced from 7.5 to 2.82 at last follow-up; ODI decreased from mean of 57.2 to 23.9	Retrospective series of patients undergoing unilateral MISS TLIFs and percutaneous screw and rod placement for MISS kyphoscoliosis correction using biplanar fluoroscopy or intraoperative CT scanning/navigation. 3 to 8 segments fused using TLIFs and facet fusion. TLIF performed using tubular access. In patients receiving short instrumentation (≤4 segments), TLIF was performed each level, whereas 3–5 segments were treated by TLIF in patients undergoing long instrumentation. Vertebral cement augmentation performed in 10 female osteopenic patients. Autologous bone chips and rhBMP-2 was used for all fusion sites	IV

Sharma et al,[63] 2011	43 patients, 25 with lumbar degenerative scoliosis	1 y	200 mL for transpsoas portion of surgery only	Mean correction of maximal Cobb angle was noted to be 10.4° (43%). VAS, ODI, and SF-12 improved significantly. Preoperatively, VAS and ODI 8.2 and 42.6; at 1 y, 4.6 and 31.5, respectively	Retrospective study. Ten patients in their series were treated with stand-alone transpsoas fusion, 9 with lateral plate and screw fixation, and 24 with pedicle screw fixation. Depending on surgeon preference, autograft or rhBMP-2 was used	IV
Wang and Mummaneni,[41] 2010	23	13.4 mo	477 mL	Decrease in mean Cobb from 31.4° to 11.5°. Thoracolumbar lordosis increased by a mean of 8°. All interbody fusions with solid arthrodesis as noted on CT scan. Two of 7 cases in which posterolateral fusions were performed alone had pseudarthrosis. Significant improvements in VAS: VAS leg averaged 4.35 and improved to 1.57; VAS back averaged 7.30 and improved to 3.35	Retrospective study. Two centers. Patients with scoliosis >20° or significant sagittal decompensation with loss of sagittal balance. Deformity correction using the transpsoas approach, along with MISS TLIF at L5-S1 if fused to the sacrum. rhBMP-2 was used for all fusion sites. Posterior fixation using percutaneous pedicle screws and rods. Posterolateral fusion at all fusion sites without interbody fusion	IV

Abbreviations: CT, computed tomography; NA, not applicable; SF-12, Short Form 12 Health Survey; SF-36, Short Form 36 Health Survey; VAS, Visual Analog Scale.

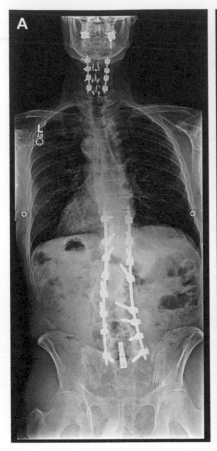
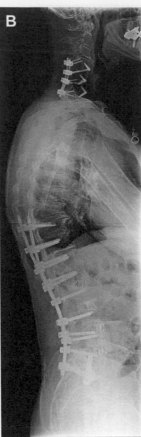

Fig. 3. (*A, B*) Anteroposterior and lateral postoperative images 3 years out from 3 stage MISS deformity correction, including AxiaLIF. The previously described curve now measures 8°. Coronal and sagittal balance is maintained.

transpsoas interbody fusion for lumbar degenerative conditions in patients with at least 6 months of follow-up. Standing preoperatively and postoperatively lumbar radiographs were used in their assessment. A total of 30 patients were included in this series, with only 6 undergoing posterior supplemental fixation: 3 with pedicle screws and 3 with interspinous process devices. Most patients underwent operations at a single level. The investigators found no effect of the procedure on sacral slope or pelvic tilt. They found lumbar lordosis not to be significantly affected by lateral transpsoas interbody fusion but Cobb angle to be significantly reduced.

Limitations exist in these studies, because the lateral transpsoas approach is typically being used for short segment deformity correction. Recent multicenter analysis of data through the International Spine Study Group and radiologic analysis of our data suggest that there are ceiling effects to both the amount of Cobb correction and the SVA, which can be corrected using circumferential MISS techniques (incorporating the lateral transpsoas approach) in spinal deformity. A

ceiling effect of 34° of Cobb correction was noted in 1 multicenter study.[65] Our study revealed a Cobb ceiling effect of 40° and an SVA ceiling effect of 10 cm.[66] Hence, the techniques do not seem to provide major correction of global lumbar lordosis or sagittal plane deformity as seen in procedures involving osteotomies. Because sagittal plane alignment is a critical parameter for outcomes in the setting of ASD,[67] patients with considerable SVA imbalance or pelvic incidence/lumbar lordosis mismatch may be better considered for appropriate osteotomy or other open techniques rather than relying solely on MISS techniques for sagittal plane deformity correction.

Nevertheless, techniques continue to involve and more lordosis may be obtainable in the future using the MISS technique. Deukmedjian and colleagues[68] reported a novel surgical technique by which release of the anterior longitudinal ligament was performed in addition to an MISS lateral retroperitoneal transpsoas approach. This technique was performed to achieve an even greater lordosis than a typical transpsoas approach. The

Table 3
Complications reported in MISS adult scoliosis series

Author, Year	Complications	MISS Complication Rate
Anand et al,[83] 2013	3 quadriceps palsy (2 made a complete recovery within 6 mo) 1 foot drop after transpsoas approach ileus Deep venous thrombosis Pulmonary embolism cerebral hemorrhage, pleural effusion and underwent thoracentesis Ureteropelvic injury, retrocapsular kidney hematoma Screw loosening Superficial sacral wound dehiscence	28% complication rate
Caputo et al,[39] 2012	Lateral incisional breakdown Pedicle fracture Hernia Atrial fibrillation 2 cases of iatrogenic anterior longitudinal ligament rupture Substantial amount of patients having thigh numbness or pain, which all resolved by 4 wk	26.6% complication rate
Dakwar et al,[40] 2010	Rhabdomyolysis, asymptomatic graft subsidence, and asymptomatic hardware failure 3 patients with thigh numbness	NA
Isaacs et al,[79] 2010	Myocardial infarction, sepsis, deep vein thrombosis, posterior wound infection, kidney laceration Motor deficit	Major complication rate of 5.8% and minor complication rate of 11.5% for those with MISS posterior instrumentation; motor deficit rate of 6.5% 33.6% of patients were noted to have some evidence of weakness after the transpsoas approach (in 86.2% this weakness was transient)
Scheufler et al,[81] 2010	13.3% with new nerve root motor disturbance 10% with worsening of preexisting neuropathic pain 5 patients with small durotomies 43.3% of patients with instrumented fusion to the sacrum with sacroiliac pain Medical complications included deep venous thrombosis, hemorrhage from an ulcer, and urinary tract infections	Major and minor complication rates were 23.4% and 59.9%, respectively
Sharma et al,[63] 2011	15 patients of 43 with thigh pain 11 patients with hip flexor weakness 4 patients with quadriceps weakness Numerous end-plate fractures in patients undergoing transpsoas interbody fusion 2 vertebral body fractures in patients undergoing lateral fixation 1 case of infection at the site of posterior instrumentation Retroperitoneal hemorrhage	NA

(continued on next page)

Table 3
(continued)

Author, Year	Complications	MISS Complication Rate
Tormenti et al,[49] 2010	2 cases of motor weakness; 1 transient Cecal perforation	NA 75% of patients to have thigh paresthesias or dysesthesias
Wang & Mummaneni,[41] 2010	Thigh numbness, pain, and weakness in 30.4% of patients undergoing the transpsoas approach, on the same side of the approach Cerebrospinal fluid leakage Hardware pullout Pneumothorax One case of significant blood loss	NA

Abbreviation: NA, not applicable.

investigators reported good results in 7 patients, in whom they noted an increase in global lumbar lordosis of 24°, segmental lordosis of 17° per level of anterior longitudinal ligament release, and a decrease in pelvic tilt of 7°. They also noted a decrease in SVA of 4.9 cm. They noted that a minimally invasive lateral retroperitoneal transpsoas approach in addition to release of the anterior longitudinal ligament might be a feasible alternative in correcting sagittal plane deformity. Wang and Madhavan[69] reported using an MISS technique in association with a miniopen approach for performance of pedicle subtraction osteotomy. These investigators described the technique as an evolution of minimally invasive techniques now being used for the treatment of fixed sagittal imbalance. Similarly, Wang[70] described using a hybrid MISS approach for deformity correction with good lordosis restoration using a combination of unilateral multilevel facet osteotomies, TLIF, expandable cages, and percutaneous screw/rod instrumentation.

From our experience, we advise in addition against using these techniques in their present form in cases of truly rigid scoliosis, for curves greater than 100° in magnitude, and for congenital and neuromuscular deformities. Osteoporosis with a T-score of less than –2.0 is also a contraindication.[6]

Other criticisms of MISS techniques in general, but specifically for deformity correction, include a larger learning curve than for open techniques, the need for specialized equipment, disorientation of the surgeon, and increased radiation exposure.[26,71–73] With proper training and experience, the disadvantages of learning curve and equipment investment are reduced with time. Disorientation may be an issue with certain deformities, especially with suboptimal imaging or poor bone density. Surgeon radiation exposure remains a serious concern regarding these procedures. When a technique is performed properly, adhering to radiation safety guidelines, many of these procedures can be performed yearly without exceeding occupational dose limits.[74] In addition, neuronavigation may be useful in increasing surgeon accuracy with instrumentation placement and reducing radiation exposure.[75–77]

SUMMARY

MISS scoliosis surgical correction continues to evolve, and its use has increased in recent years. Theoretic advantages of these techniques over open procedures include reduced blood loss, potentially reduced complication rates, and reduced tissue trauma. These techniques may be useful in their present form when up to 40° of coronal Cobb correction is desired and with fixed sagittal imbalance less than 10 cm. Questions remain as to the durability of the results and to which deformities are better served with open correction methods. Although long-term follow-up has been reported, more data are necessary to ensure that the results are comparable in the long-term with open deformity correction. Future level II or III studies should be designed to help answer what is the role of MISS technologies in the setting of scoliosis when compared with the open technique.

REFERENCES

1. Heary RF. Evaluation and treatment of adult spinal deformity. Invited submission from the Joint Section Meeting on Disorders of the Spine and Peripheral Nerves, March 2004. J Neurosurg Spine 2004; 1(1):9–18.
2. Baron EM, Albert TJ. Medical complications of surgical treatment of adult spinal deformity and how to avoid them. Spine 2006;31(Suppl 19):S106–18.

3. Hu SS. Blood loss in adult spinal surgery. Eur Spine J 2004;13(Suppl 1):S3–5.

4. Moller H, Hedlund R. Instrumented and noninstrumented posterolateral fusion in adult spondylolisthesis–a prospective randomized study: part 2. Spine 2000;25(13):1716–21.

5. Herkowitz HN, Sidhu KS. Lumbar spine fusion in the treatment of degenerative conditions: current indications and recommendations. J Am Acad Orthop Surg 1995;3(3):123–35.

6. Anand N, Baron EM. Minimally invasive approaches for the correction of adult spinal deformity. Eur Spine J 2013;22(Suppl 2):S232–41.

7. Mok JM, Hu SS. Surgical strategies and choosing levels for spinal deformity: how high, how low, front and back. Neurosurg Clin North Am 2007;18(2): 329–37.

8. Shufflebarger H, Suk SI, Mardjetko S. Debate: determining the upper instrumented vertebra in the management of adult degenerative scoliosis: stopping at T10 versus L1. Spine 2006;31(Suppl 19): S185–94.

9. Bridwell KH. Selection of instrumentation and fusion levels for scoliosis: where to start and where to stop. Invited submission from the Joint Section Meeting on Disorders of the Spine and Peripheral Nerves, March 2004. J Neurosurg Spine 2004; 1(1):1–8.

10. Kim YJ, Lenke LG, Cho SK, et al. Comparative analysis of pedicle screw versus hook instrumentation in posterior spinal fusion of adolescent idiopathic scoliosis. Spine (Phila Pa 1976) 2004; 29(18):2040–8.

11. Liljenqvist U, Lepsien U, Hackenberg L, et al. Comparative analysis of pedicle screw and hook instrumentation in posterior correction and fusion of idiopathic thoracic scoliosis. Eur Spine J 2002; 11(4):336–43.

12. Cheng I, Hay D, Iezza A, et al. Biomechanical analysis of derotation of the thoracic spine using pedicle screws. Spine (Phila Pa 1976) 2010; 35(10):1039–43.

13. Charles YP, Meyer N, Steib JP. Sagittal alignment correction of the thoracolumbar junction in idiopathic scoliosis by in situ bending technique. Stud Health Technol Inform 2008;140:72–8.

14. Vallespir GP, Flores JB, Trigueros IS, et al. Vertebral coplanar alignment: a standardized technique for three dimensional correction in scoliosis surgery: technical description and preliminary results in Lenke type 1 curves. Spine (Phila Pa 1976) 2008; 33(14):1588–97.

15. Yadla S, Maltenfort MG, Ratliff JK, et al. Adult scoliosis surgery outcomes: a systematic review. Neurosurg Focus 2010;28(3):E3.

16. Daubs MD, Lenke LG, Bridwell KH, et al. Does correction of preoperative coronal imbalance make a difference in outcomes of adult patients with deformity? Spine (Phila Pa 1976) 2013;38(6): 476–83.

17. Seo HJ, Kim HJ, Ro YJ, et al. Non-neurologic complications following surgery for scoliosis. Korean J Anesthesiol 2013;64(1):40–6.

18. Transfeldt EE, Topp R, Mehbod AA, et al. Surgical outcomes of decompression, decompression with limited fusion, and decompression with full curve fusion for degenerative scoliosis with radiculopathy. Spine (Phila Pa 1976) 2010;35(20):1872–5.

19. Akbarnia BA, Ogilvie JW, Hammerberg KW. Debate: degenerative scoliosis: to operate or not to operate. Spine 2006;31(Suppl 19):S195–201.

20. Gejo R, Matsui H, Kawaguchi Y, et al. Serial changes in trunk muscle performance after posterior lumbar surgery. Spine 1999;24(10):1023–8.

21. Kawaguchi Y, Matsui H, Tsuji H. Back muscle injury after posterior lumbar spine surgery. Part 2: histologic and histochemical analyses in humans. Spine 1994;19(22):2598–602.

22. Kawaguchi Y, Matsui H, Tsuji H. Back muscle injury after posterior lumbar spine surgery. Part 1: histologic and histochemical analyses in rats. Spine 1994;19(22):2590–7.

23. Kawaguchi Y, Yabuki S, Styf J, et al. Back muscle injury after posterior lumbar spine surgery. Topographic evaluation of intramuscular pressure and blood flow in the porcine back muscle during surgery. Spine 1996;21(22):2683–8.

24. Cervellini P, De Luca GP, Mazzetto M, et al. Microendoscopic-discectomy (MED) for far lateral disc herniation in the lumbar spine. Technical note. Acta Neurochir Suppl 2005;92:99–101.

25. Derby R, Baker RM, Lee CH. Evidence-informed management of chronic low back pain with minimally invasive nuclear decompression. Spine J 2008;8(1):150–9.

26. Eck JC, Hodges S, Humphreys SC. Minimally invasive lumbar spinal fusion. J Am Acad Orthop Surg 2007;15(6):321–9.

27. Foley KT, Holly LT, Schwender JD. Minimally invasive lumbar fusion. Spine 2003;28(Suppl 15): S26–35.

28. Foley KT, Lefkowitz MA. Advances in minimally invasive spine surgery. Clin Neurosurg 2002;49: 499–517.

29. Ivanov A, Faizan A, Sairyo K, et al. Minimally invasive decompression for lumbar spinal canal stenosis in younger age patients could lead to higher stresses in the remaining neural arch–a finite element investigation. Minim Invasive Neurosurg 2007;50(1):18–22.

30. Lidar Z, Beaumont A, Lifshutz J, et al. Clinical and radiological relationship between posterior lumbar interbody fusion and posterolateral lumbar fusion. Surg Neurol 2005;64(4):303–8 [discussion: 308].

31. Anand N, Hamilton JF, Perri B, et al. Cantilever TLIF with structural allograft and RhBMP2 for correction and maintenance of segmental sagittal lordosis: long-term clinical, radiographic, and functional outcome. Spine 2006;31(20):E748–53.

32. Christensen FB, Hansen ES, Eiskjaer SP, et al. Circumferential lumbar spinal fusion with Brantigan cage versus posterolateral fusion with titanium Cotrel-Dubousset instrumentation: a prospective, randomized clinical study of 146 patients. Spine 2002;27(23):2674–83.

33. DeBerard MS, Colledge AL, Masters KS, et al. Outcomes of posterolateral versus BAK titanium cage interbody lumbar fusion in injured workers: a retrospective cohort study. J South Orthop Assoc 2002; 11(3):157–66.

34. Yashiro K, Homma T, Hokari Y, et al. The Steffee variable screw placement system using different methods of bone grafting. Spine 1991;16(11): 1329–34.

35. Comparison of traditional midline approach versus muscle splitting paraspinal approach for posterior non-fusion stabilization of the lumbar spine–an analysis of functional outcome. 2007 AANS/CNS Section on Disorders of the Spine and Peripheral Nerves. Phoenix (AZ); 2007.

36. Anand N, Baron EM, Bray RS. Modified muscle-sparing paraspinal approach for stabilization and interlaminar decompression: a minimally invasive technique for pedicle screw-based posterior non-fusion stabilization. SAS Journal 2008;2:131–3.

37. Anand N, Baron EM, Khandehroo B, et al. Long term 2 to 5 year clinical and functional outcomes of minimally invasive surgery (MIS) for adult scoliosis. Spine (Phila Pa 1976) 2013;38(18):1566–75.

38. Anand N, Rosemann R, Khalsa B, et al. Mid-term to long-term clinical and functional outcomes of minimally invasive correction and fusion for adults with scoliosis. Neurosurg Focus 2010;28(3):E6.

39. Caputo AM, Michael KW, Chapman TM Jr, et al. Clinical outcomes of extreme lateral interbody fusion in the treatment of adult degenerative scoliosis. ScientificWorldJournal 2012;2012:680643.

40. Dakwar E, Cardona RF, Smith DA, et al. Early outcomes and safety of the minimally invasive, lateral retroperitoneal transpsoas approach for adult degenerative scoliosis. Neurosurg Focus 2010; 28(3):E8.

41. Wang MY, Mummaneni PV. Minimally invasive surgery for thoracolumbar spinal deformity: initial clinical experience with clinical and radiographic outcomes. Neurosurg Focus 2010;28(3):E9.

42. Anand N, Baron EM, Thaiyananthan G, et al. Minimally invasive multilevel percutaneous correction and fusion for adult lumbar degenerative scoliosis: a technique and feasibility study. J Spinal Disord Tech 2008;21(7):459–67.

43. Ozgur BM, Aryan HE, Pimenta L, et al. Extreme lateral interbody fusion (XLIF): a novel surgical technique for anterior lumbar interbody fusion. Spine J 2006;6(4):435–43.

44. Chung SK, Lee SH, Lim SR, et al. Comparative study of laparoscopic L5-S1 fusion versus open mini-ALIF, with a minimum 2-year follow-up. Eur Spine J 2003;12(6):613–7.

45. Kaiser MG, Haid RW Jr, Subach BR, et al. Comparison of the mini-open versus laparoscopic approach for anterior lumbar interbody fusion: a retrospective review. Neurosurgery 2002;51(1): 97–103 [discussion: 103–5].

46. Zucherman JF, Zdeblick TA, Bailey SA, et al. Instrumented laparoscopic spinal fusion. Preliminary results. Spine (Phila Pa 1976) 1995;20(18):2029–34 [discussion: 2034–5].

47. Thalgott JS, Chin AK, Ameriks JA, et al. Gasless endoscopic anterior lumbar interbody fusion utilizing the B.E.R.G. approach. Surg Endosc 2000; 14(6):546–52.

48. McAfee PC, Regan JJ, Geis WP, et al. Minimally invasive anterior retroperitoneal approach to the lumbar spine. Emphasis on the lateral BAK. Spine 1998;23(13):1476–84.

49. Tormenti MJ, Maserati MB, Bonfield CM, et al. Complications and radiographic correction in adult scoliosis following combined transpsoas extreme lateral interbody fusion and posterior pedicle screw instrumentation. Neurosurg Focus 2010;28(3):E7.

50. Rodgers WB, Gerber EJ, Patterson J. Intraoperative and early postoperative complications in extreme lateral interbody fusion: an analysis of 600 cases. Spine (Phila Pa 1976) 2011;36(1):26–32.

51. Willard FH, Vleeming A, Schuenke MD, et al. The thoracolumbar fascia: anatomy, function and clinical considerations. J Anat 2012;221(6):507–36.

52. O'Brien JR, Matteini L, Yu WD, et al. Feasibility of minimally invasive sacropelvic fixation: percutaneous S2 alar iliac fixation. Spine 2010;35(4):460–4.

53. Wang MY. Percutaneous iliac screws for minimally invasive spinal deformity surgery. Minim Invasive Surg 2012;2012:173685.

54. Aebi M. The adult scoliosis. Eur Spine J 2005; 14(10):925–48.

55. Carreon LY, Puno RM, Dimar JR 2nd, et al. Perioperative complications of posterior lumbar decompression and arthrodesis in older adults. J Bone Joint Surg Am 2003;85(11):2089–92.

56. Raffo CS, Lauerman WC. Predicting morbidity and mortality of lumbar spine arthrodesis in patients in their ninth decade. Spine 2006;31(1):99–103.

57. Zurbriggen C, Markwalder TM, Wyss S. Long-term results in patients treated with posterior instrumentation and fusion for degenerative scoliosis of the lumbar spine. Acta Neurochir (Wien) 1999;141(1): 21–6.

58. Cho KJ, Suk SI, Park SR, et al. Complications in posterior fusion and instrumentation for degenerative lumbar scoliosis. Spine 2007;32(20):2232–7.

59. Wu CH, Wong CB, Chen LH, et al. Instrumented posterior lumbar interbody fusion for patients with degenerative lumbar scoliosis. J Spinal Disord Tech 2008;21(5):310–5.

60. Bono CM, Lee CK. The influence of subdiagnosis on radiographic and clinical outcomes after lumbar fusion for degenerative disc disorders: an analysis of the literature from two decades. Spine 2005; 30(2):227–34.

61. Shaffrey CI, Smith JS. Editorial: minimally invasive spinal deformity surgery. J Neurosurg Spine 2013;18(1):1–3.

62. Acosta FL, Liu J, Slimack N, et al. Changes in coronal and sagittal plane alignment following minimally invasive direct lateral interbody fusion for the treatment of degenerative lumbar disease in adults: a radiographic study. J Neurosurg Spine 2011;15(1):92–6.

63. Sharma AK, Kepler CK, Girardi FP, et al. Lateral lumbar interbody fusion: clinical and radiographic outcomes at 1 year: a preliminary report. J Spinal Disord Tech 2011;24(4):242–50.

64. Johnson RD, Valore A, Villaminar A, et al. Pelvic parameters of sagittal balance in extreme lateral interbody fusion for degenerative lumbar disc disease. J Clin Neurosci 2013;20(4):576–81.

65. Wang M, Mummaneni P, Fu KM, et al. Less invasive surgery for treating adult spinal deformities (ASD): ceiling effects for Cobb angle correction with three different techniques. 20th International Meeting on Advanced Spine Techniques. Vancouver (Canada), July 10–13, 2013.

66. Anand N, Khanderoo B, Kahwaty S, et al. Is there a limitation to correction of sagittal balance with circumferential minimally invasive surgical (CMIS) correction of adult spinal deformity (ASD)? North American Spine Society 28th Annual Meeting. New Orleans, October 9–12, 2013.

67. Schwab F, Lafage V, Patel A, et al. Sagittal plane considerations and the pelvis in the adult patient. Spine (Phila Pa 1976) 2009;34(17):1828–33.

68. Deukmedjian AR, Dakwar E, Ahmadian A, et al. Early outcomes of minimally invasive anterior longitudinal ligament release for correction of sagittal imbalance in patients with adult spinal deformity. ScientificWorldJournal 2012;2012:789698.

69. Wang MY, Madhavan K. Mini-open pedicle subtraction osteotomy: surgical technique. World Neurosurg 2012. [Epub ahead of print].

70. Wang MY. Improvement of sagittal balance and lumbar lordosis following less invasive adult spinal deformity surgery with expandable cages and percutaneous instrumentation. J Neurosurg Spine 2013;18(1):4–12.

71. Mariscalco MW, Yamashita T, Steinmetz MP, et al. Radiation exposure to the surgeon during open lumbar microdiscectomy and minimally invasive microdiscectomy: a prospective, controlled trial. Spine (Phila Pa 1976) 2011;36(3):255–60.

72. Ropper AE, Chi JH. Maximal radiation exposure during minimally invasive spine surgery? Neurosurgery 2011;68(4):N23–4.

73. Payer M. "Minimally invasive" lumbar spine surgery: a critical review. Acta Neurochir (Wien) 2011;153(7):1455–9.

74. Taher F, Hughes AP, Sama AA, et al. How safe is lateral lumbar interbody fusion for the surgeon? A prospective in-vivo radiation exposure study. Spine (Phila Pa 1976) 2013;38(16):1386–92.

75. Houten JK, Nasser R, Baxi N. Clinical assessment of percutaneous lumbar pedicle screw placement using the O-arm multidimensional surgical imaging system. Neurosurgery 2012;70(4):990–5.

76. Cho JY, Chan CK, Lee SH, et al. The accuracy of 3D image navigation with a cutaneously fixed dynamic reference frame in minimally invasive transforaminal lumbar interbody fusion. Comput Aided Surg 2012;17(6):300–9.

77. Kim CW, Lee YP, Taylor W, et al. Use of navigation-assisted fluoroscopy to decrease radiation exposure during minimally invasive spine surgery. Spine J 2008;8(4):584–90.

78. Dorward IG, Lenke LG, Bridwell KH, et al. Transforaminal versus anterior lumbar interbody fusion in long deformity constructs: a matched cohort analysis. Spine (Phila Pa 1976) 2013. [Epub ahead of print].

79. Isaacs RE, Hyde J, Goodrich JA, et al. A prospective, nonrandomized, multicenter evaluation of extreme lateral interbody fusion for the treatment of adult degenerative scoliosis: perioperative outcomes and complications. Spine (Phila Pa 1976) 2010;35(Suppl 26):S322–30.

80. Karikari IO, Nimjee SM, Hardin CA, et al. Extreme lateral interbody fusion approach for isolated thoracic and thoracolumbar spine diseases: initial clinical experience and early outcomes. J Spinal Disord Tech 2011;24(6):368–75.

81. Scheufler KM, Cyron D, Dohmen H, et al. Less invasive surgical correction of adult degenerative scoliosis. Part II: complications and clinical outcome. Neurosurgery 2010;67(6):1609–21 [discussion: 1621].

82. Scheufler KM, Cyron D, Dohmen H, et al. Less invasive surgical correction of adult degenerative scoliosis, part I: technique and radiographic results. Neurosurgery 2010;67(3):696–710.

83. Anand N, Khanderoo B, Kahwaty S, et al. Complications of minimally invasive spinal surgery (MISS) for correction of spinal deformity–a 5 year experience. Chicago (IL): American Academy of Orthopaedic Surgeons; 2013.

Intraoperative Navigation in Minimally Invasive Transforaminal Lumbar Interbody Fusion and Lateral Interbody Fusion

James A. Stadler III, MD, Nader S. Dahdaleh, MD*,
Zachary A. Smith, MD, Tyler R. Koski, MD

KEYWORDS

- Minimally invasive • Transforaminal lumbar interbody fusion
- Minimally invasive pedicle screw placement • Intraoperative navigation

KEY POINTS

- Advanced intraoperative navigation technologies are currently being applied to a wide variety of minimally invasive spine surgical procedures.
- These advanced intraoperative navigation technologies carry many advantages with decreased radiation exposure and improved accuracy of hardware placement.
- The technique for use of neural navigation for minimally invasive placement of pedicle screws is discussed.

INTRODUCTION

Minimally invasive spine techniques have been developed with the aim of preserving the surrounding anatomy and avoiding unnecessary muscle disruption and damage, which has translated clinically into decreased blood loss, infection rates, length of hospitalization, narcotic use, and physiologic stress.[1] Importantly, outcomes following minimally invasive approaches are favorable compared with open techniques for many procedures, as increasingly demonstrated in the literature.[1–5]

Similarly, advances in intraoperative navigation technology have increased the safety and efficacy of spine surgery. Navigation is critical for a wide range of spinal procedures to facilitate localization and instrumentation. Traditional 2-dimensional techniques like fluoroscopy are progressively being augmented or replaced by advanced systems, such as cone-beam computed tomography (CT) or 3-dimensional fluoroscopy. As with traditional navigation, advanced imaging guidance can be used for multiple applications in any area of the spine.[6] Navigation has been applied during minimally invasive transforaminal interbody fusion, and there is to date only one report demonstrating feasibility of navigation during lateral interbody fusion.[7]

Advanced intraoperative navigation techniques carry many advantages when applied to minimally invasive spine surgeries, which are primarily driven by radiographic anatomy.[8] Beyond localization, an important advantage of advanced navigation is the

Sources of Support: None.
Department of Neurological Surgery, Northwestern University Feinberg School of Medicine, 676 North Saint Clair Street, Suite 2210, Chicago, IL 60611, USA
* Corresponding author.
E-mail address: nsdahdaleh@gmail.com

Neurosurg Clin N Am 25 (2014) 377–382
http://dx.doi.org/10.1016/j.nec.2013.12.015
1042-3680/14/$ – see front matter © 2014 Elsevier Inc. All rights reserved.

increased accuracy of pedicle screw placement and instrumentation.[9] Critical structures, including neural elements, major vessels, and viscera, can be avoided with real-time feedback. A meta-analysis of nonnavigated pedicle screws in the thoracolumbar spine showed a satisfactory pedicle screw position of only 79%.[10] In a separate meta-analysis of traditional fluoroscopic navigation, this rate improved to 87%.[11] However, individual reports of nonnavigated and traditional fluoroscopic techniques achieved have demonstrated satisfactory pedicle screw placement rates of up to 98.3% and 93.8%, suggesting variability between individual surgical results.[12,13] These rates compare to a reported accuracy of 98.2% and 98.8% with the use of advanced intraoperative navigation in recent studies.[14,15] Although the current data have largely focused on navigation in open cases, consideration of these findings seems appropriate for minimally invasive approaches as well.[4,6,16]

A significant concern in any spinal fusion is optimization of instrumentation biomechanics. It has been demonstrated that pedicle screw medialization, greater screw outer diameter, and greater cortical engagement contribute to improved screw pullout strength; increased screw inner diameter separately improves fatigue strength.[17] Advanced navigation allows the surgeon to maximize these variables intraoperatively with direct pedicle measurements and real-time adjustments to obtain biocortical or tricortical purchase.

Radiation exposure, to both the patient and the surgeon, during minimally invasive spine surgery is not insignificant. Multiple studies have demonstrated significant decreases in surgeon and staff radiation exposure with the use of intraoperative navigation.[4,14,18,19] Although the dose of radiation delivered to the patient intraoperatively may be similar or higher with these techniques, this difference becomes somewhat mitigated if routine postoperative CT scans are used to confirm the accuracy of nonnavigated instrumentation.[20]

There are additional notable benefits of advanced intraoperative navigation. Approach planning may be optimized to reduce incision length. This technique is a useful adjunct for resident training, because it provides real-time feedback to both the surgeon and the trainee. Beyond pedicle screw placement, navigation is also useful during decompression, in approaching and exploring of the disc space, and for interbody measurements.

Although minimally invasive surgical approaches were initially limited to a few procedures, the scope of applications continues to expand.[1,21,22] Advanced reconstructive imaging helps safely advance the indications as these interventions become more complex.[23]

SURGICAL TECHNIQUE FOR THE USE OF NAVIGATION FOR MINIMALLY INVASIVE OR MINI-OPEN PEDICLE SCREW PLACEMENT

Preparation and Patient Positioning

The patient is positioned on an OSI open Jackson table to maintain appropriate lumbar lordosis. All pressure points are appropriately padded.

Surgical Procedure

The patient presented underwent an anterior lumbar interbody fusion at L4/5 and L5/S1.

Step 1

The base of navigation reference frame is embedded firmly into posterior superior iliac crest following a small stab incision (**Fig. 1**). Two paraspinal incisions are marked 4.5 cm away from the midline on both sides.

Step 2

The camera of the navigation system recognizes the reference frame, and the surgical instruments to be used in the operation are registered for intraoperative navigation onto the station by placing them on the reference frame (**Fig. 2**).

Step 3

With the camera recognizing the reference frame and the O-Arm, the O-Arm is used to generate a 3-dimensional intraoperative CT of the lumbar spine level of interest (**Fig. 3**).

Step 4

Live intraoperative images in the axial, sagittal, and coronal planes are generated. The smallest dilator (attached to spherical sensors) is recognized by

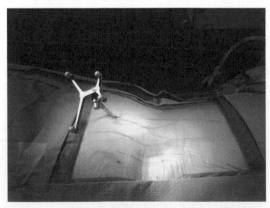

Fig. 1. The reference frame is embedded in the posterior superior iliac crest.

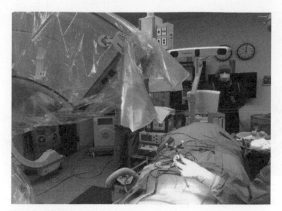

Fig. 2. The surgical instruments are registered for intraoperative navigation.

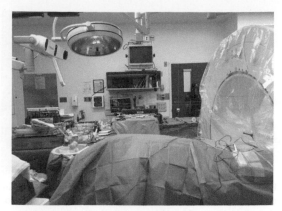

Fig. 3. O-Arm is used to generate a3-dimensional intraoperative CT of the lumbar spine level of interest.

the station and can be navigated (**Fig. 4**A). Through a small stab incision, the dilator is advanced and docked on the facet or pars interarticularis under live navigation (see **Fig. 4**B).

Step 5
A K-wire is advanced through the cannulated dilator embedded firmly into bone and the navigable dilator is withdrawn (**Fig. 5**A). Sequential nonnavigable dilators are used to dilate through the paraspinal muscles (see **Fig. 5**B), followed by the placement of a table-mounted retractor system. The same steps are repeated on the contralateral side so that the operation can proceed on both sides concomitantly.

Step 6
After selecting the appropriate entry point for the pedicle screw, the navigable tap is then used to cannulate the pedicle under live image guidance (**Fig. 6**).

Step 7
Using a probe, the created pathway can be palpated to rule out any pedicle wall violations (**Fig. 7**A). The appropriate screw length can be measured as well by gauging the depth of the probe (see **Fig. 7**B).

Step 8
Using a navigable screwdriver, the screw is introduced into the pedicle under image guidance (**Fig. 8**).

Step 9
An appropriately sized and contoured rod is placed connecting the screw heads on both sides of the construct (**Fig. 9**). Before rod placement, a transforaminal interbody fusion can be performed through the working channel or retractor system.

Step 10
Both incisions are approximated in layers (**Fig. 10**).

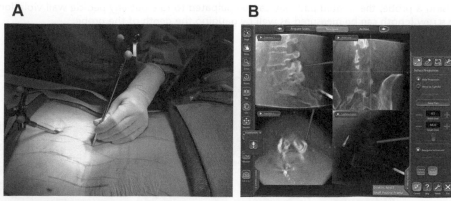

Fig. 4. Through a small stab incision, the dilator is advanced and docked on the facet or pars interarticularis (*A*) under live navigation (*B*).

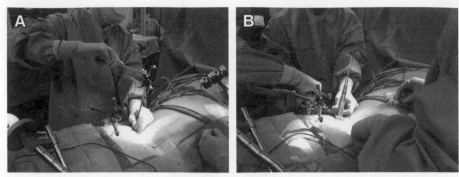

Fig. 5. (*A*) A K-wire is advanced through the cannulated dilator embedded firmly into bone and the navigable dilator is withdrawn. Sequential dilators are used to dilate through the paraspinal muscles, (*B*) followed by the placement of a table-mounted retractor system.

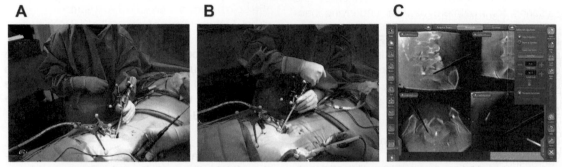

Fig. 6. The navigable tap is then used to cannulate the pedicle under live image guidance (*A, B, C*).

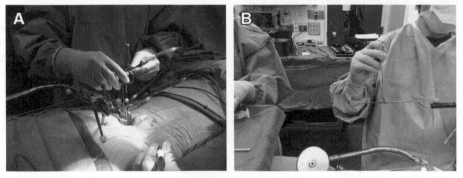

Fig. 7. (*A*) Using a probe, the created pathway can be palpated to rule out any pedicle wall violations. (*B*) The appropriate screw length can be measured as well by gauging the depth of the probe.

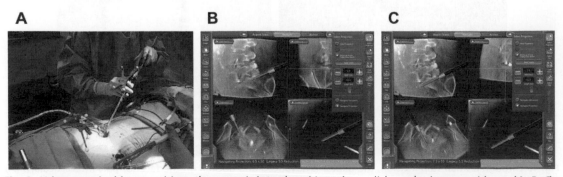

Fig. 8. Using a navigable screwdriver, the screw is introduced into the pedicle under image guidance (*A, B, C*).

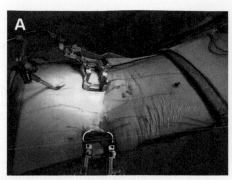
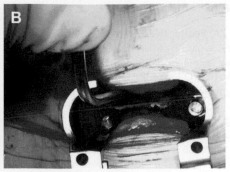

Fig. 9. An appropriately sized and contoured rod is placed connecting the screw heads on both sides of the construct (*A*, *B*).

LIMITATIONS

As with any surgery, the potential complications of this surgical approach must be understood by both surgeons and patients. In addition to intraoperative and perioperative medical risks associated with general anesthesia, the risks of posterior percutaneous surgery for transforaminal lumbar interbody fusion or pedicle screw placement include pain, infection, failure to improve, durotomy, malpositioned instrumentation, and pseudoarthrosis; although some risks may be decreased with use of advanced navigation, they cannot be completely obviated.

There are limitations to the use of advanced intraoperative navigation. This technique does include a small incision for placement of the reference frame, and this may incur slight additional postoperative pain. Despite rigid bony attachment, the reference frame is at risk for movement during the case. Care must be taken intraoperatively not to disrupt the frame during the course of the operation, and it is helpful to confirm registration to known anatomic bony landmarks periodically. In a large multicenter prospective study, the rate of intraoperative

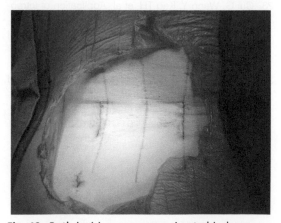

Fig. 10. Both incisions are approximated in layers.

cone-beam CT failure was found to be 5.1%, emphasizing the need for surgeon comfort in safely proceeding with other available forms of navigation as well.[14]

Although advanced intraoperative navigation has improved rates of satisfactory pedicle screw placement, malpositioned instrumentation remains a consideration with these surgeries. Despite high accuracy rates, it may be helpful to assess screw position intraoperatively so that correction can be accomplished at the time of initial surgery.[14] Some variability between virtual and actual screw placement does exist, with a reported difference in angulation of 2.8° ± 1.9°.[24]

As previously discussed, the use of intraoperative CT scanning may increase intraoperative radiation exposure to the patient. Optimal radiation dose delivery, with consideration of image quality and therefore navigation accuracy, is difficult to define and is likely variable according to patient body habitus, prior instrumentation, and surgeon preference.[14,19,20]

Overall, these limitations compared favorably with current alternative techniques. Direct, comprehensive comparison of surgical options in the form of well-designed studies would provide greater understanding and aid clinical decision-making. Ultimately, however, as intraoperative technologies improve, the surgical techniques, benefits, and risk profiles for these procedures will continue to evolve as well.

SUMMARY

Advanced intraoperative navigation technologies are applicable to a wide variety of minimally invasive spine surgical procedures and carry the advantages of decreased radiation exposure and improved accuracy of hardware placement with minimal soft tissue disruption, thus meeting the classic outcomes and reduced complication rates of percutaneous spine surgery.

REFERENCES

1. Smith ZA, Fessler RG. Paradigm changes in spine surgery: evolution of minimally invasive techniques. Nat Rev Neurol 2012;8(8):443–50.
2. Fessler RG, O'Toole JE, Eichholz KM, et al. The development of minimally invasive spine surgery. Neurosurg Clin N Am 2006;17(4):401–9.
3. Rodriguez-Vela J, Lobo-Escolar A, Joven E, et al. Clinical outcomes of minimally invasive versus open approach for one-level transforaminal lumbar interbody fusion at the 3- to 4-year follow-up. Eur Spine J 2013;22(12):2857–63.
4. Scheufler KM, Franke J, Eckardt A, et al. Accuracy of image-guided pedicle screw placement using intraoperative computed tomography-based navigation with automated referencing. Part II: Thoracolumbar spine. Neurosurgery 2011;69(6):1307–16.
5. Scheufler KM, Cyron D, Dohmen H, et al. Less invasive surgical correction of adult degenerative scoliosis, part I: technique and radiographic results. Neurosurgery 2010;67(3):696–710.
6. Moses ZB, Mayer RR, Strickland BA, et al. Neuronavigation in minimally invasive spine surgery. Neurosurg Focus 2013;35(2):E12.
7. Drazin D, Liu JC, Acosta FL. CT navigated lateral interbody fusion. J Clin Neurosci 2013;20(10):1438–41.
8. Holly LT, Foley KT. Image guidance in spine surgery. Orthop Clin North Am 2007;38(3):451–61 [abstract viii].
9. Kazemi N, Crew LK, Tredway TL. The future of spine surgery: new horizons in the treatment of spinal disorders. Surg Neurol Int 2013;4(Suppl 1):S15–21.
10. Kosmopoulos V, Schizas C. Pedicle screw placement accuracy: a meta-analysis. Spine 2007;32(3):E111–20.
11. Tian NF, Xu HZ. Image-guided pedicle screw insertion accuracy: a meta-analysis. Int Orthop 2009;33(4):895–903.
12. Smith ZA, Sugimoto K, Lawton CD, et al. Incidence of lumbar spine pedicle breach following percutaneous screw fixation: a radiographic evaluation of 601 screws in 151 patients. J Spinal Disord Tech 2012. [Epub ahead of print].
13. Parker SL, McGirt MJ, Farber SH, et al. Accuracy of free-hand pedicle screws in the thoracic and lumbar spine: analysis of 6816 consecutive screws. Neurosurgery 2011;68(1):170–8 [discussion: 178].
14. Van de Kelft E, Costa F, Van der Planken D, et al. A prospective multicenter registry on the accuracy of pedicle screw placement in the thoracic, lumbar, and sacral levels with the use of the O-arm imaging system and StealthStation Navigation. Spine 2012;37(25):E1580–7.
15. Tormenti MJ, Kostov DB, Gardner PA, et al. Intraoperative computed tomography image-guided navigation for posterior thoracolumbar spinal instrumentation in spinal deformity surgery. Neurosurg Focus 2010;28(3):E11.
16. Waschke A, Walter J, Duenisch P, et al. CT-navigation versus fluoroscopy-guided placement of pedicle screws at the thoracolumbar spine: single center experience of 4,500 screws. Eur Spine J 2013;22(3):654–60.
17. Cho W, Cho SK, Wu C. The biomechanics of pedicle screw-based instrumentation. J Bone Joint Surg Br 2010;92(8):1061–5.
18. Schafer S, Nithiananthan S, Mirota DJ, et al. Mobile C-arm cone-beam CT for guidance of spine surgery: image quality, radiation dose, and integration with interventional guidance. Med Phys 2011;38(8):4563–74.
19. Smith HE, Welsch MD, Sasso RC, et al. Comparison of radiation exposure in lumbar pedicle screw placement with fluoroscopy vs computer-assisted image guidance with intraoperative three-dimensional imaging. J Spinal Cord Med 2008;31(5):532–7.
20. Tabaraee E, Gibson AG, Karahalios DG, et al. Intraoperative cone beam computed tomography with navigation (O-ARM) versus conventional fluoroscopy (C-ARM): a cadaveric study comparing accuracy, efficiency, and safety for spinal instrumentation. Spine (Phila Pa 1976) 2013;38(22):1953–8.
21. Jaikumar S, Kim DH, Kam AC. History of minimally invasive spine surgery. Neurosurgery 2002;51(Suppl 5):S1–14.
22. Hsieh PC, Koski TR, Sciubba DM, et al. Maximizing the potential of minimally invasive spine surgery in complex spinal disorders. Neurosurg Focus 2008;25(2):E19.
23. Cui G, Wang Y, Kao TH, et al. Application of intraoperative computed tomography with or without navigation system in surgical correction of spinal deformity: a preliminary result of 59 consecutive human cases. Spine 2012;37(10):891–900.
24. Oertel MF, Hobart J, Stein M, et al. Clinical and methodological precision of spinal navigation assisted by 3D intraoperative O-arm radiographic imaging. J Neurosurg Spine 2011;14(4):532–6.

Index

Note: Page numbers of article titles are in **boldface** type.

A

Abdominal wall dissection, in lateral lumbar intervertebral fusion, 212–214
Annulus, penetration of, in LLIF procedure, 216
Anterior lumbar interbody fusion
    for scoliosis, 363–364
    versus lateral transpsoas approach, 220
Anterolateral corpectomy, for spinal tumors, **317–325**
As Low As Reasonably Achievable principle, 248
Astrocytomas, spinal, 327–336
Axia-LIF technique, for scoliosis, 363–364, 366–367

B

Bone morphogenetic protein, 364
Bowel perforation, in lateral transpsoas approach, 225–226

C

Cerebrospinal fluid leaks, in TLIF, 296, 300
Cervical myelopathy and radiculopathy, techniques for, **261–270**
Collimation, for radiation exposure control, 250
Coronal deformities, lateral transpsoas lumbar interbody fusion for, **353–360**
Corpectomy
    anterolateral, for spinal tumors, **317–325**
    transpedicular, for spinal tumors, **305–315**

D

Decompressive procedures
    extracavitary transpedicular corpectomy, **305–315**
    posterior
        complications of. *See* Posterior approaches, complications of.
        for cervical myelopathy and radiculopathy, **261–270**
    TLIF, **279–304**
Degenerative disease, lateral transpsoas lumbar interbody fusion for, **353–360**
Direct lateral interbody fusion. *See* Lateral transpsoas approach.
Discectomy
    cervical, **261–270**
    complications of. *See* Posterior approaches, complications of.
    for scoliosis, 363, 366
    in LLIF procedure, 216
    in TLIF, 284–289
Disk herniation, recurrent, in posterior approaches, 241–242
Diskitis, in posterior approaches, 242–243
Durotomy, in posterior approaches, 235, 238–239

E

Electromyography, for complication prevention, 228–229
Endoscopic thoracic disc removal, 273
Engineering controls, for radiation exposure, 250
Ependymomas, spinal, 327–336
Extracavitary transpedicular corpectomy, for spinal tumors, **305–315**
Extreme lateral interbody fusion. *See* Lateral transpsoas approach.
Eyewear, for radiation exposure control, 252

F

Flat-back syndrome, 361
Foraminotomy
    cervical, **261–270**
    complications of. *See* Posterior approaches, complications of.
Fractures, thoracolumbar, percutaneous pedicle screw fixation for, **337–346**

G

Gangliogliomas, spinal, 327–336
Germinomas, spinal, 327–336
Gloves, lead, for radiation exposure control, 252
Goggles, for radiation exposure control, 252

H

Hardware, complications from, in lateral transpsoas approach, 226, 229
Hemangioblastomas, spinal, 327–336
Hematoma, in lateral transpsoas approach, 223
Hernias, surgical, in lateral transpsoas approach, 223
Hyperlordosis, in scoliosis, 361

I

Iliohypogastric nerve, protection of, in LLIF procedure, 212–213

Neurosurg Clin N Am 25 (2014) 383–385
http://dx.doi.org/10.1016/S1042-3680(14)00010-2
1042-3680/14/$ – see front matter © 2014 Elsevier Inc. All rights reserved.

Moving?

Make sure your subscription moves with you!

To notify us of your new address, find your **Clinics Account Number** (located on your mailing label above your name), and contact customer service at:

Email: journalscustomerservice-usa@elsevier.com

800-654-2452 (subscribers in the U.S. & Canada)
314-447-8871 (subscribers outside of the U.S. & Canada)

Fax number: 314-447-8029

**Elsevier Health Sciences Division
Subscription Customer Service
3251 Riverport Lane
Maryland Heights, MO 63043**

*To ensure uninterrupted delivery of your subscription, please notify us at least 4 weeks in advance of move.

Printed and bound by CPI Group (UK) Ltd, Croydon, CR0 4YY

03/10/2024

01040375-0017